McMinn's Concise
Human Anatomy

Second Edition

McMinn's Concise Human Anatomy

Second Edition

David Heylings
Honorary Senior Fellow at the
    University of East Anglia
University of East Anglia
Norwich, UK

Stephen Carmichael
Professor Emeritus of Anatomy
    and Orthopedic Surgery
Mayo Clinic
Rochester, Minnesota, USA

Samuel Leinster
Emeritus Professor of Medical
    Education
University of East Anglia
Norwich, UK

Janak Saada
Consultant Radiologist
Norfolk and Norwich University
    Hospitals NHS Foundation Trust
Norwich, UK

With anatomical preparations by:
Bari M. Logan
Formerly University Prosector
Department of Anatomy
University of Cambridge
Cambridge, UK
and
Formerly Prosector
Department of Anatomy
The Royal College of Surgeons
    of England
London, UK

And photography by:
Ralph T. Hutchings
Formerly Chief Medical Laboratory
    Scientific Officer
The Royal College of Surgeons
    of England
London, UK

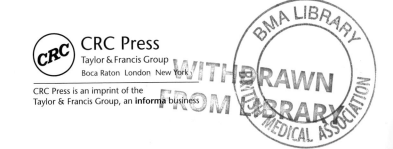
CRC Press
Taylor & Francis Group
Boca Raton London New York

CRC Press is an imprint of the
Taylor & Francis Group, an **informa** business

BMA LIBRARY
BRITISH MEDICAL ASSOCIATION
WITHDRAWN
FROM LIBRARY

CRC Press
Taylor & Francis Group
6000 Broken Sound Parkway NW, Suite 300
Boca Raton, FL 33487-2742

© 2018 by Taylor & Francis Group, LLC
CRC Press is an imprint of Taylor & Francis Group, an Informa business

No claim to original U.S. Government works

Printed and bound in India by Replika Press Pvt. Ltd.

Printed on acid-free paper

International Standard Book Number-13: 978-1-4987-8774-1 (Paperback)
International Standard Book Number-13: 978-1-138-03310-8 (Hardback)

Visit the Taylor & Francis Web site at
http://www.taylorandfrancis.com

and the CRC Press Web site at
http://www.crcpress.com

Contents

Foreword

In the preface to the 1st edition of this book, Professor McMinn described the need for a book that provides a short synopsis intended for those who need the essential facts of Human Anatomy without the mass of detail that occupies so much of most anatomy texts. The need is even greater now, with the continuing erosion of the time allotted for the study of Anatomy in many medical schools. He also stated that the surface of the body is all that most people (except surgeons) see of it. How things have changed. The development and availability of modern medical imaging mean that more clinicians than ever before have access to and, therefore, need to know the internal anatomy of the human body. The authors of the 2nd edition have ensured that its text remains concise and easy to read, providing a basis for *understanding* the structure of the human body and not simply learning a list of anatomical facts. Although the text remains concise, the 2nd edition contains welcome and valuable additions. A strength of the 1st edition was the quality of the dissections illustrating the structure of the human body and their photographic reproduction. These illustrations have now

been augmented, often in juxtaposition, with relevant radiological images (plain X-rays, CT, MR and 3-D reconstructions) that introduce the student to radiological anatomy in preparation for their clinical studies. All illustrations are very well laid out and clearly labelled. The 2nd edition now introduces students to the Anatomy relevant to common minimally invasive interventional techniques, and students will find that the Summary at the end of most sections provides extremely useful pointers towards the essential knowledge that they need to acquire. Furthermore, the 'clinical boxes' clearly inform students why they need to know the information presented and how it is used. In short, this is a text for a student to realistically read all of, and not simply dip into as a reference. It provides a sound basis for developing an understanding of Human Anatomy, well suited to students of contemporary healthcare-related courses.

D. Ceri Davies
Professor of Anatomy
Imperial College London
London, UK

Preface to the first edition

Despite all the wonders of 'microchippery', there will always be a need for books that can be perused and provide a welcome relief from staring at a rectangular screen. This short synopsis is intended for those who need the essential facts of Human Anatomy without becoming lost in the mass of detail that occupies so much of most anatomical texts. We have attempted to sort out the wood from the trees and to give a concise account of the more important anatomical facts, without becoming bogged down in academic details which, although necessary for some, only hinder the understanding of the things that really matter for most people beginning the study of anatomy. Of course, there are endless arguments as to what is regarded as essential or basic, but we offer this as a presentation based on long experience of teaching at medical and paramedical levels.

The surface of the body is all that most people (except surgeons!) ever see of it, and much of 'learning anatomy' is really an exercise in being able to visualise exactly what is below each part of the surface, and then to think of the practical implications; there are numerous illustrations of surface anatomy in this book. When looking at the surface it is necessary to be able to 'mentally X-ray' every bit of the body, especially the chest and abdomen. Conventional radiology and modern imaging techniques are powerful aids to 'looking below the surface', and selected examples are included here to supplement dissections and explanatory drawings.

We hope this small volume will be helpful to all who are seeking a concise account of Human Anatomy as a basis for medical and paramedical studies.

R.M.H. McMinn
R.T. Hutchings
B.M. Logan

Preface to the second edition

In preparing the second edition of this very popular text, the authors have built upon the original concept to maintain it as a concise text for any student who is undertaking his or her study of the human body. Whereas many anatomy textbooks offer considerably more detail, this text offers a very readable account of human anatomy in an easily understood format, providing a firm basis to which extra detail can be added as the student becomes more experienced and detail becomes important. This emphasis on basic concepts is made possible by the extensive collective experience of the authors who have worked for several decades to introduce students to the marvelous structure of the human body.

While still keeping the text concise, clinical relevance is presented throughout with clinical hints and radiological imaging. Differences in spelling between that used in the United Kingdom and that used in the United States of America are highlighted in Appendix B (Glossary: derivation of anatomical and other terms). Short practice examination exercises have been added to most chapters to stress anatomical concepts in order to reinforce the knowledge gained by students from the text.

Two relatively recent clinical advances are given further emphasis. As radiological advances have occurred, more methods are now available to allow the clinician to easily visualise anatomical structure in a living individual. The authors have demonstrated this by adding appropriate radiological images alongside cadaveric illustrations to help the reader make the connection. In doing this we have accounted for the expansion of radiological imaging within the text and have used terminology to match that used clinically. Secondly, clinical techniques have developed considerably with minimally invasive clinical procedures now more prominent and these are referred to as appropriate. These two advances in particular will become increasingly abundant in clinical practice of the future and shape learning of human anatomy.

David Heylings
Stephen Carmichael
Samuel Leinster
Janak Saada

Acknowledgements

We are much indebted to Lynette Nearn for assistance with the preparation of dissections. We are also grateful for the advice and assistance given by colleagues Dr. Hilmar Spohr and Dr. Sarah Abdulla of the Norfolk and Norwich University Hospital Department of Radiology in the preparation of the radiological images.

We would also like to thank Norfolk and Norwich University NHS trust for their support with this project.

We would also like to thank Peter Beynon for his editorial help and Paul Bennett and Joanna Koster for taking this project on to publication.

Dissection credits

The following individuals are credited for their many hours of skilled and meticulous work in the art of preparing the anatomical material illustrated:

Bari M. Logan 3.1, 3.3, 3.4, 3.5, 3.6, 3.7, 3.8, 3.10, 3.11A, 3.12, 3.22, 3.23, 3.24, 3.26, 3.29A, 3.30, 3.37, 3.38A, 3.40, 4.2, 4.3, 4.5A, 4.6, 4.7, 4.9A, 4.11, 4.13, 4.14, 4.15A, 5.1, 5.4A, 5.5A, 5.7, 5.9, 5.10, 5.11, 5.12, 5.13, 6.4A, 6.10, 6.12A, 6.13, 7.4, 7.5A, 8.6A, 8.10, 8.11, 8.15A, 8.16A, 8.17, 8.18, 8.20

Professor R.M.H. McMinn 3.9A

Lynette Nearn 6.9, 7.6, 7.7, 8.3, 8.4, 8.5

Chapter 1
Body form and function

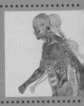

Introduction

The study of anatomy, from the Greek meaning to cut up, refers to the study of the structure of the body allied to its function as seen with the naked eye (in contrast to various kinds of microscopy). It is often referred to as gross or topographical anatomy – the geography of the body. Traditionally gross anatomy is learned through dissection, the Latin equivalent of the Greek for cutting. Although many current students do not carry out dissection themselves, they are usually able to study through the use of appropriate specimens prepared by their teachers and through the use of textbooks or other visual material. Study therefore tends to give the impression that deep to the skin human anatomy is identical, although our eyes show that everyone, externally at least, is different.

Dissection shows that under the skin, while we have the same structures, their size and relationship to each other may vary, creating differences known as anatomical variation, something that causes confusion for the novice dissector but for the experienced dissector is normal anatomy. Most variations do not lead directly to disease, but they can complicate clinical presentations and treatment. This text will highlight as appropriate some of the more common variations that are well noted by the dissector or have clinical implications.

Modern imaging techniques allow all parts of the body to be examined without a knife or even a finger being laid on the body. As this area develops, the resolution of the images and the level of detail visible is growing rapidly. Today it is seen as the best way to visualise living anatomy in the clinical situation, and in this text such images are used to demonstrate living anatomy alongside the images of cadaveric dissection. Radiographs using X-rays provide excellent detail about bones, joints and soft tissues. Images can be obtained in the three orthogonal planes – axial, coronal and sagittal – in a superficially similar way to the use of a conventional camera, which uses light instead of X-rays, for image production in the three orthogonal directions (frontal, side and bird's-eye views). More sophisticated, computer generated, cross-sectional images are obtained using X-rays (computerised tomography [CT] scanner) or radio frequency (magnetic resonance imaging [MRI] scanner) to provide high-detail multiplanar anatomical studies. The physical basis of CT and MRI is vastly different but they are considered to be complementary techniques with a wide range of applications. CT and radiography, both X-ray based techniques, exploit differences in physical densities for image generation, with denser objects (e.g. bone) appearing whiter than less dense objects such as fat or air. The MR image signal is much more difficult to interpret, giving an extraordinary range of signal intensities that are peculiar to the many different pulse sequences used to generate images. Both CT and MRI can be used to generate images of blood vessels using iodinated contrast agents and flow sensitive pulse sequences, respectively.

Anatomical terms

Anatomical terminology has its origins in the past when it was common to study Latin and Greek, and it is from these languages that the names of most structures have their origin. While study of these ancient languages is no longer needed, it does help to understand where many words have their origin.

Structural relationships

To describe how structures lie in relation to one another, an agreed standard position of the body, the anatomical position (**Fig. 1.1**), is used. This is where the body is standing upright with the feet together, the head and eyes facing forwards and the arms straight at the sides with the palms of the hands facing forwards. It does not matter whether you are standing up, lying down or standing on your head – the terms are always used to refer to this standard anatomical position.

Superior (cranial) and inferior (caudal) – towards the upper and lower ends of the body (e.g. the head is superior to the neck, the hip is inferior to the shoulder). These terms are usually used with the head, neck and trunk.

Anterior (ventral) and posterior (dorsal) – nearer the front and back of the body (e.g. the eyes are anterior to the ears, the ears are posterior to the eyes).

Proximal and distal – nearer to and further from the root of the structure (e.g. the elbow is proximal to the forearm, the hand is distal to the forearm). These terms are usually used in the limbs.

Medial and lateral – nearer to and further from the median plane (e.g. the great toe is on the medial side of the foot, the little toe on the lateral side).

Superficial and deep – nearer to and further from the skin surface.

Planes

The body can be divided by planes. The planes most commonly used in modern imaging are: (1) the coronal plane, which passes from the right side through to the left side of a body part (**Fig. 1.1A**); (2) the sagittal plane, which passes from anterior to posterior through a body part (**Fig. 1.1B**); and (3) the axial or transverse plane, which is an axial slice through a body part (**Fig. 1.1C**).

Special terms

Some special terms apply to the hand and foot. In the hand the palm is the anterior (palmar) surface and the dorsum is the posterior (dorsal) surface. In the foot the upper surface is the dorsum (dorsal surface) and the lower surface is the sole or plantar surface.

For joints of the limbs, flexion means bending and extension means straightening out. Special terms are used for certain forearm movements (p. 112).

Flexion and extension are also used for movements of the head and trunk. Bending the head or trunk forwards is flexion and the opposite is extension. Bending sideways (but still looking straight ahead) is lateral flexion.

Medial and lateral rotation applied to the limbs means rotation in the long axis of the limb. Putting a hand behind your back involves medial rotation of the arm, while putting it behind your head involves lateral rotation of the arm.

The Glossary (Appendix B, p. 253) explains the derivation of these and other terms.

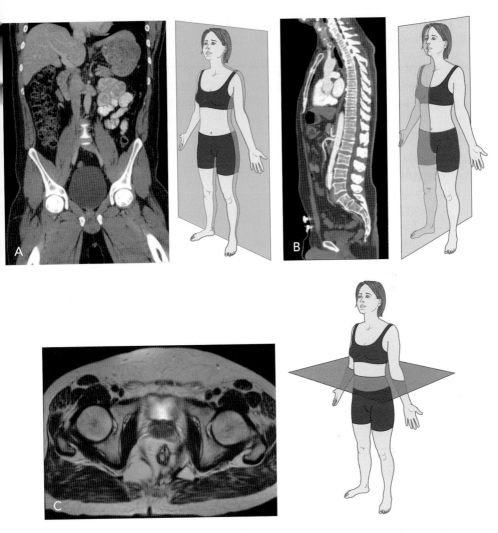

Fig. 1.1 Anatomical position and key anatomical planes: (A) coronal plane (CT image), (B) sagittal plane (CT image), (C) axial plane (MR image).

Systems

In the main this book discusses the anatomy of the body according to its various parts or regions (e.g. head, hand, thorax, pelvis [regional anatomy]). However, the various structures of the body can also be grouped together according to their common function, to make up what are commonly called systems (systemic anatomy). These are briefly summarised below and tend to involve more than one gross regional boundary, although the nervous system has a rather longer explanation in order to provide an adequate background to the later descriptions of the brain and spinal cord.

Musculoskeletal system

The skeleton, consisting of bones and cartilages, gives support to the body and provides protection for some organs, especially the brain and spinal cord. It also acts as a storehouse for minerals and the marrow cavities of some bones are the sites of formation of blood cells. The voluntary or skeletal muscles (muscular system) usually pull on their bony attachments and, through the joints, create movement.

Integumentary system (integument)

The integument – commonly known as the skin – forms the protective visible outer covering of the body and includes specialised derivatives – nails, hair, sebaceous glands (which lubricate the surface) and sweat glands (**Fig. 1.2**) which, in association with the blood flow through the skin, play a vital part in controlling body temperature (by surface evaporation). The breasts (mammary glands) are modified sweat glands, designed to secrete milk for the newborn (p. 132). Through its sensory nerve supply (cutaneous nerves, with specialised endings or receptors) the skin assesses the body's environment. Certain kinds of skin cells are concerned with pigmentation, immune responses and the synthesis of vitamin D.

Cardiovascular (circulatory) system

The cardiovascular system includes the heart as a muscular pump (**Fig. 1.3**), blood vessels as pipes and the blood that circulates through them to form a transport system (**Fig. 1.4**) for many substances, including blood gases. Arteries conduct blood away from the heart and veins conduct it back to the heart. Through branches of arteries of ever decreasing size, blood reaches the capillary bed, microscopic vessels forming a vast network in organs and tissues through which fluid and many substances can be exchanged. From the capillaries blood is gathered into veins of ever increasing size to be returned to the heart. Blood consists of a fluid (plasma) containing red cells (erythrocytes, for the transport of blood gases), various types of white cells (leucocytes) associated with defence and platelets (thrombocytes, concerned with blood clotting).

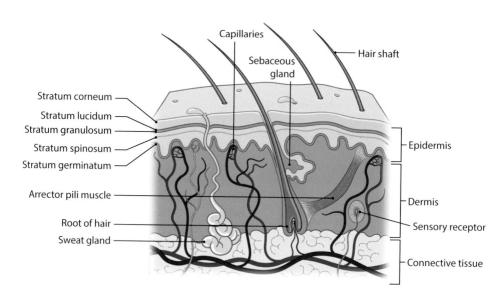

Fig. 1.2 Diagram of a transverse section of skin.

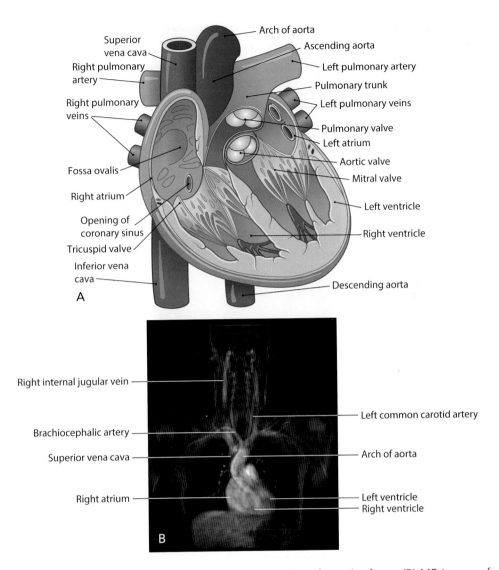

Fig. 1.3 (A) Heart and great vessels, model opened up from the front, (B) MR image of the heart and great vessels.

Lymphatic system

The lymphatic system is closely allied to the cardiovascular system. It consists of the lymphoid organs (thymus, spleen, tonsils) and lymph nodes, lymphoid follicles scattered in certain non-lymphoid organs (especially in parts of the digestive tract) and lymphatic channels (lymphatics), which drain lymphocytes and fluid (lymph) from the lymphoid organs and follicles, as well as tissue fluid from other components of the body. The lymph nodes are sites for lymph filtration and as a result may become the sites for infections or cancerous deposits derived from any part of the drainage area. The cervical, axillary and inguinal nodes are those most readily palpable and routinely examined. Apart from

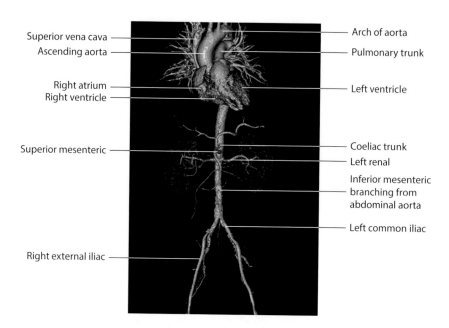

Superior vena cava — Arch of aorta
Ascending aorta — Pulmonary trunk

Right atrium — Left ventricle
Right ventricle

Superior mesenteric — Coeliac trunk
— Left renal

Inferior mesenteric branching from abdominal aorta

— Left common iliac

Right external iliac

Fig. 1.4 Reconstructed CT angiogram of the heart and main trunk arterial branches.

drainage, the system is concerned with the manufacture and transport of lymphocytes for the body's immune responses. Part of it also transports fat absorbed from the intestine.

Respiratory system

The respiratory system is concerned with the exchange of oxygen and carbon dioxide between blood and air, which takes place in the lungs (**Fig. 1.5**). The rest of this system is the respiratory tract and is simply a conducting pathway for air and includes the nose and paranasal sinuses, pharynx, larynx, trachea and bronchi. Part of the larynx acts as a respiratory sphincter, concerned with the production of voice (p. 91).

Digestive system

The digestive system is concerned with the digestion and absorption of the foodstuffs necessary to provide the chemical energy for all body functions. The digestive or alimentary tract is composed of the mouth, pharynx, oesophagus, stomach, small

intestine and large intestine (**Fig. 1.6**). The digestive processes of the stomach and intestines are assisted by the secretions of the major digestive glands – the liver (with the gallbladder) and pancreas (pp. 175–180).

Urinary system

The urinary system in both sexes consists of the paired kidneys and ureters, the single urinary bladder and the urethra. The system is concerned with the production, storage and elimination of urine in order to maintain the body's proper content of water and dissolved substances (pp. 181).

Reproductive system

The reproductive system in the female provides the female germ cells (ova [singular, ovum]) from the paired ovaries, whereas the uterus and vagina are organs for the conception, development and birth of a new individual. In the male reproductive system the paired testes provide the

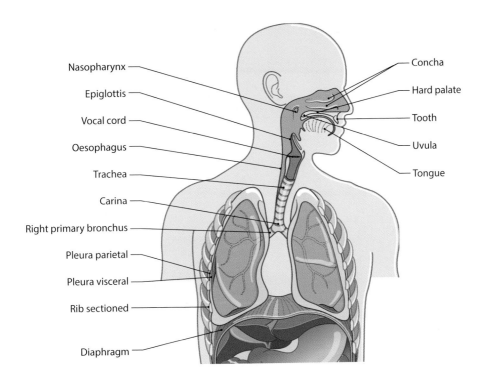

Nasopharynx
Epiglottis
Vocal cord
Oesophagus
Trachea
Carina
Right primary bronchus
Pleura parietal
Pleura visceral
Rib sectioned
Diaphragm

Concha
Hard palate
Tooth
Uvula
Tongue

Fig. 1.5 Parts of the respiratory system.

male germ cells (sperm or spermatozoa [singular, spermatozoon]). Since some of the male genital organs are shared with some urinary organs, the combined systems are often called the genitourinary system (see Chapter 7).

Endocrine system

Like the nervous system, the endocrine system is for communication, but it acts at a much slower rate via the hormones secreted by its various components and is mostly distributed through the bloodstream. It consists of the main endocrine organs (the pituitary gland and the adjacent part of the brain [p. 37], the adrenal [p. 182], thyroid and parathyroid glands [p. 90]) and various other groups of endocrine cells that are found in other organs, especially in the pancreas (the islets of Langerhans) (p. 179) and digestive tract, testis and ovary (p. 200–202).

Nervous system

The nervous system is a communication system designed to receive information from the outside world and from the body itself (sensory input), and then make appropriate responses (motor output). Topographically, it is divided into the central nervous system (CNS), composed of the brain and spinal cord (**Fig. 1.7**), and the peripheral nervous system (PNS), composed of cranial nerves that exit/pass through cranial foramina and spinal nerves that pass through intervertebral foramina.

Motor nerves that supply skeletal (voluntary) muscle constitute the voluntary or somatic nervous system, whereas others supply cardiac muscle, smooth (involuntary) muscle and glands to form the autonomic nervous system (ANS), which is concerned with automatic or involuntary activities such as heart rate, constriction of blood vessels,

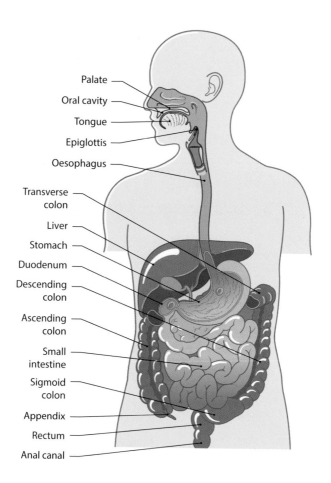

Fig. 1.6 Parts of the digestive system.

sweating, secretion in the stomach and the size of the pupil. Importantly, the ANS maintains the homeostasis of the body mainly through the parasympathetic and sympathetic nervous systems. Nerve cells (neurons) have filamentous processes (nerve fibres) that are collected into bundles to form the nerves as seen in dissection of the PNS and the various tracts in the brain and spinal cord.

Fibres that convey nerve impulses away from their own cell bodies (the part of the nerve cell containing the nucleus) or from the CNS are *efferent* fibres; these include the motor fibres that supply muscles and glands. Those that convey impulses towards their own cell bodies or to the CNS are *afferent*

fibres; these include the sensory fibres that convey general or special types of sensation, as well as those unconscious impulses concerned with reflexes. General sensations are those of touch, pain, pressure, temperature and proprioception (muscle–joint sense, which gives information on position and movement) and the special sensations are vision, smell, taste, hearing and balance (equilibrium).

The transmission of nerve impulses from one neuron to another occurs at specialised sites, known as synapses, and depends on the release of a transmitter substance, which sets off an impulse in the receiving cell. The synaptic connections between neurons complete the neuronal pathways that control bodily

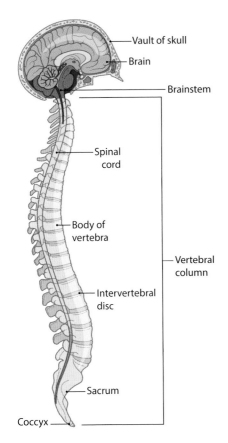

Fig. 1.7 Left half of brain and the spinal cord within part of the skull and vertebral column.

activities. Neuromuscular junctions are sites on skeletal muscle fibres that are similar to synapses; at these sites the impulse for contraction is passed on from nerve to muscle, again by a transmitter substance. At these junctions and at parasympathetic synapses the transmitter is acetylcholine; at sympathetic synapses it is noradrenaline (norepinephrine). Elsewhere there may be other transmitters.

The majority of neurons within the CNS have microscopically short processes and are collectively called interneurons. They vastly outnumber the main motor and sensory neurons, and form intercommunicating networks between themselves and the larger neurons.

As far as motor activity is concerned it is essential to understand the difference between somatic and autonomic innervation. In somatic motor nerves the fibres run directly from their cells of origin in the CNS to skeletal muscle fibres without interruption. In autonomic innervation there are two sets of neurons in series:

- Preganglionic, with cell bodies in the CNS whose fibres run to ganglion cells outside the CNS.
- Postganglionic, with ganglion cells in the PNS whose fibres run to the target organ.

If **sympathetic** (**Fig. 1.8**), the preganglionic cell bodies are in the thoracic and upper lumbar parts of the spinal cord. Their fibres run out in the thoracic and upper lumbar spinal nerves to synapse with the postganglionic cells, which are either in the ganglia of the sympathetic trunks lying beside the vertebral column (paravertebral) or in other ganglia anterior to the vertebral column (prevertebral). (A few fibres pass directly to cells of the medulla of the adrenal glands.) The postganglionic fibres are widely distributed to all parts of the body by peripheral nerves and/or blood vessels; for the body surface they supply blood vessels, sweat glands and the arrector pili muscles (the ones attached to hair follicles that cause 'goose pimples' on a cold day).

If **parasympathetic** (**Fig. 1.8**), the preganglionic cells are in certain cell groups in the brainstem (cranial nerves III, VII, IX and X and the sacral part (S2, 3 and 4) of the spinal cord. Their fibres run out in cranial or sacral nerves to postganglionic cells, which are within or very near the walls of some organs (in particular the heart, stomach and pelvic viscera) or in the head and neck in four small discrete ganglia (ciliary, otic, pterygopalatine and submandibular) to supply the pupil or salivary and lacrimal glands. Parasympathetic nerves are more localised in their distribution than are sympathetic nerves and do not supply any part of the limbs or body surface.

Labels for Fig. 1.7:
Vault of skull
Brain
Brainstem
Spinal cord
Body of vertebra
Vertebral column
Intervertebral disc
Sacrum
Coccyx

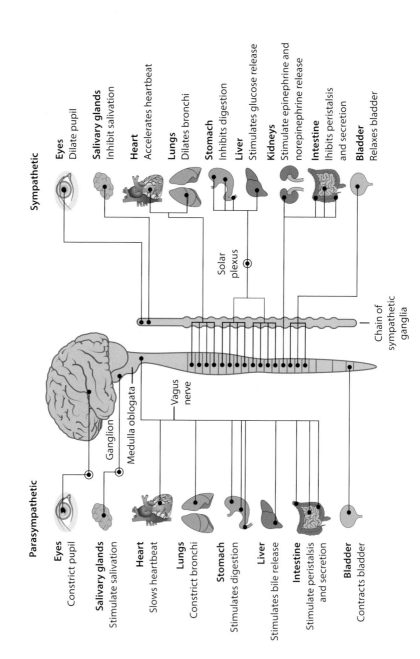

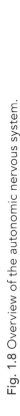

Fig. 1.8 Overview of the autonomic nervous system.

Chapter 2
Bones and joints

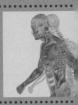

Introduction

The bones of the body (**Figs. 2.1–2.7**) make up its internal supporting framework or skeleton without which the body would collapse like a jellyfish out of water.

Through the course of human evolution, the more general four-legged support of the mammalian body concerned entirely with locomotion has given place to locomotion confined to the lower limbs, with the upper limbs becoming specialised for prehensile activities.

The common diseases of joints (arthritis) are not life-threatening but can result in varying degrees of disability, ranging from interference with the commonplace hand movements, which are so essential for the activities of daily living, to severe mobility problems that prevent people from getting about in the normal way.

Bones can be classified as those of the axial skeleton (head, neck and trunk) and those of the appendicular skeleton (limbs). Bones can also be classified according to their shape as long (the main limb bones), short (as in fingers and toes), flat (like the scapula-shoulder blade), irregular (as in the skull, vertebral column, hand and foot) and sesamoid (found in some tendons; the largest is the patella or kneecap).

A few bones (clavicle, mandible and some other skull bones) develop in foetal life by groups of connective-tissue cells becoming transformed into bone-forming cells (osteoblasts); this is 'ossification in membrane', or intramembranous ossification, and the site where the bone is first formed is a primary centre of ossification. However, most bones are formed first as cartilage, which is destroyed in an orderly manner and then replaced by bone in the process known as endochondral ossification ('ossification in cartilage'). The cartilaginous shaft of a long bone, for example, develops in early foetal life a primary ossification centre from which bone formation spreads throughout the length of the shaft, but the ends of the bone remain cartilaginous until about the time of birth or later; only then do the ends (called epiphyses) develop their own or secondary centres of ossification. Although subject to some variation, each bone has its own characteristic time pattern for the appearance of ossification centres. Radiographs in children and adolescents show that epiphyses are separated from the shaft by a gap, the epiphyseal line/plate (**Fig. 2.8**), which is due to the remaining cartilage (the epiphyseal plate, being radiolucent, not radiopaque like bone, and must not be mistaken for a fracture line). It is the site where much of the growth in length of the bone occurs. When the epiphyseal cartilage disappears, growth is complete.

Bones are held together to form joints, most of which are mobile, so enabling the whole or selected parts of the body to move as required by the muscles acting upon them. These joints, also known as articulations, are of three types: fibrous, cartilaginous and synovial.

- **Fibrous joints** – bones united by fibrous tissue, allowing no movement, as in skull sutures.
- **Cartilaginous joints** – bones united by plates of cartilage, sometimes allowing limited movement, as at intervertebral discs between the bodies of vertebrae and the pubic symphysis between the front ends of the two hip bones. The junctions between the shafts and epiphyses of developing bones are also a type of cartilaginous joint, although they disappear as growth ceases.
- **Synovial joints** – typical joints of the limbs, and what most people understand by the word joint. The bone ends are covered by cartilage and surrounded by a fibrous capsule that encloses a joint cavity. The capsule is reinforced by ligaments on the outside and sometimes has other ligaments inside. The inside of the capsule is lined by synovial membrane, which secretes a minute amount of synovial fluid (the knee joint, the largest, has only 0.5 ml). Synovial joints allow varying degrees of movement and, depending on the shape of the articulating surfaces, can be classified into various types: ball-and-socket (hip, shoulder), hinge (elbow, interphalangeal joints of fingers and toes), condylar (modified hinge, as at the knee and temporomandibular, or jaw, joint), ellipsoid (modified ball-and-socket, as at the wrist), saddle (saddle-shaped surfaces, as at the base of the thumb) and plane (rather flat surfaces, as between some wrist and foot bones).

The details of individual joints are considered in the chapters for the appropriate regions. There is a general principle that governs innervation of each joint known as Hilton's Law: this states that 'a joint is innervated by the same nerves that innervate the muscles acting across that joint'.

Axial skeleton

The axial skeleton consists of the skull, hyoid bone, vertebrae, ribs and costal cartilages, and the sternum (**Figs. 2.1–2.3**).

Skull

The skull (**Figs. 2.1, 2.2**) consists of paired and unpaired bones (a total of 22), most of which are firmly connected by sutures (fibrous joints), except for the mandible, which forms the movable synovial temporomandibular joint (jaw joint) with the lower surface of the temporal bone on each side. In radiographs, suture lines must not be mistaken for fracture lines.

Cranium – strictly means the skull without the mandible, but is often used to mean the upper part of the skull that encloses the brain; it is made up of paired parietal and temporal bones and of single occipital, sphenoid, ethmoid and frontal bones. The uppermost part is the cranial vault, the rest is the base of the skull. External features are considered below and internal features in Chapter 3 (Head, neck and vertebral column, p. 35).

Pterion – region where parietal, frontal, sphenoid and temporal bones meet to give an H-shaped pattern of suture lines (**Figs. 2.1B, 2.2B**). It lies about 5 cm above the midpoint of the zygomatic arch. Underlying it on the inside is a branch of the middle meningeal artery, liable to be

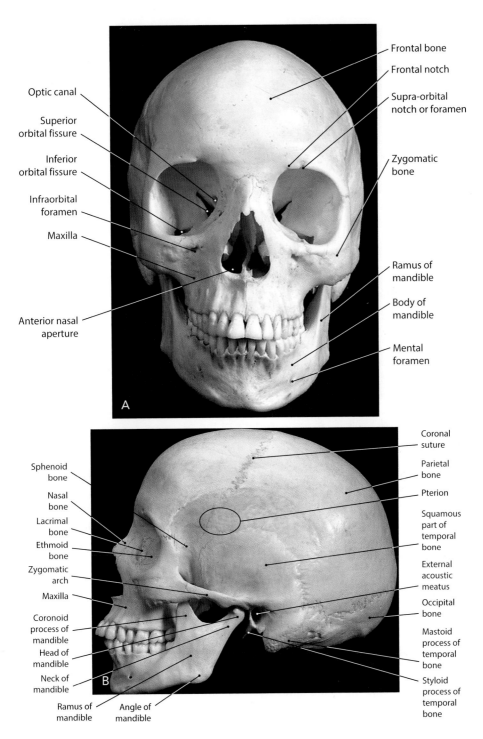

Fig. 2.1 Skull: (A) from the front, (B) from the left.

(Continued)

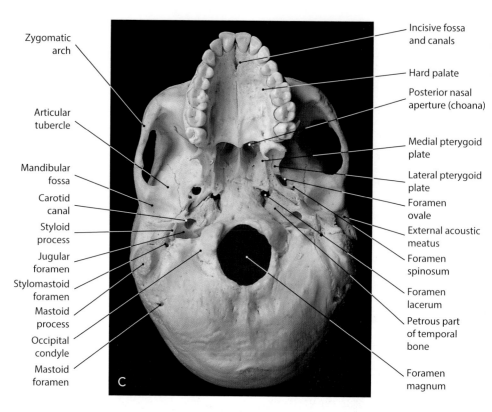

Zygomatic arch

Articular tubercle

Mandibular fossa

Carotid canal

Styloid process

Jugular foramen

Stylomastoid foramen

Mastoid process

Occipital condyle

Mastoid foramen

Incisive fossa and canals

Hard palate

Posterior nasal aperture (choana)

Medial pterygoid plate

Lateral pterygoid plate

Foramen ovale

External acoustic meatus

Foramen spinosum

Foramen lacerum

Petrous part of temporal bone

Foramen magnum

C

Fig. 2.1 *(Continued)* Skull: (C) external surface of the base.

damaged in skull fractures of this area and cause haemorrhage, with resulting pressure on the brain. Bone can be drilled away to relieve pressure and ligate the damaged vessel.

Facial skeleton – the front (anterior) part of the skull, containing the orbital and nasal cavities. The principal bones are the single mandible (lower jaw with lower teeth) and paired zygomatic bones and maxillae (forming the upper jaw with upper teeth), with the frontal bone forming the forehead. The margins of each orbit are formed by the frontal and zygomatic bones and maxilla. The zygomatic bone is often called the cheek bone. The frontal, ethmoid and sphenoid bones and the maxillae contain the paranasal air sinuses (**Fig. 3.25**).

External surface of the base of the skull

Hard palate – forms the floor of the nasal cavity and roof of the mouth (**Figs. 2.1C, 2.2B**).

Posterior nasal apertures (choanae) – above the back of the hard palate, opening into the nasal part of the pharynx.

Mandibular fossa – in the temporal bone, forming the temporomandibular joint (jaw joint) with the head of the mandible.

Occipital condyles – on either side of the foramen magnum, forming atlanto-occipital joints with C1 vertebra (atlas).

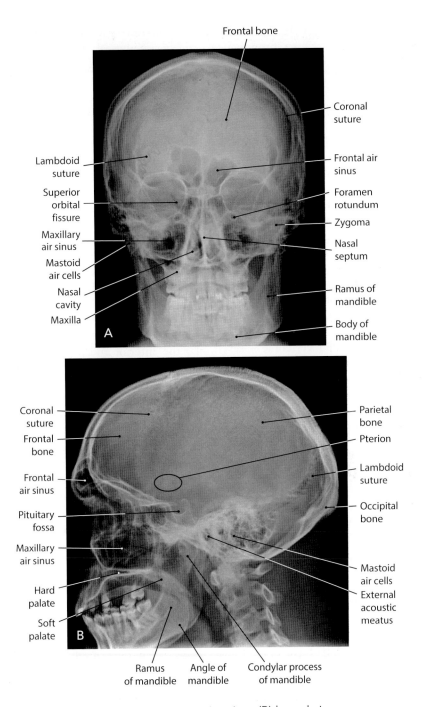

Fig. 2.2 Skull radiographs: (A) anteroposterior view, (B) lateral view.

Mastoid process – part of the temporal bone, forming the bony prominence behind the ear, and containing mastoid air cells, which communicate with the middle ear (**Fig. 3.33C**).

Hyoid bone

The hyoid bone is a small U-shaped bone in the anterior (front) of the neck just inferior to the mandible and above the thyroid cartilage of the larynx (**Figs. 3.38B, 3.41**). It consists of a central body and a greater horn on each side, with a much smaller lesser horn projecting up from the junction between the body and greater horn. Various muscles and ligaments are attached to it, but it is unique in that it makes no joint with any other bone.

Vertebrae

There are normally 33 vertebrae – seven cervical, 12 thoracic, five lumbar, five sacral (fused together forming the sacrum), and four coccygeal (fused as the coccyx), all linked to form the vertebral column (spinal column, spine, or backbone, 'the back') (**Figs. 2.3, 2.4**).

Each vertebra typically consists of a body anteriorly, with a vertebral (neural) arch posterior to the body. The space between the body and arch is the vertebral foramen; in the articulated vertebral column the foramina collectively form the vertebral or spinal canal (**Fig. 3.16B**), within which lies the thecal sac, which contains the spinal cord and the surrounding membranes (p. 55). The arch is made up of a pedicle (attached to the body) on each side and a lamina posteriorly; two laminae unite in the midline to form the spinous process. Where the pedicle and lamina join, a transverse process projects laterally, and there are also superior and inferior articular processes projecting upwards and downwards, respectively (**Fig. 2.4**). When articulated, the gap between the pedicles of adjacent vertebrae, bounded posteriorly by the zygapophyseal (commonly called facet) joints and anteriorly by the intervertebral disc, forms the intervertebral foramen, the important opening through which each spinal nerve emerges (p. 59).

The first cervical vertebra is also called the atlas (unique in that is has no body), which makes joints on each side with the skull above (atlanto-occipital joints) and with the second cervical vertebra, the axis, below (lateral atlanto-axial joints). The unique feature of the axis is the dens (odontoid process), projecting upwards from the body to articulate with the anterior arch of the atlas (median atlanto-axial joint, **Figs. 3.5, 3.11B**).

The remaining cervical vertebrae and the thoracic and lumbar vertebrae are united by various ligaments, in particular the anterior and posterior longitudinal ligaments (each of which is a long continuous band on the anterior and posterior surfaces, respectively, of the vertebral bodies) and small joints between the adjacent articular processes (zygapophyseal or facet joints). Ligaments with a high content of elastic tissue, the ligamenta flava ('yellow ligaments'), unite adjacent laminae. The most extensive connections between vertebrae are the intervertebral discs (**Figs. 2.5, 3.16B**), which act like slightly compressible rubber cushions between adjacent vertebral bodies. Each consists of outer concentric rings of fibrocartilage that form the annulus fibrosus, with a more centrally located gelatinous mass, the nucleus pulposus.

In a prolapsed or 'slipped' disc the nucleus becomes displaced through part of the annulus and may impinge on nerve roots passing from the vertebral canal into the intervertebral foramen (**Fig. 3.16A**).

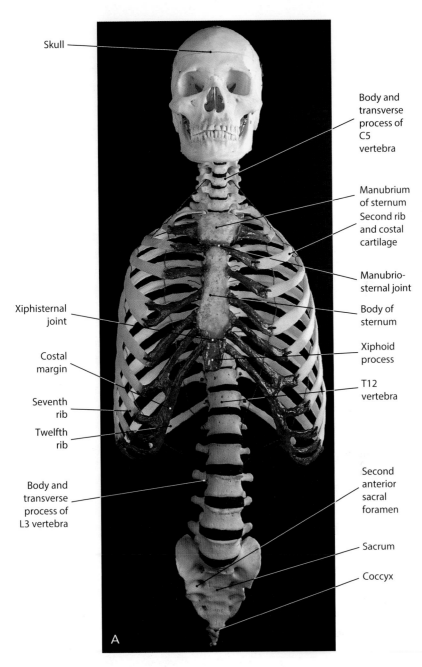

Skull

Body and transverse process of C5 vertebra

Manubrium of sternum

Second rib and costal cartilage

Manubrio-sternal joint

Body of sternum

Xiphoid process

T12 vertebra

Xiphisternal joint

Costal margin

Seventh rib

Twelfth rib

Body and transverse process of L3 vertebra

Second anterior sacral foramen

Sacrum

Coccyx

A

Fig. 2.3 Axial skeleton: (A) from the front.   (Continued)

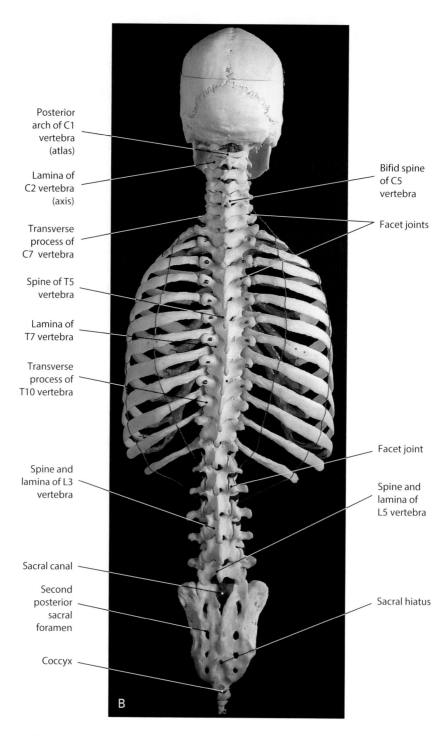

Posterior arch of C1 vertebra (atlas)

Lamina of C2 vertebra (axis)

Transverse process of C7 vertebra

Spine of T5 vertebra

Lamina of T7 vertebra

Transverse process of T10 vertebra

Spine and lamina of L3 vertebra

Sacral canal

Second posterior sacral foramen

Coccyx

Bifid spine of C5 vertebra

Facet joints

Facet joint

Spine and lamina of L5 vertebra

Sacral hiatus

B

Fig. 2.3 *(Continued)* Axial skeleton: (B) from behind.

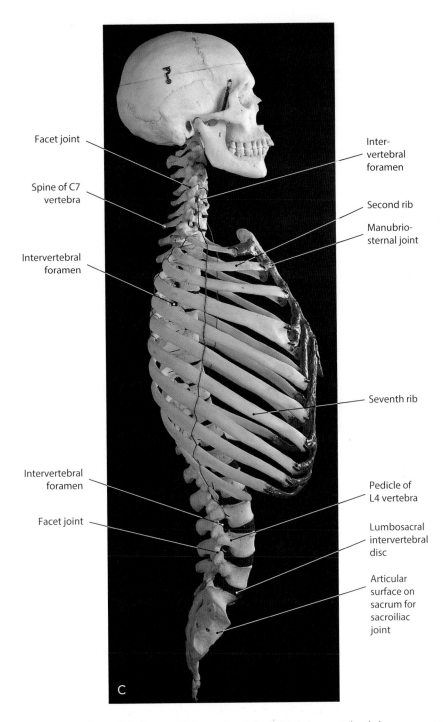

Facet joint

Spine of C7
vertebra

Intervertebral
foramen

Intervertebral
foramen

Facet joint

Inter-
vertebral
foramen

Second rib

Manubrio-
sternal joint

Seventh rib

Pedicle of
L4 vertebra

Lumbosacral
intervertebral
disc

Articular
surface on
sacrum for
sacroiliac
joint

C

Fig. 2.3 *(Continued)* Axial skeleton: (C) from the right (with intervertebral discs represented by felt pads between the vertebral bodies). (For the hyoid bone see Figs. 3.38B and 3.41.)

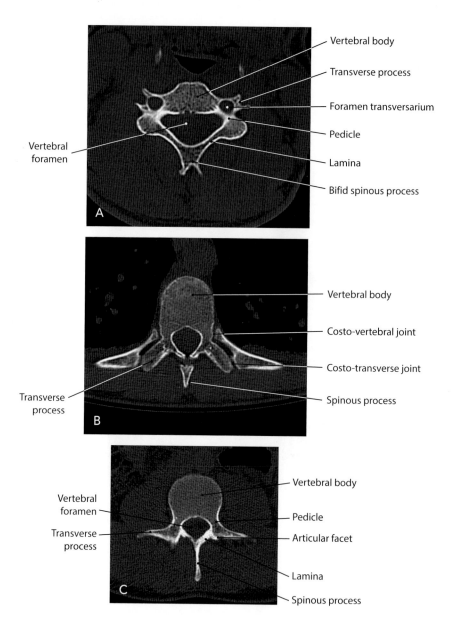

Fig. 2.4 CT axial views of a typical vertebra: (A) cervical, (B) thoracic showing rib articulation, (C) lumbar.

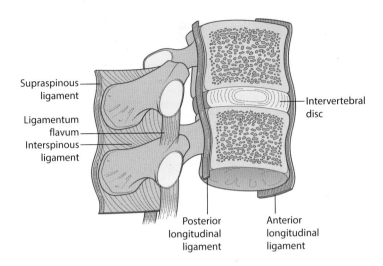

Fig. 2.5 Drawing of upper lumbar spinal column.

The highest disc is the one between the C2 (axis) and the C3 vertebrae; the lowest (the one most commonly prolapsed) is between the L5 vertebra and S1 of the sacrum.

The sacrum consists of the five fused sacral vertebrae (**Figs. 2.3A & B, 7.1, 7.2**), and has four pairs of anterior and posterior sacral foramina (corresponding to the intervertebral foramina in other regions). It is joined above to the fifth lumbar vertebra by an intervertebral disc and ligaments and laterally to the hip bones through the sacroiliac joints to form the bony pelvis, and at its lower end it is joined with the coccyx (of four rudimentary coccygeal vertebrae) through the sacrococcygeal joint.

Ribs and sternum

There are 12 pairs of ribs (**Figs. 2.3, 2.4B**), articulating with vertebrae posteriorly and with costal cartilage anteriorly. Each rib has a head, which typically articulates with the bodies of two adjacent vertebrae, a neck, a tubercle (which articulates with the transverse process of its own vertebra) and

a body or shaft of variable length that forms the curved chest wall. The first seven pairs of ribs (true ribs) are joined to the sternum by their costal cartilages. The next three pairs (false ribs) are joined by their cartilages to the cartilage above. The last two pairs (floating ribs) are short and not joined to others.

The sternum consists of the manubrium (at the top cranial end), body and xiphoid process (at the lower caudal end). Together the ribs, costal cartilages and the 12 thoracic vertebrae form the skeleton of the thorax. The manubrium and body are not quite in a vertical line, but unite at a slight angle (the sternal angle of Louis) to each other, forming the cartilaginous manubriosternal joint. It may become ossified in later life.

> The important manubriosternal joint locates the articulation of the second costal cartilage, which is useful when clinically locating specific intercostal spaces.

Appendicular skeleton

The appendicular skeleton consists of the bones of the upper limbs (**Fig. 2.6**) and lower limbs (**Fig. 2.7**), including those of the limb girdles, which are the bones that attach the limb to the axial skeleton (clavicle and scapula, forming the pectoral or shoulder girdle, and the hip bone, consisting of the ilium, ischium and pubis fused together to form the pelvic or hip girdle).

Upper limb bones

Clavicle – rather S-shaped, with a bulbous medial end for the sternoclavicular joint and a flattened lateral end for the acromioclavicular joint, and a groove on the under surface. The clavicle is the first bone to begin to ossify, between the fifth and sixth week of embryonic life, by intramembranous ossification.

Scapula – shaped roughly like a triangle, with a prominent spine projecting from the posterior (dorsal) surface that ends laterally as the flattened acromion. The upper outer angle is expanded to form the glenoid cavity, which accommodates the head of the humerus to form the shoulder (glenohumeral) joint. Projecting anteriorly above the glenoid cavity is the palpable coracoid process located just inferior to the acromioclavicular joint.

Humerus – bone of the arm, with a rounded head at the proximal end: the greater tubercle (tuberosity) at the outer lateral side of the head, the lesser tubercle (tuberosity) anteriorly, with the intertubercular (bicipital) groove between them located anteriorly on the proximal end of the shaft (**Fig. 2.6**). The margin of the smooth head is the anatomical neck; between the proximal part of the shaft and the head (and tubercles) is the surgical neck (as this is the commoner site for fractures in this region of the humerus). At the distal end there is a prominent medial epicondyle and a less obvious lateral epicondyle. Between the two are the smooth articular surfaces for the elbow joint: medially, the pulley-shaped trochlea (for the ulna) with a prominent medial lip; and laterally, the rounded capitulum (for the radius). Posteriorly at the distal end is the deep olecranon fossa, which accommodates the olecranon of the ulna when the elbow is extended.

Radius – lateral bone of the forearm: has a rounded proximal end, the radial head, which articulates with the capitulum of the humerus and a notch on the ulna. The shaft immediately distal to the head is the neck, distal to which on the medial side, is the radial tuberosity (for attachment of the biceps tendon). Distally, the radial shaft is expanded to articulate with the carpal bones to form part of the wrist joint, and it ends by forming the point-like styloid process.

Ulna – medial bone of the forearm, with the proximal end deeply depressed anteriorly, forming the trochlear notch (whose posterior boundary is the olecranon) for articulation with the trochlea of the humerus. The small rounded distal end comprises the head, with a styloid process on its medial side. (**Note:** The head of the radius is located proximally while the head of the ulna is at its distal end.)

Carpal bones – bones of the wrist. The eight small carpal bones each have their own characteristic sizes and shapes, details of which need not be learned. The important point is to remember the order of the bones in the two rows of four from the lateral to the medial side: in the proximal row, the scaphoid, lunate, triquetral

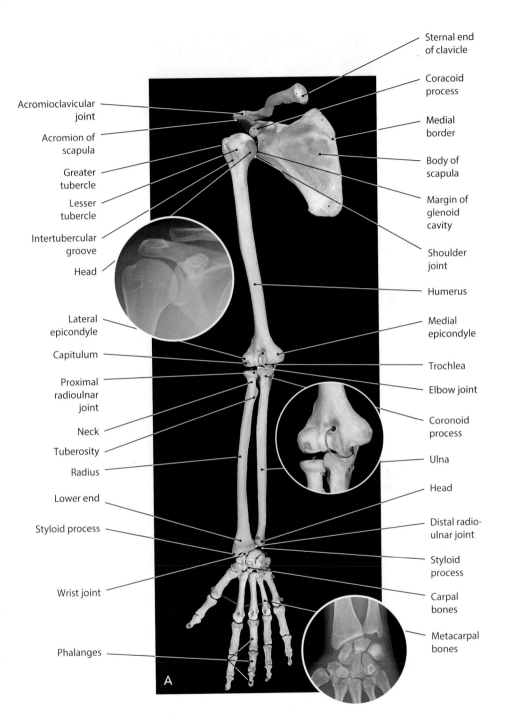

Sternal end
of clavicle

Coracoid
process

Acromioclavicular
joint

Acromion of
scapula

Greater
tubercle

Lesser
tubercle

Intertubercular
groove

Head

Lateral
epicondyle

Capitulum

Proximal
radioulnar
joint

Neck

Tuberosity

Radius

Lower end

Styloid process

Wrist joint

Phalanges

Medial
border

Body of
scapula

Margin of
glenoid
cavity

Shoulder
joint

Humerus

Medial
epicondyle

Trochlea

Elbow joint

Coronoid
process

Ulna

Head

Distal radio-
ulnar joint

Styloid
process

Carpal
bones

Metacarpal
bones

A

Fig. 2.6 Bones of the right upper limb: (A) from the front.   *(Continued)*

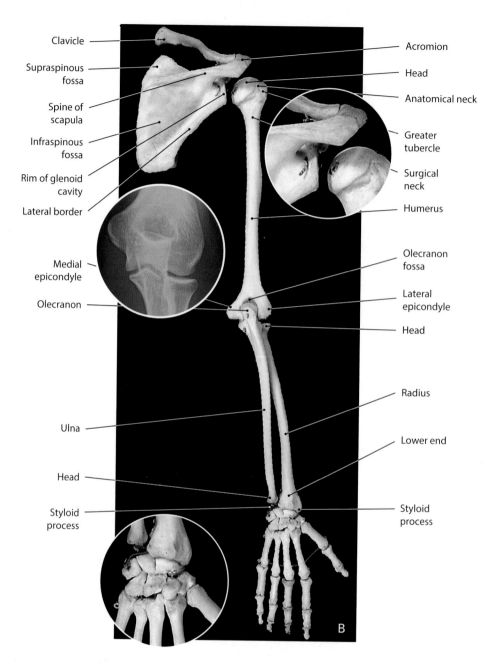

Clavicle

Supraspinous fossa

Spine of scapula

Infraspinous fossa

Rim of glenoid cavity

Lateral border

Medial epicondyle

Olecranon

Ulna

Head

Styloid process

Acromion

Head

Anatomical neck

Greater tubercle

Surgical neck

Humerus

Olecranon fossa

Lateral epicondyle

Head

Radius

Lower end

Styloid process

B

Fig. 2.6 (*Continued*) Bones of the right upper limb: (B) from behind.   (*Continued*)

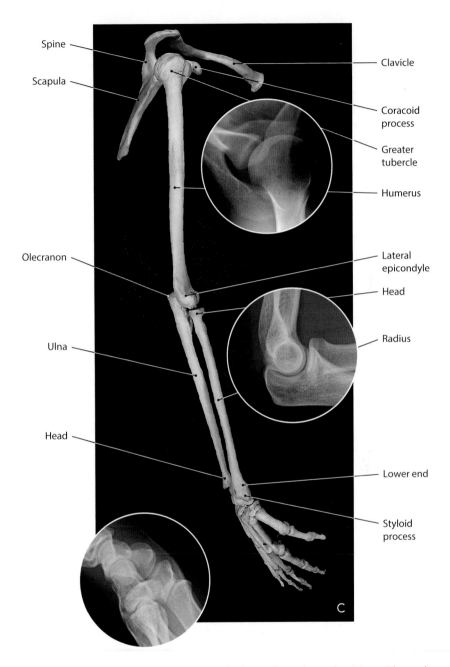

Fig. 2.6 (*Continued*) Bones of the right upper limb: (C) from the right. (Note: The radiograph of the shoulder is viewed from above down rather than laterally.)

and pisiform bones; and in the distal row, the trapezium, trapezoid, capitate and hamate bones. The scaphoid, lunate and triquetral bones articulate with the distal radius, forming the wrist joint (**Fig. 4.15**). The most important carpal bones are the scaphoid (most commonly fractured) and the lunate (most commonly dislocated). The trapezium and the base of the first metacarpal make the carpometacarpal joint of the thumb the most important of the carpometacarpal joints.

Metacarpal bones and phalanges – bones of the hand and fingers. Each has a shaft with a base at the proximal end and a head at the distal end, so that the heads and bases of adjacent bones make metacarpophalangeal and interphalangeal joints for each digit. Metacarpal bases articulate with the distal carpal bones to form the carpometacarpal joints.

Lower limb bones

Hip bone – three bones fused together: the ilium, ischium and pubis. Parts of all three form the cup-shaped acetabulum on the outer surface, for the hip joint. The proximal (upper) part is the ilium, whose upper margin is the iliac crest, ending anteriorly as the anterior superior iliac spine (ASIS). The medial surface forms the sacroiliac joint with the sacrum. The rough distal lowest part of the hip bone is the tuberosity of the ischium, and the anterior part is the body of the pubis (which in the intact pelvis unites with its fellow at the midline pubic symphysis). The large hole inferior to the acetabulum is the obturator foramen. The ischial spine projects medially from the ischium between the greater and lesser sciatic notches (**Figs. 2.7C, 7.1, 7.2**), which are converted into the greater and

lesser sciatic foramina by the transversely placed sacrospinous ligament and by the larger and tough, almost vertical, sacrotuberous ligament. The sacrum (with the coccyx at its lower end) and the two hip bones form the bony pelvis.

Femur – bone of the thigh, with the ball-shaped head at the proximal end for the hip joint; it is joined to the shaft by the neck at an angle of about 125°. The greater trochanter is the large prominence located laterally at the junction of the shaft and neck; the lesser trochanter is the smaller cone-shaped projection at the distal part of the neck and adjacent shaft, facing medially and posteriorly. The expanded distal end has curved medial and lateral condyles for the knee joint and on either side palpable prominences known as the medial and lateral epicondyles. The epiphysis at the distal end usually begins to ossify in the ninth foetal month, a fact of possible medicolegal significance as an indication of maturity.

Patella – kneecap, of which the posterior surface is smooth with facets for articulating with the condyles of the femur, and the distal end is rather pointed compared with the upper end for attachment of the patellar ligament (**Figs. 2.7, 8.8A & B, 8.10**).

Tibia – medial and main bone of the leg, of which the large proximal end has flat medial and lateral condyles for the knee joint, with the tibial tuberosity in the centre of the anterior of the shaft just distal to the condyles. The medial surface of the shaft is flat and subcutaneous and commonly called the shin. The smaller distal end terminates with an articular surface for the talus and is extended medially to form the medial malleolus with an articular facet on its lateral surface.

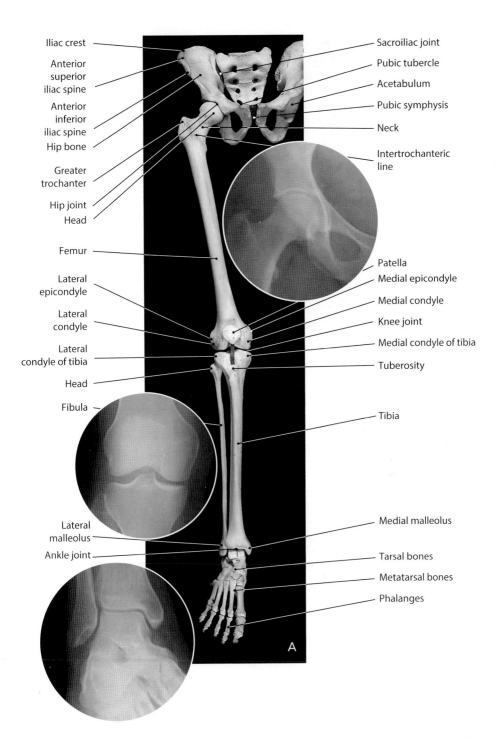

Iliac crest

Anterior superior iliac spine

Anterior inferior iliac spine

Hip bone

Greater trochanter

Hip joint

Head

Femur

Lateral epicondyle

Lateral condyle

Lateral condyle of tibia

Head

Fibula

Lateral malleolus

Ankle joint

Sacroiliac joint

Pubic tubercle

Acetabulum

Pubic symphysis

Neck

Intertrochanteric line

Patella

Medial epicondyle

Medial condyle

Knee joint

Medial condyle of tibia

Tuberosity

Tibia

Medial malleolus

Tarsal bones

Metatarsal bones

Phalanges

A

Fig. 2.7 Bones of the right lower limb: (A) from the front, with the sacrum and part of the left hip bone. *(Continued)*

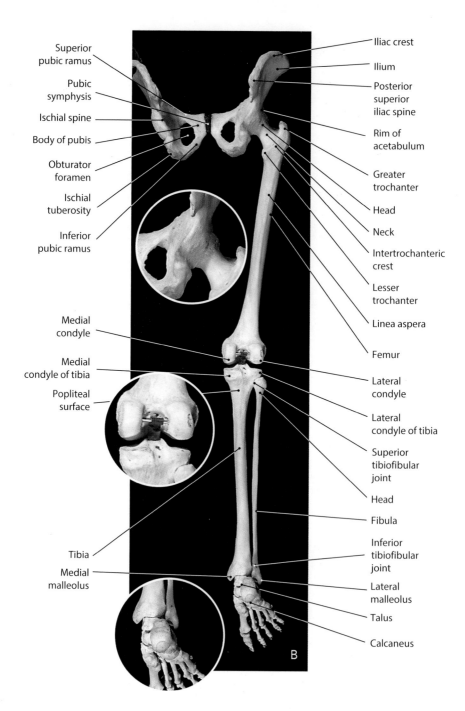

Superior pubic ramus

Pubic symphysis

Ischial spine

Body of pubis

Obturator foramen

Ischial tuberosity

Inferior pubic ramus

Medial condyle

Medial condyle of tibia

Popliteal surface

Tibia

Medial malleolus

Iliac crest

Ilium

Posterior superior iliac spine

Rim of acetabulum

Greater trochanter

Head

Neck

Intertrochanteric crest

Lesser trochanter

Linea aspera

Femur

Lateral condyle

Lateral condyle of tibia

Superior tibiofibular joint

Head

Fibula

Inferior tibiofibular joint

Lateral malleolus

Talus

Calcaneus

B

Fig. 2.7 (Continued) Bones of the right lower limb: (B) from behind, with part of the left hip bone.   (Continued)

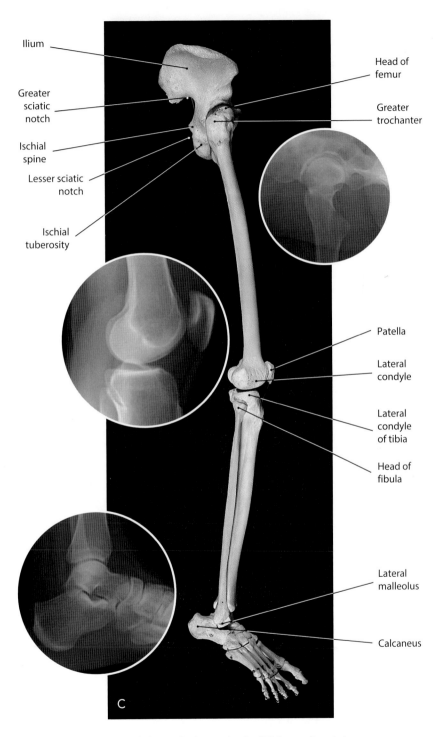

Ilium

Greater
sciatic
notch

Ischial
spine

Lesser sciatic
notch

Ischial
tuberosity

Head of
femur

Greater
trochanter

Patella

Lateral
condyle

Lateral
condyle
of tibia

Head of
fibula

Lateral
malleolus

Calcaneus

C

Fig. 2.7 *(Continued)* Bones of the right lower limb: (C) from the right.

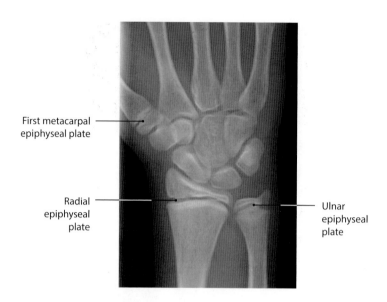

First metacarpal
epiphyseal plate

Radial
epiphyseal
plate

Ulnar
epiphyseal
plate

Fig. 2.8 Radiograph (anteroposterior view) of the right wrist of a 17 year old demonstrating cartilaginous growth (epiphyseal) plates.

Fibula – lateral and non-weight-bearing bone of the leg, with the slightly expanded head proximally having an oblique articular facet on its upper surface for the superior tibiofibular joint. Separating the head and shaft is the narrow neck. The thin shaft has a rather flattened distal end, the lateral malleolus, which has a vertical articular facet on its medial surface for the ankle joint.

Tarsal bones – bones of the hind foot. The talus and calcaneus are the most important of the seven tarsal bones. The talus, with a convex upper surface (wider anteriorly than posteriorly), articulates with the tibia and is gripped between the two malleoli to form the anatomical ankle joint. The rounded head of the talus faces forwards to articulate with the navicular bone and the calcaneus (talocalcaneonavicular joint), and there is a concave articular facet on the under surface for another joint with the calcaneus (subtalar joint) (**Fig. 8.15**).

> The talocalcaneonavicular and subtalar joints facilitate inversion and eversion of the ankle joint, and together with the anatomical ankle joint form the clinical ankle joint.

The calcaneus is the largest foot bone, forming the heel, with facets on the upper surface for joints with the talus; it is the only tarsal bone with an epiphysis (on the posterior surface). The projection on the medial side is the sustentaculum tali, which forms part of the support and articulation for the head of the talus. The navicular bone is distal to the talus on the medial side, with the three cuneiform bones distal to the navicular bone. On the lateral side, the cuboid bone lies distal to the calcaneus.

Metatarsal bones and phalanges – like the corresponding metacarpal bones and phalanges in the hand, each metatarsal bone and phalanx has a shaft with a base at the proximal end and a head at the distal end, to make tarsometatarsal, metatarsophalangeal and interphalangeal joints. The most important is the metatarsophalangeal joint of the great toe.

Arches of the foot – medial and lateral, longitudinal and transverse. Because of the orientation of the calcaneus, which does not lie flat but is angled upwards, and of the shapes of other bones, the articulated foot has an arched form (**Fig. 8.14B**). The higher medial longitudinal arch is composed of the calcaneus, talus, navicular, the three cuneiforms and the three medial metatarsals (with two sesamoid bones under the head of the first metatarsal); the lower lateral longitudinal arch is formed by the calcaneus, the cuboid and the two lateral metatarsals. The transverse arch (really a half arch in each foot) is made up by the cuneiforms, the cuboid and the bases of the metatarsals. These arches are maintained by ligaments and muscle action.

Summary

- The *backbone* of the body is the spine or vertebral column. Its component vertebrae are held together by various small joints and ligaments, including the intervertebral discs, which act like shock absorbers between the bodies of individual vertebrae.
- The *skull* sits on top of the cervical part of the spine, with one of its largest bones, the mandible, making the temporomandibular or jaw joint on each side.
- The thoracic part of the spine, with ribs and cartilages, and the sternum anteriorly, form the *thorax*.
- The lumbar part of the spine forms the *central part of the abdomen*, with the two hip bones forming the *bony pelvis*.
- The *main bones of the upper limb* are the humerus, radius and ulna, with the clavicle and scapula forming the pectoral girdle.
- The most important of the small *wrist bones* is the scaphoid bone (the one most frequently fractured).
- The *main bones of the lower limb* are the femur, tibia and fibula, with the hip bone (fused ilium, ischium and pubis) articulating with the sacrum to form the pelvic girdle.
- The largest *foot bone* is the calcaneus or heel bone.

Questions

Answers can be found in Appendix A, p. 243.

Question 1

Which of the following statements is anatomically accurate with regard to the wrist?

(a) The scaphoid, lunate, trapezium and pisiform from medial to lateral form the proximal row of carpal bones.

(b) The scaphoid, lunate, trapezoid and pisiform from lateral to medial form the distal row of carpal bones.

(c) The trapezium, trapezoid, capitate and hamate from lateral to medial form the distal row of carpal bones.

(d) The trapezium, capitate, trapezoid and hamate from lateral to medial form the distal row of carpal bones.

(e) The scaphoid, trapezium and lunate articulate with the distal radius.

Question 2

Which of the following statements is anatomically accurate with regard to the ankle region?

(a) The calcaneus, talus and cuboid form the medial longitudinal arch.

(b) The upper surface of the calcaneus and sustentaculum tali articulate with the head and lower aspect of the body of head of talus to facilitate inversion and eversion.

(c) The upper surface of the calcaneus and sustentaculum tali articulate with the two malleoli to form the joint that facilitates the movements of inversion and eversion.

(d) The calcaneus and cuboid and cuneiform bones form the lateral longitudinal arch.

(e) The talus and calcaneus both articulate with the two malleoli to form the joint that facilitates inversion and eversion.

Question 3

Which of the following statements about the spinal column is anatomically accurate?

(a) The posterior longitudinal ligament joins the posterior aspect of the vertebral arches together.

(b) The zygapophyseal (facet) joints form the anterior boundary of the intervertebral foramina.

(c) The intervertebral discs are pads of tissue that cannot be compressed, forming a rigid junction between adjacent vertebral bodies.

(d) The lamina of adjacent vertebral arches are united by the elastic ligamentum flavum.

(e) Each spinal nerve emerge from the spinal canal through a vertebral foramen.

Question 4

When studying the origin of the bones of the adult skeleton, which of the following statements is anatomically accurate?

(a) The bones of the skull form through a process of intracartilagenous ossification.

(b) The ossification of the epiphyseal plate results in the cessation of bone growth in the axial skeleton.

(c) The distal epiphyseal plate of the humerus is classically used to estimate foetal maturity.

(d) The cartilaginous type of joint seen in long bones of the foetus disappear before birth without affecting bone growth.

(e) The synovial type of joint is only seen to develop after the long bones have matured.

Question 5

Concerning the skeleton, which of the following statements is anatomically accurate?

(a) Long bones grow as osteoblasts replace a cartilaginous precursor.

(b) Bone growth occurs with a single centre of ossification in all bones of the axial skeleton.

(c) The clavicle is a good example of intracartilagenous ossification.

(d) Sutures seen in the adult skull are good examples of cartilaginous joints.

(e) The primary centre of ossification is always located at the proximal end of a long bone and is present at birth.

Question 6

A 27-year-old man slips while walking and falls on his outstretched left hand as he hits concrete. He experiences severe pain in the left wrist. The pain is exacerbated when the 'anatomical snuff box' is palpated. Radiographs are most likely to reveal a fracture in which of the following bones?

(a) Scaphoid.

(b) Lunate.

(c) Capitate.

(d) Trapezium.

(e) Styloid process of the ulna.

Question 7

A 24-year-old man has a cancerous tumour in a radius bone. The tumour is surgically resected leaving a 10 cm (4 inch) gap in the mid-shaft of the radius. Which of the following bones could be used as a graft to repair this defect?

(a) Ulna.

(b) The contralateral radius.

(c) Fibula.

(d) Tibia.

(e) Femur.

Question 8

A 22-year-old man sustains trauma to his shoulder in a motorcycle crash. Physical examination in the local Emergency Department reveals a marked 'step down' from the clavicle to the acromion. A diagnosis of a dislocated shoulder is made and this is confirmed by a plain radiograph. Which of the following most likely occurred in this injury?

(a) The costoclavicular ligament was torn.

(b) The capsule of the acromioclavicular joint ruptured.

(c) The coracoclavicular ligament was torn.

(d) The anterior glenohumeral ligament was torn.

(e) The capsule of the glenohumeral joint ruptured.

Introduction

The head and neck are the most intricate regions of the body, with many major nerves and blood vessels in close proximity to one another. Within the cranial cavity of the skull lies the brain and its extension, the spinal cord, extends through the foramen magnum to the cervical and thoracic parts of the vertebral column down to the level of L1 in the adult. Protected by the skull itself are found such vital structures as the eye and ear. The head contains the beginning of the alimentary and respiratory tracts, with the pharynx extending into the neck and the larynx (voice box) branching off the lower pharynx.

Cranial cavity

In life the cranial cavity is lined by the dura mater (**Fig. 3.1**), the outermost and toughest of the three membranes or meninges that cover the brain (p. 50). The dura is firmly adherent to the periosteal (endocranial) lining of the cranial cavity, so there is normally no patent extradural space. This space is normally only created when bleeding occurs after a skull fracture, especially in the middle cranial fossa (see below). In places the dura forms partitions that help to keep the brain in place: the falx cerebri between the two cerebral hemispheres, and the tentorium cerebelli between the cerebral hemispheres above and the cerebellum below. The dura also forms the venous sinuses of the skull (see below).

Anterior cranial fossa – front (anterior) part of the interior of the skull base (**Figs. 3.2, 3.3**) which, on each side, forms the roofs of the orbits and, centrally, the roof of the nose. The inferior surfaces of the frontal lobes of the cerebral hemispheres of the brain lie in this fossa. Adjacent to the midline, where the crista galli projects upwards anteriorly, the cribriform plates of the ethmoid bone are pierced by the filaments of the olfactory nerve, passing upwards to the olfactory bulb on the under surface of the frontal lobes.

> Fractures in this location may cause loss of smell (anosmia) (see below).

Middle cranial fossa – middle part of the base, the butterfly-shaped sphenoid bone, has a central part containing the midline pituitary fossa (usually indenting one or both sphenoidal air sinuses) containing the pituitary gland and the optic canals (**Figs. 3.1, 3.2, 3.4**).

> The pituitary fossa (also called the sella turcica) is a key landmark in lateral radiographs of the head (**Fig. 2.2B**).

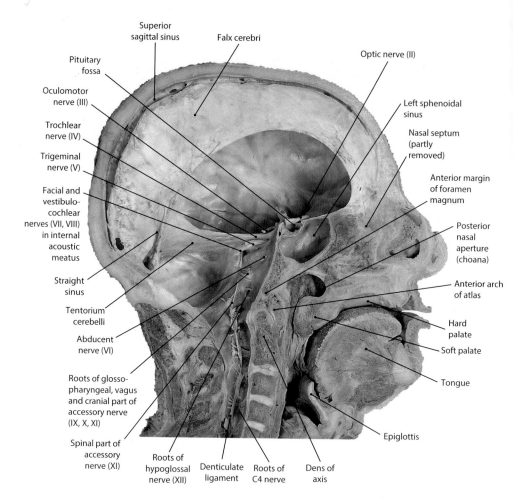

Fig. 3.1 Left half of the head and cranial cavity (sagittal section), with the dura mater intact, after removal of the brain and spinal cord (compare with Fig. 3.4A).

On each side is a lateral part where the temporal lobe of the brain lies, separated by the cavernous venous sinus from the pituitary fossa; the internal carotid artery emerges from the roof of the cavernous sinus and divides into the anterior and middle cerebral arteries. More laterally, there are grooves for the middle meningeal vessels, the superior orbital fissure, foramen rotundum, foramen ovale and foramen spinosum. The grooves for the middle meningeal vessels are visible on radiographs and may be mistaken by the unwary for fractures of the skull.

A fracture of the skull laterally (especially in the region of the pterion) may cause haemorrhage from a middle meningeal artery, resulting in an extradural (referred to as epidural in the USA) haematoma (a collection of blood between the skull and the dura), which causes an increase in pressure on the motor area of the cerebral cortex and eventually unconsciousness and death. (*Continued*)

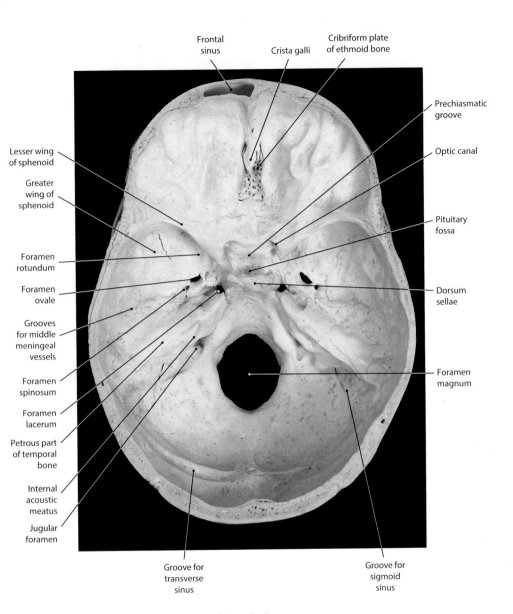

Fig. 3.2 Internal surface of the base of the skull.

Pituitary gland – properly called the hypophysis cerebri (**Figs. 3.4A & B**), this is a major organ of the endocrine system and is itself under the control of the hypothalamus (p. 44). It is connected to the floor of the third ventricle by the pituitary stalk, and consists mainly of posterior and anterior lobes. Superior to the gland lies the optic chiasma.

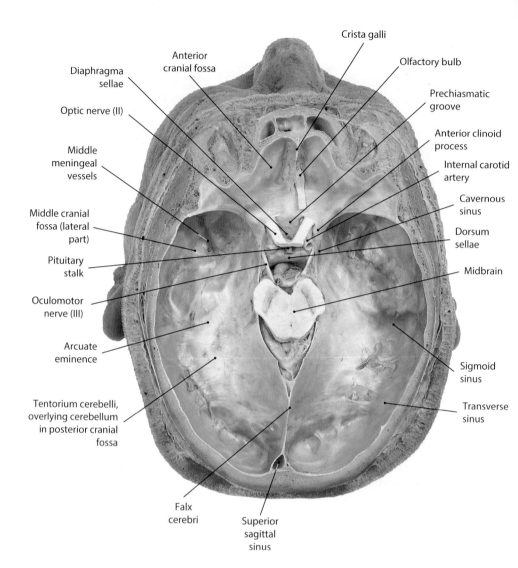

Fig. 3.3 Cranial fossae, after removal of the brain by cutting through the midbrain part of the brainstem.

Tumours of the pituitary growing upwards and backwards may press on the optic chiasma, causing visual defects.

The hormones of the posterior pituitary – antidiuretic hormone (influencing urine production by the kidneys) and oxytocin (which stimulates uterine contraction and milk ejection from the breasts) – are produced by hypothalamic neurosecretory cells whose fibres store the secretion and run down the pituitary stalk. Although the anterior pituitary is also connected to the stalk, the factors that control it (produced by different hypothalamic cells) pass into a network of very small veins that surround the stalk – the hypophyseal portal system (like a miniature hepatic portal system) and so reach the anterior pituitary to deliver the stimuli for hormone production by its own cells. The main anterior pituitary hormones are growth hormones and those that control the thyroid and adrenal cortices, ovaries, testes, and breasts.

Posterior cranial fossa – posterior part of the skull base, containing the foramen magnum below and the tentorium cerebelli above with its large central gap for the midbrain to pass through. It contains the brainstem and cerebellum, the basilar artery and some large venous sinuses. The petrous part of the temporal bone makes a ridge, to which the tentorium attaches, to separate the middle from the posterior fossa. Posteriorly and to the sides of the posterior fossa are grooves for the transverse and sigmoid sinuses. The hypoglossal canal is just above the foramen magnum, while more laterally are the jugular foramen and the internal auditory meatus.

Venous sinuses – veins within the skull formed by a double layer of dura mater normally located where dural folds meet the bones of the skull (**Figs. 3.1, 3.3, 3.4**). The superior sagittal sinus (in the superior edge of the falx cerebri) runs posteriorly below the midline of the cranial vault to the confluence of sinuses. Most of the blood normally flows to the right, becoming the right transverse sinus, which in turn runs down as the right sigmoid sinus to pass through the jugular foramen on the right and emerging inferior to the skull as the right internal jugular vein. The straight sinus receives the inferior sagittal sinus (lying in the lower edge of the falx cerebri) and the great cerebral vein and runs posteriorly to the confluence of sinuses at the junction of the falx cerebri and tentorium cerebelli. Most of this blood normally flows

to the left as the left transverse sinus, which continues as the left sigmoid sinus and, via the left jugular foramen, becomes the left internal jugular vein. The paired cavernous sinuses lie on either side of the pituitary gland and body of the sphenoid bone.

> The cavernous venous sinuses communicate with the facial vein via the superior ophthalmic vein. As a result, infections of the nose and central part of the face can result in infection of the venous sinuses, leading to the very serious condition cavernous venous sinus thrombosis.

Passing through each cavernous sinus are the internal carotid artery and the abducent nerve. The other two nerves of the extraocular muscles (oculomotor and trochlear nerves) and the ophthalmic and maxillary branches of the trigeminal nerve run in the walls of each cavernous sinus. Other sinuses include the superior petrosal sinus, which runs posteriorly from the cavernous sinus, along the top of the petrous part of the temporal bone, to join the transverse sinus, and the inferior petrosal sinus, which also runs posteriorly from the cavernous sinus, but at a lower level, in the groove between the petrous temporal and occipital bones to pass through the jugular foramen, becoming the highest tributary of the internal jugular vein.

Nasal septum – formed primarily by the vomer and the ethmoid bone, but the anterior part is of cartilage (**Fig. 3.4A**) and so not present in the dry bony skull.

Petrous part of temporal bone – commonly called the petrous temporal, forming the prominent ridge (**Fig. 3.2**) marking the boundary between the middle and posterior cranial fossae. It contains the internal acoustic meatus.

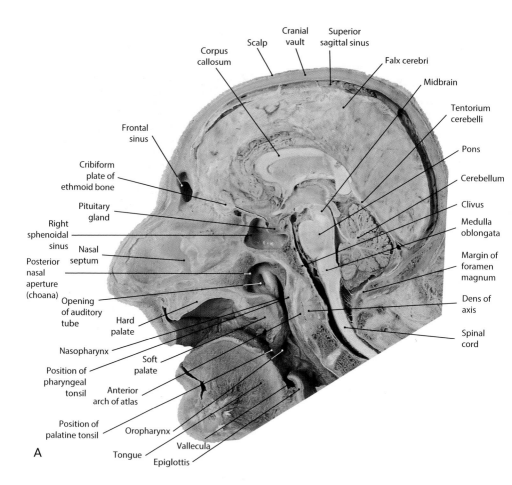

Fig. 3.4 Right half of the head and neck: (A) sagittal section.

(Continued)

Hypoglossal canal – lies above the occipital condyle, which forms the lateral aspect of the foramen magnum.

Osteological features of the mandible

Mandibular foramen – in the medial surface of the ramus of the mandible and guarded anteriorly by the spike-like lingula.

Mylohyoid line – oblique ridge on the medial surface of the body of the mandible, for attachment of the mylohyoid muscle, below which lies the groove for the mylohyoid nerve running from the mandibular foramen.

Skull foramina

Only the most important skull foramina are listed here, with the principal structures that pass through them (**Figs. 2.1C, 3.2**).

Optic canal – optic nerve and ophthalmic artery.

Superior orbital fissure – oculomotor, trochlear and abducent nerves, and lacrimal, frontal and nasociliary branches of ophthalmic branch of the trigeminal nerve.

Foramen rotundum – maxillary branch of the trigeminal nerve.

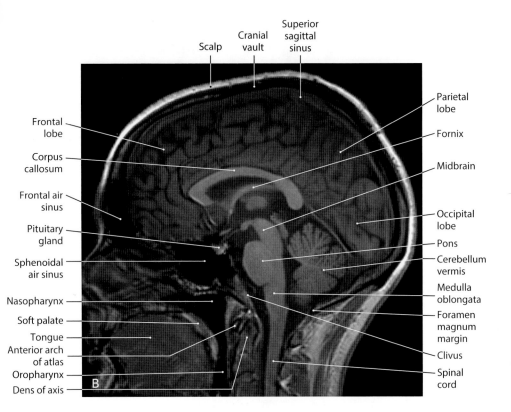

Scalp
Cranial vault
Superior sagittal sinus
Parietal lobe
Frontal lobe
Fornix
Corpus callosum
Midbrain
Frontal air sinus
Occipital lobe
Pituitary gland
Pons
Sphenoidal air sinus
Cerebellum vermis
Nasopharynx
Medulla oblongata
Soft palate
Foramen magnum margin
Tongue
Anterior arch of atlas
Clivus
Oropharynx
Spinal cord
Dens of axis

Fig. 3.4 (Continued) Right half of the head and neck: (B) sagittal MR image.

Foramen ovale – mandibular branch of the trigeminal nerve.

Foramen spinosum – middle meningeal artery and accompanying veins.

Foramen lacerum – internal carotid artery, entering laterally from the carotid canal to emerge from its upper part.

Carotid canal – only visible externally, internal carotid artery, entering on the lateral aspect of the foramen lacerum internally.

Internal acoustic meatus – facial and vestibulocochlear nerves.

Jugular foramen – sigmoid sinus (emerging inferiorly as the internal jugular vein), and glossopharyngeal, vagus and accessory nerves.

Hypoglossal canal – hypoglossal nerve.

Stylomastoid foramen – only visible externally, facial nerve.

Foramen magnum – medulla oblongata, vertebral arteries and spinal parts of accessory nerves.

Head and neck in sagittal section

Much useful anatomy can be viewed from a sagittal section in or very near the midline

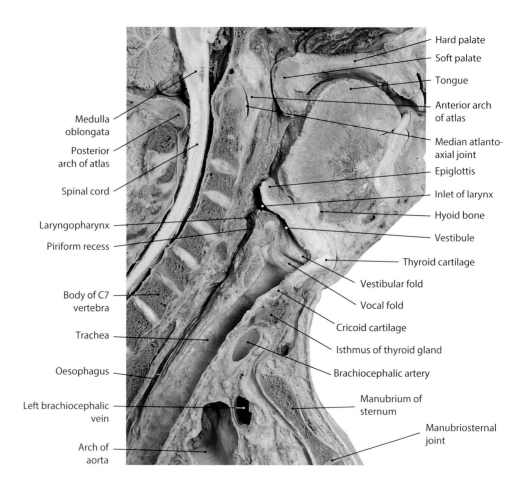

Hard palate
Soft palate
Tongue
Anterior arch of atlas
Median atlanto-axial joint
Epiglottis
Inlet of larynx
Hyoid bone
Vestibule
Thyroid cartilage
Vestibular fold
Vocal fold
Cricoid cartilage
Isthmus of thyroid gland
Brachiocephalic artery
Manubrium of sternum
Manubriosternal joint

Medulla oblongata
Posterior arch of atlas
Spinal cord
Laryngopharynx
Piriform recess
Body of C7 vertebra
Trachea
Oesophagus
Left brachiocephalic vein
Arch of aorta

Fig. 3.5 Left half of neck and upper thorax (superior mediastinum) in a median sagittal section.

(Figs. 3.4, 3.5), and the features listed below should be especially noted.

Nose – is at approximately the same horizontal level anteriorly as the cerebellum posteriorly.

Hard palate – is at approximately the same horizontal level as the foramen magnum.

Posterior nasal aperture (choana) – opens into the nasopharynx (nasal part of the pharynx), which has the pharyngeal tonsil (adenoids) on the posterior wall.

Mouth (oral cavity) – with the tongue in its floor, opens into the oropharynx (oral part of the pharynx), between the soft palate and epiglottis.

Inlet of the larynx – inferior to the epiglottis, opens into the laryngopharynx (laryngeal part of the pharynx).

Hyoid bone – is at the horizontal level of the C3 vertebra.

Thyroid cartilage – is at the level of the C4 and C5 vertebrae.

Cricoid cartilage – is at the level of the C6 vertebra.

Vocal folds (vocal cords) – are at a level midway between the laryngeal prominence (Adam's apple) and the lower border of the thyroid cartilage.

Frontal lobe of the brain – rests on the floor of the anterior cranial fossa.

Falx cerebri – part of the dura mater (p. 35), lies between the cerebral hemispheres; here (**Fig. 3.4A**) the left hemisphere has been removed to show the surface of the falx, which covers most of the medial surface of the right hemisphere.

Tentorium cerebelli – part of the dura mater, separating the lower posterior parts of the cerebral hemispheres from the cerebellum and forms the roof of the posterior cranial fossa.

Midbrain – upper part of the brainstem (p. 48), passing through the central gap in the tentorium cerebelli.

Pons – middle part of the brainstem, posterior to the clivus of the skull.

Medulla oblongata – lower end of the brainstem, passing through the foramen magnum to become the spinal cord at the level of the atlas (C1 vertebra).

Brain, spinal cord and nerves

Brain

The brain (**Figs. 3.6, 3.7**), consisting of the cerebrum (forebrain), brainstem and cerebellum (together the hindbrain) joined together by the midbrain, is the part of the central nervous system that lies within the cranial cavity of the skull. The functions of certain areas are clearly defined; among the most important are those that control the movements of skeletal muscles (voluntary movement) and those at which various kinds of sensory impressions reach consciousness. Other parts are concerned with the body's own internal control mechanisms (often closely associated with the endocrine system), and with such functions

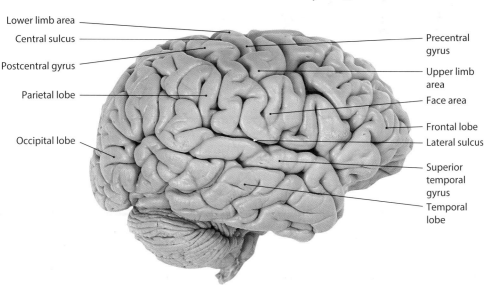

Lower limb area
Central sulcus
Postcentral gyrus
Parietal lobe
Occipital lobe

Precentral gyrus
Upper limb area
Face area
Frontal lobe
Lateral sulcus
Superior temporal gyrus
Temporal lobe

Fig. 3.6 Right side of the brain, after removal of the arachnoid mater and surface vessels (compare with Fig. 3.12).

as memory, thought, emotion and all the vast gamut of behaviour. Attention is focused here only on neurons concerned with major motor and sensory activities.

Grey matter – predominantly nerve cell bodies and glia (glial cells outnumber neurons about 50:1), concentrated in the cortex on the surface of the cerebral and cerebellar hemispheres (see below) and in subcortical groups or nuclei (**Fig. 3.8**). In each cerebral hemisphere these include the caudate and lentiform nuclei (collectively called the corpus striatum), which, with some other groups, form the basal nuclei, still often called by their old name, basal ganglia, and mainly concerned with helping to coordinate muscular activity. One of the largest and most important cellular masses is the thalamus, the main relay station for conscious sensations on the way to the cerebral cortex. The thalamus forms a slight bulge in the lateral wall of the third ventricle (see below), and the region just below, the hypothalamus, which contains the neurosecretory cells that control the pituitary gland.

White matter – predominantly nerve fibres and oligodendrocytes, concentrated deep to the cortex and forming communicating networks. Some fibres form well-recognised tracts with specific functions; many have come from or go to the spinal cord (e.g. the main motor tracts, as well as tracts for the different types of sensation and special senses).

Cerebrum – forebrain, with a central part and two cerebral hemispheres, whose surface is thrown into folds or gyri (singular, gyrus), with intervening grooves or sulci (singular, sulcus) (**Fig. 3.6**). The main connection between the hemispheres is the corpus callosum, a bundle of approximately 200 million nerve fibres, best seen when the brain is bisected in the sagittal plane (**Fig. 3.7**).

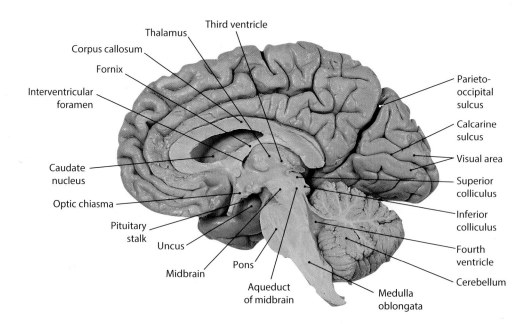

Fig. 3.7 Right half of a median sagittal section of the brain.

Central sulcus – one of the key features of the whole brain separating the anterior frontal and the central parietal lobes (thus separating motor and sensory areas – see below), runs down the lateral surface from near the middle of the upper margin towards the lateral sulcus (but not continuing directly into it, an identifying feature) (**Fig. 3.6**).

Precentral gyrus – anterior to the central sulcus, lying posteriorly in the frontal lobe. This is the *main motor area of cortex* and contains nerve cells responsible for controlling skeletal muscles via connections with the motor nuclei of cranial nerves and anterior horn cells of the spinal cord, with coordinating connections through basal nuclei, thalamus and cerebellum. The parts of the body are represented 'upside down' in the motor cortex: the lower limb is controlled from the uppermost part (supplied by the anterior cerebral artery), the upper limb from the middle, and the face, larynx, etc., from the lower part (all supplied by the middle cerebral artery). The precise regions concerned with highly important functions, such as finger, thumb and lip movements, occupy comparatively large areas of cortex.

> Vascular damage to, or pressure on, the motor cortex and the fibres leading from it causes upper motor neuron (spastic) paralysis. This is commonly known as a stroke.

Postcentral gyrus – posterior to the central sulcus, anteriorly in the parietal lobe. It is the *main sensory area of cortex*, where sensations, such as touch, reach consciousness. The representation of body parts is upside down, similar to that in the motor cortex.

Lateral sulcus – prominent longitudinal sulcus on the lateral surface, separating frontal and temporal lobes. Some cortex of the (usually) left frontal lobe near the front end of the sulcus is the main speech area (Broca's area).

Superior temporal gyrus – in the temporal lobe below the lateral sulcus, it contains the auditory area of cortex, which is for the conscious appreciation of sound.

Calcarine sulcus – on the medial surface of the posterior occipital lobe (**Fig. 3.7**). The adjacent cortex is the visual area (supplied by the posterior cerebral artery), where visual impulses reach consciousness.

> Thrombosis of the posterior cerebral artery may cause visual defects.

Internal capsule – area of white matter between the thalamus and caudate and lentiform nuclei (**Figs. 3.8, 3.9**). In horizontal sections of the hemisphere it appears rather like a capital L on its side, with an anterior limb, genu and posterior limb. *It is one of the supremely important areas of the whole brain and, indeed, of the whole body*: through the genu run corticonuclear fibres from the cerebral cortex to the motor nuclei of cranial nerves, and through the posterior limb run corticospinal fibres from the cortex to the anterior horn cells of the spinal cord. Other internal capsule fibres include those that run from the thalamus to sensory areas of the cortex (thalamocortical fibres).

> Damage to these internal capsule fibres by haemorrhage or thrombosis of the striate arteries (p. 52) results in a 'stroke' (or cerebral vascular accident), with paralysis of the *opposite* side of the body (hemiplegia), because in the medulla of the brainstem most fibres cross over (deccusate) to the opposite side to form the corticospinal tracts (see below) This is the commonest cause of upper motor neuron paralysis.

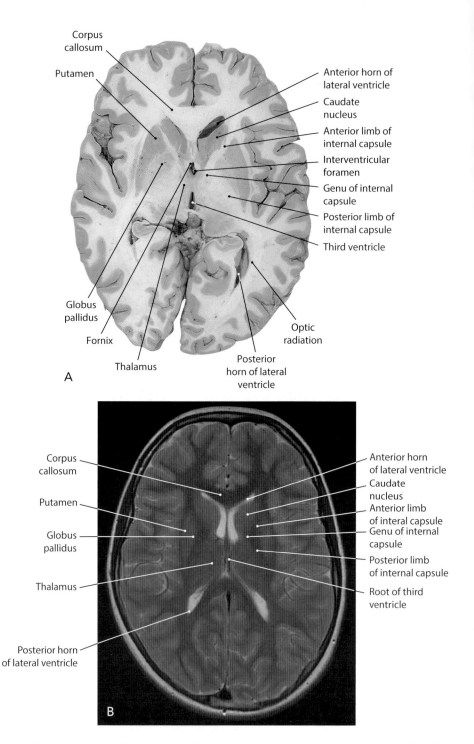

Fig. 3.8 Axial sections of the brain: (A) section at the level of the pineal body, (B) MR image at a similar level.

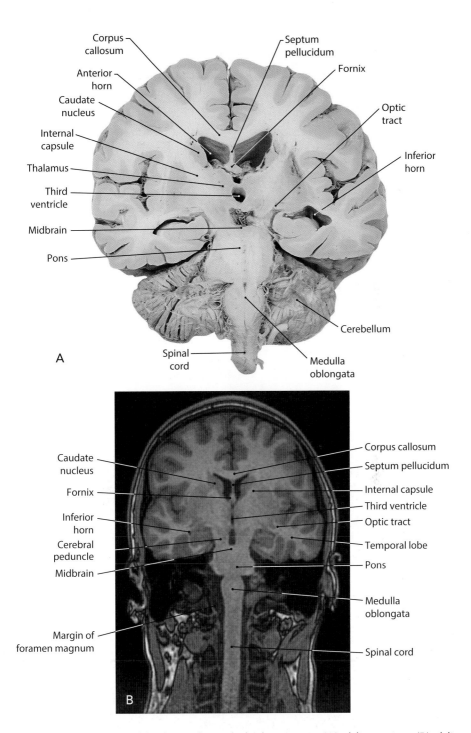

Fig. 3.9 Coronal sections of the brain through the brainstem: (A) oblique view, (B) oblique MR image at a similar level.

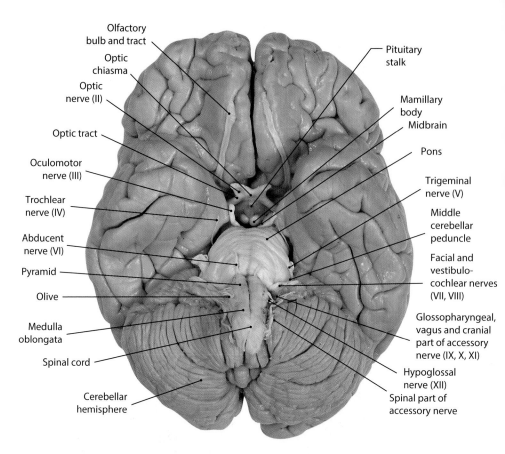

Fig. 3.10 Inferior surface (base) of the brain.

Cerebellum – connected by the superior, middle and inferior cerebellar peduncles to the midbrain, pons and medulla, respectively. Through them it has multiple connections with the rest of the brain and spinal cord. Concerned with muscular coordination, it does not *initiate* movements (that depends on the cerebral cortex), but it helps movements to be carried out in a smooth and controlled manner. The cerebellum has nothing to do with conscious sensation.

Cerebellar disease causes jerky and uncoordinated movements (but not paralysis), tremors and speech defects.

Brainstem – extends down from the central part of the cerebrum (**Figs. 3.7–3.11**) and consists from above downwards of the midbrain, pons and medulla oblongata. In the brainstem are groups of nerve cells (cranial nerve *nuclei*), which either give rise to the motor (efferent) fibres of cranial nerves (p. 52) or receive sensory (afferent) fibres from cranial nerve *ganglia*, situated on the nerves outside the brainstem (corresponding to the posterior root ganglia of spinal nerves, p. 59). Among the fibres that pass through the brainstem to and from other parts of the brain and spinal cord are the motor fibres from the cerebral cortex. They become grouped together to form a

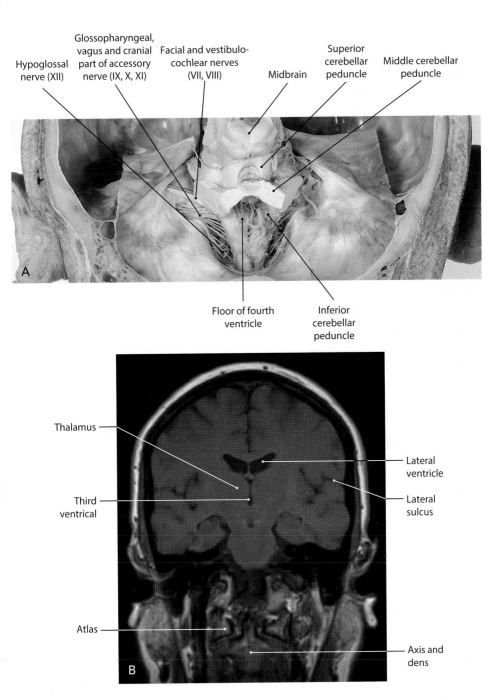

Fig. 3.11 (A) Brainstem *in situ*, from behind after removal of the cerebrum and cerebellum, (B) coronal MR image through the pons and just anterior to the medulla oblongata (compare with more posterior image in Fig. 3.9B).

bulge, the pyramid, on either side of the midline of the medulla; here, most of the fibres cross to the opposite side (motor decussation or decussation of the pyramids) to form the lateral corticospinal tract that continues into the spinal cord (p. 58).

Respiratory and cardiac centres – certain cell groups in the medulla that are associated with the glossopharyngeal and vagus nerves, they control breathing and heart rate. Death occurs when such control ceases irreversibly; tests carried out to establish whether death has, indeed, occurred are tests of function of different parts of the brainstem, assessed by electrical activity (or rather the lack of activity) in certain cranial nerves and their interconnections within the brainstem. Tests for brainstem death are necessary to determine whether organs can be removed for transplantation.

> These tests include a loss of pupillary reflex, loss of oculovestibular reflex, loss of cough reflex, loss of respiratory reflex, low pO_2 or high pCO_2 and whole brain death as evidenced by a flat electro-encephalography (EEG) recording.

Ventricles of the brain – cavities within various parts of the brain (**Figs. 3.7–3.9, 3.11**) that contain cerebrospinal fluid (CSF). Each cerebral hemisphere has a lateral ventricle (with anterior, posterior and inferior horns), which communicates through an interventricular foramen with a narrow central cavity, the third ventricle. This in turn passes posteriorly through the aqueduct of the midbrain to the fourth ventricle, located posterior to the brainstem with a tent-like bulge towards the cerebellum.

Cerebrospinal fluid – total volume about 130 ml, it acts as a protective 'waterbath' to support and protect the brain and spinal cord, and also as a medium for exchange of materials to and from nervous tissue. It is constantly secreted from specialised blood capillaries, the choroid plexuses, within parts of the lateral, third and fourth ventricles. From each lateral ventricle, CSF passes through the interventricular foramen into the third ventricle, and then through the aqueduct of the midbrain into the fourth ventricle. From the posterior of the fourth ventricle below the cerebellum, CSF escapes from the ventricular system into the subarachnoid space (see text below) through three small apertures in the arachnoid – one median and two lateral.

> Obstruction to the outflow of CSF results in hydrocephalus (enlargement of the ventricular system).

Since it is continuously secreted, CSF must be constantly absorbed; this occurs into the bloodstream through arachnoid granulations that project into the superior sagittal sinus at the top of the cranial cavity.

Meninges – membranes that enclose the brain and spinal cord. The outermost is the dura mater (**Fig. 3.1**) (p. 35). Lying in contact with the inside of the dura is the arachnoid mater (**Fig. 3.12**), a much thinner membrane with thin processes resembling spider webs that connect it to the even thinner pia mater, which is directly applied to the brain surface. In life, the subarachnoid space between the arachnoid and pia is filled with CSF. When the brain is removed from the skull, the arachnoid (not the dura) should come with it, although it may be torn in places (e.g. when cutting through cranial nerves and brainstem). These same three meninges continue through the foramen magnum to surround the spinal cord within the vertebral canal.

Blood supply of the brain – by the vertebral and internal carotid arteries, whose branches form the arterial circle (of Willis) on the base of the brain (**Fig. 3.13**).

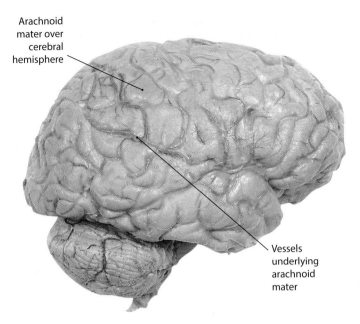

Arachnoid mater over cerebral hemisphere

Vessels underlying arachnoid mater

Fig. 3.12 Right side of the brain, as removed from the skull with the arachnoid mater intact.

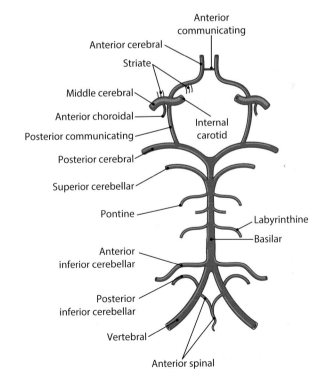

Anterior communicating

Anterior cerebral

Striate

Middle cerebral

Anterior choroidal

Posterior communicating

Internal carotid

Posterior cerebral

Superior cerebellar

Pontine

Labyrinthine

Basilar

Anterior inferior cerebellar

Posterior inferior cerebellar

Vertebral

Anterior spinal

Fig. 3.13 Arterial circle at the base of the brain. The vessels 'fit on' to Fig. 3.10, with the basilar artery lying over the pons and the anterior cerebral arteries lying deep to the optic nerves.

Should one of these branches rupture within the cranial cavity, usually a result of weakness in the vessel wall (aneurysm), as the vessels are contained between the arachnoid and the pia, there will be a bleed into the subarachnoid space known as a subarachnoid haemorrhage, a very serious clinical condition.

Falls and blunt trauma to the front or back of the head, usually without evidence of a skull fracture, create a shearing action where the veins drain into the dural venous sinus and a resultant tear may create a haemorrhage within the subdural space. Such a subdural haemorrhage is clinically serious as it results in a more gradual deterioration of cerebral function than is usually seen in the arterial extradural haemorrhage.

The vertebral artery (from the subclavian, runs cranially up through the foramina in the transverse processes of the upper six cervical vertebrae) enters the skull through the foramen magnum and unites with its fellow to form the single midline basilar artery, which lies on the ventral (anterior) surface of the pons. It divides into the two posterior cerebral arteries – each is joined by the posterior communicating artery to the internal carotid where that vessel divides into its two main branches. The internal carotid artery terminates as the middle cerebral artery (which runs laterally in the lateral sulcus to emerge on the lateral surface of the cerebral cortex) and the anterior cerebral artery (which is united to its fellow by the very short anterior communicating artery and runs on to the medial surface of the cerebral hemisphere). Anterior and middle cerebral vascular lesions cause paralysis; posterior cerebral lesions cause visual defects. Apart from cortical, brainstem and cerebellar branches, there are very small but highly important striate branches of the anterior and middle cerebral arteries that penetrate the brain substance to supply the internal capsule (p. 45).

Various cerebral veins, which usually do not accompany arteries, drain into adjacent venous sinuses. Like veins of the heart, they are usually unaffected by disease.

Cranial nerves

The cranial nerves as seen within the cranial cavity (**Figs. 3.10, 3.11A**) can be referred to by their names or numbers (by long tradition in Roman numerals, or as first, second, third, etc.).

The cranial nerves most commonly damaged are I, II, III, VI and VII (the commonest of all).

I Olfactory – the nerve for smell (olfaction), it is formed by about 20 nerve filaments (or fascicles), which pierce the roof of the nose to pass through the cribriform plate of the ethmoid bone to enter the olfactory bulb of the brain in the anterior cranial fossa.

Fractures here through the base of the skull may tear all nerve filaments of one side to give complete anosmia (loss of smell) on that side and occasionally a leakage of cerebrospinal fluid into the nasal cavity.

From the bulb fibres pass directly to the cerebral cortex (the uncus of the temporal lobe) without synapse in the thalamus – an afferent pathway unique to olfaction, since all other senses involve the thalamus on their way to the cortex.

II Optic – the nerve for vision, it is formed by fibres from the retina of the eye and passes posteriorly through the optic canal to the optic chiasma (see Visual pathway, p. 76).

> A complete lesion of one optic nerve causes total blindness in that eye.

III Oculomotor – the motor nerve to four of the six muscles that move the eye (medial, superior and inferior rectus, and inferior oblique) and to the levator muscle of the upper eyelid (levator palpebrae superioris). It also carries parasympathetic fibres via the ciliary ganglion to constrict the pupil for light reflexes and accommodation (adjusting the shape of the lens and pupil for near vision, p. 78). It leaves the brainstem near the midline of the midbrain and runs through the cavernous sinus to enter the orbit through the superior orbital fissure.

> Paralysis of each of the three 'eye nerves' (III, IV and VI) gives squint (strabismus) and double vision (diplopia), and the eye takes up a characteristic position for each nerve affected.

IV Trochlear – the smallest cranial nerve and the only one to emerge from the dorsal surface of the brainstem (from the midbrain behind the inferior colliculus). It is the motor nerve to the superior oblique muscle (the tendon of which passes through a trochlea or pulley) of the eye, and runs through the lateral wall of the cavernous sinus to enter the orbit through the superior orbital fissure.

> Due to its long course it can be damaged, especially if the tentorium is displaced, as with a tumour of the brainstem.

V Trigeminal – the largest cranial nerve, it supplies through its three branches sensory fibres for many structures in the head, including much of the skin of the face and scalp, and the mucous membranes of the nose, mouth, palate and pharynx, the teeth, the conjunctiva and (most important of all) the cornea of the eye, and motor fibres for the muscles of mastication located in the mandibular division (see below). The main nerve leaves the brainstem at the junction of the pons and middle cerebellar peduncle and passes over the apex of the petrous part of the temporal bone to enter a pocket of dura (known as the trigeminal or Meckel's cave), where the trigeminal ganglion (with cell bodies of afferent nerves) is situated. The three branches of the trigeminal nerve diverging from the ganglion are: the ophthalmic nerve (V_1) passing through the lateral wall of the cavernous sinus to enter the orbit through the superior orbital fissure; the maxillary nerve (V_2), passing through the floor of the sinus and then through the foramen rotundum; and the mandibular nerve (V_3), which runs downwards through the foramen ovale.

VI Abducent – the motor nerve to the lateral rectus muscle of the eye. It leaves the brainstem at the junction of the pons and the pyramid of the medulla, and is the only nerve that passes within the cavernous sinus to enter the orbit through the superior orbital fissure.

VII Facial – the motor nerve for the muscles of the face (but not the skin, which is the trigeminal nerve), with some fibres for the special sensation of taste from the anterior part of the tongue, parasympathetic secretomotor fibres for the submandibular and sublingual glands (via the submandibular ganglion) and for the lacrimal gland (via the pterygopalatine ganglion) via fibres distributed along branches of the trigeminal nerve.

Lower motor neuron paralysis of the facial nerve (Bell's palsy, damage usually in the facial canal) causes drooping of the mouth on the affected side, with uncontrolled dribbling of saliva, inability to close the eye and wrinkle the forehead, and inability to blow or whistle properly. When the facial nerve is affected by upper motor neuron paralysis, the ability to wrinkle the forehead is preserved because there is innervation of the upper part of the cranial nerve VII nucleus by an ipsilateral corticobulbar tract.

The facial nerve leaves the brainstem at the junction of the pons and medulla to enter the internal acoustic meatus and run to the genu (bend), where the geniculate ganglion is located, before passing through the facial canal within the temporal bone, lying medial to and then behind the middle ear. It then emerges through the stylomastoid foramen without its sensory and autonomic fibres, which branch off between the dura and this skull foramen. (The sensory fibres for taste, with cell bodies in the geniculate ganglion, leave just proximal to this foramen, cross the tympanic membrane and leave through the small petrotympanic fissure before the chorda tympani crosses to join the lingual nerve, p. 66).

VIII Vestibulocochlear – really two nerves in one that supply the inner ear: the vestibular part is concerned with balance (equilibrium) and the cochlear part with hearing. The combined nerve leaves the brainstem with the facial nerve at the junction of the pons and medulla to enter the internal acoustic meatus, innervating the inner ear.

IX Glossopharyngeal – a mixed nerve that supplies only one small muscle of the pharynx (stylopharyngeus), sensory fibres to the palate and tongue (including taste from the posterior third) and highly important sensory fibres to monitor blood pressure and blood carbon dioxide levels from special receptors associated with the carotid arteries. Also parasympathetic secretomotor fibres for the parotid gland (via the otic ganglion by fibres that join the auriculotemporal nerve, a branch of the mandibular branch of the trigeminal nerve). The nerve rootlets that form the glossopharyngeal, vagus and cranial part of the accessory nerves leave the side of the brainstem lateral to the olive of the medulla and pass through the jugular foramen.

X Vagus – a mixed nerve with wide distribution not only in the head and neck, but also (uniquely for a cranial nerve) in the thorax and abdomen (vagus means wandering). It contains efferent fibres to supply muscles of the palate, pharynx, oesophagus and larynx, the heart, smooth muscle of the bronchi, much of the alimentary tract all the way to the transverse colon near the splenic flexure (most importantly, the stomach and its glands) and afferent fibres from all these structures. For its cranial course, see Glossopharyngeal nerve above.

XI Accessory – in two parts: the cranial part, which joins the vagus, provides the skeletal muscle supply to the palate, pharynx, oesophagus and larynx; and the spinal part (what is usually meant by the term accessory nerve), whose cells of origin are in the upper cervical segments of the spinal cord and which supply the sternocleidomastoid and trapezius muscles.

Operations on the neck (e.g. to remove cancerous lymph nodes) may damage the accessory nerve, causing paralysis of trapezius and inability to shrug the shoulder.

The cranial part leaves the brainstem as described for the glossopharyngeal nerve; the rootlets of the spinal part leave the cervical part of the spinal cord behind the denticulate ligament and unite to run up through the foramen magnum and join the cranial part before leaving through the jugular foramen.

XII Hypoglossal – motor nerve to muscles of the tongue. It leaves the brainstem by two roots between the pyramid and olive of the medulla, and the roots unite as they pass through the hypoglossal canal.

Spinal cord

The spinal cord, continuous with the medulla oblongata of the brainstem (**Fig. 3.5**), is the part of the CNS that lies within the vertebral (spinal) canal. It extends from the C1 vertebra to the L1 vertebra (in the adult; in the newborn it reaches the L3 vertebra, but the vertebral column grows at a greater rate than does the cord, a process called differential growth). The spinal nerves (see below) emerge from the side of the cord; the part of the cord that gives attachment to a pair of spinal nerves is referred to as a segment of the cord. Like the brain, the cord is surrounded by the same three meninges, but unlike the brain the grey matter is concentrated centrally, with no 'cortex'.

Meninges – dura mater, continuous with that inside the skull, lines the vertebral canal down as far as the second segment of the sacrum. However, unlike the dura inside the skull where it is firmly adherent to the endocranium (periosteum), in the spinal canal it is only tethered where it forms a sleeve around each spinal nerve as it leaves the vertebral canal through its own intervertebral foramen. Therefore, there is a patent extradural space around the spinal cord that does not exist inside the cranial cavity. Inside the dura is the arachnoid mater and the subarachnoid space containing CSF; pia mater adheres to the surface of the cord and the emerging nerve roots.

Specimens of CSF can be obtained by lumbar puncture – passing a needle into the subarachnoid space through the midline of the back, usually between the spines of L3 and L4 vertebrae (level with the highest points of the iliac crests). The spinal cord, having ended at the L1 level in the adult, is not in danger of being damaged by the needle, and the nerve roots that form the lower spinal nerves (see below) are simply displaced, not impaled.

Grey matter – nerve cell bodies that are concentrated in the cord's central part (which on cross-section is H-shaped); the extremities of the H are the horns of grey matter (**Fig. 3.14**). Some posterior horn cells are concerned with transmission of pain and temperature sensations, while anterior horn cells give rise to motor fibres that supply skeletal muscles. All segments of the cord have anterior and posterior horns, but a more limited number of segments have smaller lateral horns, whose cells are part of the autonomic nervous system: from segments T1 down to L2 they are sympathetic, and in segments S2–S4 they are parasympathetic. (**Note:** These are spinal cord segments giving nerve roots to form the nerves exiting the spinal canal at these stated levels.)

Between and around the cells and fibres mentioned above there are masses of interneurons. Some take part in spinal reflexes – the neuronal circuits within the spinal cord concerned with such involuntary activities as the sudden withdrawal on touching something hot. However, the

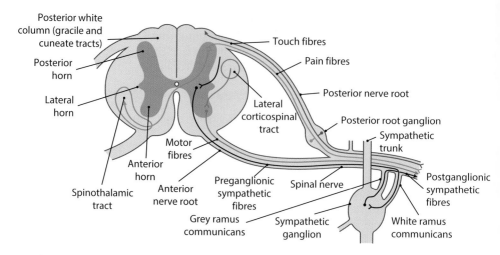

Fig. 3.14 Major tracts of the spinal cord and fibre components of the spinal nerves.

stretch reflexes, commonly called tendon jerks (such as the knee jerk that occurs on tapping the patellar tendon with the knee flexed, the biceps jerk in the arm and the Achilles' tendon jerk in the leg) do not involve interneurons; there is a direct synaptic connection between the afferent fibres from the muscle that has been stretched momentarily (by tapping the tendon) and the motor nerve cells and their fibres that produce the momentary muscle contraction or 'jerk' of the appropriate joint (**Fig. 3.15**).

White matter – nerve fibres that are arranged around the periphery of the cord and referred to as columns of white matter (**Fig. 3.14**). The posterior white columns are entirely occupied by the (ascending) gracile and cuneate tracts, which form the main pathway for touch and associated sensations. The lateral and anterior white columns contain various ascending and descending tracts, of which the most important are the (descending) corticospinal and other associated motor tracts, the (ascending) spinothalamic tracts for pain and temperature,

and the (ascending) spinocerebellar tracts that assist in muscular coordination.

Gracile and cuneate tracts – from cell bodies in the posterior root ganglia (see below) of all the spinal nerves of the same side; the gracile tract is composed of fibres from sacral, lumbar and lower thoracic nerves, and the cuneate tract from upper thoracic and cervical nerves.

> Damage to the gracile and cuneate tracts of one side causes loss of touch sensation on the same side of the body.

Fibres run up in the posterior white column (**Fig. 3.14**) to end in the medulla by synapsing with cells of the gracile and cuneate nuclei, from whence fibres that form the medial lemniscus cross to the opposite side of the brainstem to pass to the thalamus, where there are further synapses with cells whose fibres pass to the appropriate sensory areas of the cerebral cortex. The tracts form the *main pathway* for touch, proprioception, vibration sense and the sensation of fullness of the bladder and rectum.

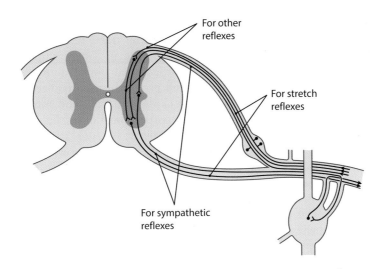

For other
reflexes

For stretch
reflexes

For sympathetic
reflexes

Fig. 3.15 Reflex pathways in the cord. The stretch reflexes (tendon jerks) depend on direct synaptic connections between afferent and efferent fibres, but for others there are intervening neurons.

Lateral and anterior spinothalamic tracts – formed by fibres from posterior horn cells of the *opposite* side (i.e. they are crossed tracts) (**Fig. 3.14**). These posterior horn cells are in synaptic connection with incoming fibres from posterior root ganglion cells of their own side.

> Damage to spinothalamic tracts of one side causes loss of pain and temperature sensations on the opposite side of the body.

The tracts run up in the anterior part of the lateral white column and in the anterior white column. In the brainstem many fibres end by synapsing with cell groups there, which in turn send their fibres to the thalamus, while other fibres pass directly to the thalamus. From the thalamus, fibres pass to the appropriate areas of the cerebral cortex. These tracts are the *main pathway* for pain and temperature sensations.

Note that the pathway for touch (which crosses over in the medulla of the brainstem) is different from that for pain and temperature (which crosses in the spinal cord). Thus, disease or injury of the posterior columns may interrupt the transmission of touch sensation while leaving pain and temperature sensation intact ('dissociated sensation'), and vice versa. Note also that each pathway has essentially three groups of neurons: the first with cell bodies in posterior root ganglia; the second with cell bodies in the medulla (touch) or posterior horns (pain and temperature); and the third with cell bodies in the thalamus.

Anterior and posterior spinocerebellar tracts – from posterior horn cells, which give rise to crossed and uncrossed fibres that run at the periphery of the lateral white column to the cerebellum. They assist with muscular coordination and have nothing to do with conscious sensation.

Lateral corticospinal tract – this is the *supremely important motor tract*; it is the downward continuation of the crossed fibres from the motor decussation in the medulla and occupies the posterior part of the lateral white column (**Fig. 3.14**). The fibres end by synapsing (usually via interneurons) with the anterior horn cells, whose axons supply skeletal muscles. The smaller anterior corticospinal tract, which contains uncrossed fibres, runs in the anterior white column, near the median fissure, but the fibres eventually cross to anterior horn cells of the opposite side.

> Damage to corticospinal tracts of one side above their motor decussation causes upper motor neuron paralysis of muscles on the opposite side of the body.

Extrapyramidal tracts – collective name for several tracts (e.g. vestibulospinal and reticulospinal, often intermingled with corticospinal fibres) derived from various cell groups in the brainstem. Their fibres synapse with the same anterior horn cells as corticospinal fibres, but are called extrapyramidal because (unlike corticospinal fibres) they do not run through the pyramid of the medulla. Anterior horn cells are thus subject to many influences from both cortical and subcortical cell groups.

Upper and lower motor neurons – corticospinal (and corticonuclear) and extrapyramidal fibres constitute the upper motor neurons. Anterior horn cells with their fibres running to skeletal muscles constitute the lower motor neurons. Typical causes of damage to upper motor neurons are birth

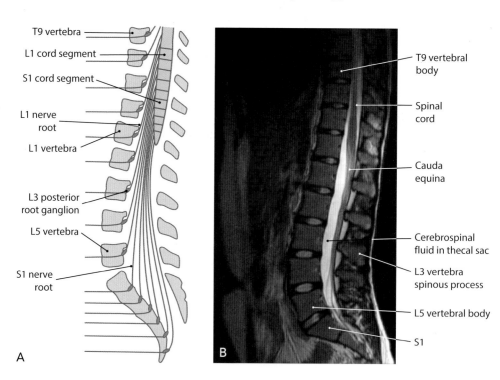

T9 vertebra
L1 cord segment
S1 cord segment
L1 nerve root
L1 vertebra
L3 posterior root ganglion
L5 vertebra
S1 nerve root

A

T9 vertebral body
Spinal cord
Cauda equina
Cerebrospinal fluid in thecal sac
L3 vertebra spinous process
L5 vertebral body
S1

B

Fig. 3.16 Lower end of the spinal cord and cauda equina: (A) diagram with only anterior nerve roots shown, (B) comparable sagittal MR image.

injury to the brain (cerebral palsy), vascular damage to the internal capsule (stroke, see above), or spinal cord injury that damages the tracts. Polio (anterior poliomyelitis, a virus infection of anterior horn cells) and a severed peripheral nerve are examples of lower motor neuron damage.

> Damage to upper motor neurons leads to spastic paralysis, with increased stretch reflexes; damage to lower motor neurons leads to flaccid paralysis with reduced or absent reflexes.

Blood supply of the spinal cord – by (single) anterior and (paired) posterior spinal arteries, derived at the upper end from the vertebral arteries and forming longitudinal trunks that are supplemented at various, but variable, segmental levels by small radicular arteries that run along the spinal nerve roots. There are corresponding veins.

Spinal nerves

There are 31 pairs of spinal nerves – eight cervical (C), twelve thoracic (T), five lumbar (L), five sacral (S) and one coccygeal (Co). Each one of each pair is attached to its own side of its own segment of the cord by a posterior (dorsal) and an anterior (ventral) root (**Fig. 3.14**), each root in turn being formed by bundles of nerve fibres known as rootlets. Thus, the fourth cervical nerves (C4 nerves) are attached to the fourth cervical segment (C4 segment).

> Posterior nerve roots contain afferent (sensory) nerve fibres; anterior nerve roots contain efferent (motor) nerve fibres.

The sites of the cell bodies that give origin to the fibres in each nerve root are different. The posterior root contains afferent (sensory) fibres, whose cell bodies are in the posterior (dorsal) root ganglion, which is the slight swelling on the posterior nerve root situated in the intervertebral foramen, just before the two roots unite to form the spinal nerve itself. The anterior root contains efferent (motor) fibres, whose cells of origin are in the anterior horns of the spinal cord (lower motor neurons – see above), for the supply of skeletal muscle fibres or, in the lateral horns, as the source of preganglionic autonomic fibres (p. 9). The lateral horn cells in segments T1 down to L2 are sympathetic and those in segments S2–S4 are parasympathetic. A typical spinal nerve thus contains motor, sensory and autonomic fibres.

The different lengths of the spinal cord and vertebral column mean that the lower nerve roots must become longer and longer in order to reach their own intervertebral foramina. Thus, below L1 vertebra (where the cord ends) there is a sheaf of nerve roots, the cauda equina ('horse's tail', **Fig. 3.16**). It follows that injury to the lumbar part of the vertebral column can only damage nerve roots (i.e. lower motor neurons), with flaccid paralysis of the muscles supplied; it cannot cause spastic paralysis (p. 58), because the upper motor neurons in the spinal cord are not involved.

Each spinal nerve emerges from its own intervertebral foramen and immediately divides into two branches (rami), which both contain motor and sensory fibres. The posterior ramus is the smaller and supplies muscles and skin of the back near the midline. The anterior ramus is larger and more important, and is what is commonly meant by the term spinal nerve; some rami join their fellows as the roots of the great nerve plexuses – cervical, brachial, lumbar and sacral. The last three provide the innervation of the limbs.

Because of the way nerves unite and divide in plexuses, any given peripheral nerve may contain fibres from more than one spinal nerve. Knowledge of the distribution of dermatomes (the areas of skin supplied by any one peripheral nerve, **Fig. 3.17**) is often useful clinically (e.g. in determining the level of a spinal cord injury) and also assists in understanding the phenomenon of referred pain. Thus, irritation of part of the diaphragm, innervated through the phrenic nerve, mainly by the C4 nerve, may give rise to pain that appears to come from above the shoulder, which is the area of skin supplied by the C4 nerve.

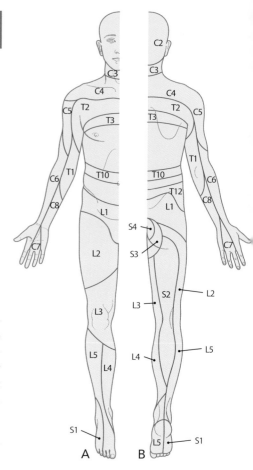

Fig. 3.17 Dermatomes of the body: (A) front, (B) back.

Cervical plexus – roots from C1–C4 anterior rami, it gives small motor branches to deep neck muscles and forms some cutaneous nerves for the neck and head, but by far the most important branch is the phrenic nerve, which supplies its own half of the diaphragm (p. 132).

Brachial plexus – roots from C5–T1 anterior rami (**Fig. 3.18**), it forms the nerves of the upper limb to supply muscles, joints and skin. The parts of the plexus are the roots, trunks, divisions and cords, in that order. Classically, the roots are anterior rami that unite to form upper (C5 and 6), middle (C7) and lower (C8 and T1) trunks. Each trunk gives rise to anterior and posterior divisions. The three posterior divisions unite to form the posterior cord, while the anterior divisions form the lateral and medial cords; it is these cords that give rise to the largest branches of the plexus (**Fig. 3.18**). It is of note here that many variations of the branching pattern have been described during dissection, normally with no clinical significance.

Lumbar plexus – roots from L1–L5 anterior rami (**Fig. 3.19**), it supplies the lowest part of the anterior abdominal wall and muscles of the anterior and medial parts of the thigh. The largest branches are the femoral and obturator nerves and the lumbosacral trunk, which is the contribution that the lumbar plexus makes to the sacral plexus.

Sacral plexus – roots from L4–S3 anterior rami (**Fig. 3.20**), it supplies the rest of the lower limb and structures of the pelvis and perineum. The largest branches are the sciatic (typically, the largest nerve in the body), posterior femoral cutaneous, pudendal and superior and inferior gluteal nerves.

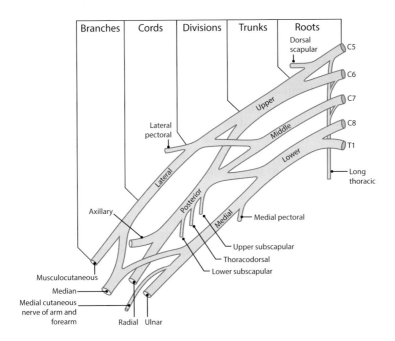

Fig. 3.18 Right brachial plexus and main branches.

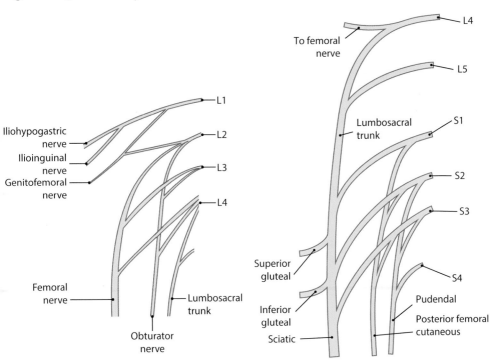

Fig. 3.19 Right lumbar plexus and principal branches.

Fig. 3.20 Sacral plexus and principal branches.

Segmental supply of muscles – although most muscles are supplied by nerves whose motor fibres come from more than one spinal cord segment, there is usually one segment that predominates. The following list indicates which segments of the cord supply certain key muscles and which are involved in the stretch reflexes (the 'jerks' that occur when tapping tendons, such as the patellar tendon to induce the knee jerk):

C4 – diaphragm
C5 – deltoid
C6 – biceps (and biceps jerk)
C7 – triceps (and triceps jerk)
C8 – wrist flexors and extensors
T1 – small muscles of the hand
L2 – psoas major
L3 – quadriceps femoris (and knee jerk)
L4 – tibialis anterior and posterior
L5 – fibularis (peroneus) longus and brevis
S1 – gastrocnemius (and ankle jerk)
S2 – small muscles of the foot

Face and scalp

The face (**Figs. 3.21, 3.22**), the front part of the head, extends between both ears and from the hairline (or where the hairline originally was) to the chin. The scalp covers the vault of the skull and includes the forehead (common to face and scalp).

Face – the obvious features of the face are the openings of the eyes, ears (posteriorly), nose and mouth, while posteriorly, below and in front of the ear, lies the parotid gland. Most of the facial muscles, commonly called as a group 'muscles of facial expression', typically pass from various parts of the facial skeleton or deep fascia to skin and often blend with one another; hence, they are unlike most muscles, which pass from bone to bone. The three most important muscles are orbicularis oculi,

orbicularis oris and buccinator. The whole group is innervated by the facial nerve and must not be confused with the other group of muscles located in the face, 'the muscles of mastication', which are designed to act on and move the mandible – the temporalis, masseter and the lateral and medial pterygoids, all innervated by the mandibular branch of the trigeminal nerve.

Scalp – the main components are hairy skin, thin muscles anteriorly (frontalis, which has no bony attachment) and posteriorly (occipitalis, attached to the back of the occipital bone) and a tough connective tissue layer (galea aponeurotica) connecting the two muscles, which are both innervated by the facial nerve and are collectively known as occipitofrontalis. Only some very loose tissue connects the muscles and aponeurosis to the cranial vault, hence the scalp can move freely on the underlying bone, and there is a plane of cleavage here where the scalp can be dragged off the bone.

> Wounds of the scalp bleed profusely because the dense connective tissue surrounding the vessels prevents the transected vessels from constricting.

The main arterial supplies are the supraorbital, superficial temporal and occipital arteries (see below). A handy mnemonic for the five layers of the scalp is:

Skin
Connective tissue (dense)
Aponeurosis
Loose connective tissue
Periosteum (pericranium)

Cutaneous nerves of the face and scalp – largely from the three divisions of the trigeminal nerve: the ophthalmic nerve supplies skin above the level of the eye

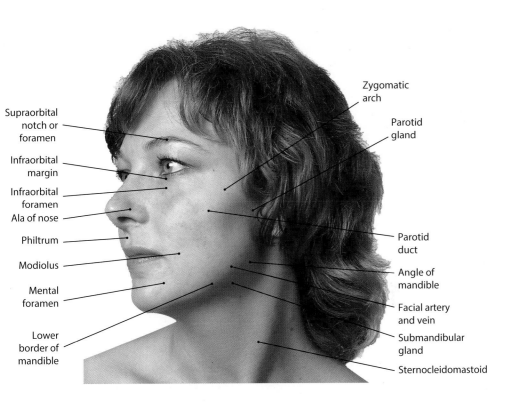

Fig. 3.21 Surface features of the left side of the face (see also Fig. 3.35).

and the anterior of the nose, and extends far posteriorly over the vault of the skull; the maxillary nerve supplies the triangular area between the ear, eye and corner of the mouth (including the upper lip and teeth); and the mandibular nerve supplies the skin over the mandible (including the lower lip and teeth), continuing up into a strip just anterior to the ear.

> Branches of the maxillary nerve provide the sensory supply for the upper lip and branches of the mandibular nerve for the lower lip.

The only facial skin not supplied by the trigeminal nerve is that over the angle of the mandible, which is supplied by the great auricular nerve (cervical plexus). Branches from C2 and C3 nerves supply the back

of the scalp (the C1 nerve does not supply any skin).

Orbicularis oculi – encircles the eye, running through both lids, and is responsible for 'screwing up' and closing the eye. The upper eyelid has its own muscle, the levator palpebrae superioris, for opening the eye, which is supplied by the oculomotor nerve (p. 53).

> Facial nerve paralysis (p. 53) does not lead to ptosis (drooping) of the upper lid but the lesion does prevent blinking, which can allow the cornea to become dry and ulcerated, leading to blindness.

Orbicularis oris – encircles the opening of the mouth, to form the muscle of the lips along with several other muscles that blend with it.

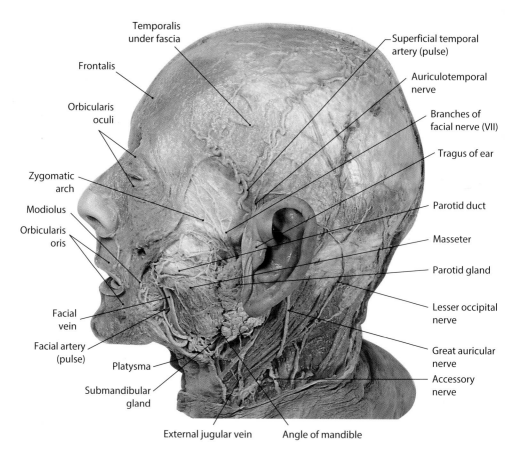

Temporalis under fascia

Frontalis

Orbicularis oculi

Zygomatic arch

Modiolus

Orbicularis oris

Facial vein

Facial artery (pulse)

Platysma

Submandibular gland

Superficial temporal artery (pulse)

Auriculotemporal nerve

Branches of facial nerve (VII)

Tragus of ear

Parotid duct

Masseter

Parotid gland

Lesser occipital nerve

Great auricular nerve

Accessory nerve

External jugular vein

Angle of mandible

Fig. 3.22 Superficial dissection of the left side of the face and upper neck.

Buccinator – attached to the bone of maxilla and mandible opposite the three molar teeth, it blends anteriorly with muscles round the mouth and posteriorly with the superior constrictor of the pharynx and the pterygomandibular raphe (p. 93). It is important for blowing and sucking (particularly in infants) and for keeping food between the teeth, although it must not be classified as a muscle of mastication (it does not move the jaw), and it is innervated, like other facial muscles, by the facial nerve.

Parotid gland – the largest salivary gland, named for its position next to the ear, is on the side of the face overlapping the deeper masseter muscle and with the ear and the sternocleidomastoid posterior to it; its deep lobe extends deep to the ramus of the mandible towards the styloid process and lies within a tough connective tissue capsule. Embedded within the gland, from superficial to deep, are branches of the facial nerve, retromandibular vein and the end of the external carotid artery and its terminal branches (superficial temporal and maxillary). Also embedded are some lymph nodes and secretory nerve fibres from the auriculotemporal nerve via the (parasympathetic) otic ganglion, situated on the medial side of the mandibular nerve just inferior to the foramen ovale.

Mumps, a viral infection, causes painful swelling of the parotid gland.

Parotid duct – runs forwards superficially from the anterior border of the gland and lies along the middle third of a line drawn from the tragus of the ear to the midpoint of the philtrum (the rectangular area above the middle of the upper lip). The duct turns sharply around the anterior edge of masseter to pierce buccinator obliquely and opens into the mouth opposite the second upper molar tooth.

Facial nerve – after emerging from the stylomastoid foramen and running superficially between the deep and superficial lobes within the parotid gland, its branches fan out from the front of the parotid gland to supply the facial muscles. Note that this nerve *does not supply facial skin*, although it does supply a very small area of the tympanic membrane and external acoustic meatus via a branch given during its course through the temporal bone.

The facial nerve may be damaged during surgery for tumours arising in the superficial lobe of the parotid gland unless it is first identified at the stylomastoid foramen. The superficial lobe can then be carefully dissected off the nerve along with the tumour.

Facial artery and vein – the artery ascends from the neck onto the face 3 cm anterior to the angle of the mandible by the anterior border of masseter, where the facial pulse can be felt. The artery runs upwards deep to facial muscles towards the inner canthus (angle) of the eye; it is a tortuous vessel, in contrast to the straight facial vein lying just deep to it, and runs into the upper neck, draining into the internal jugular vein.

The facial artery pulse is felt where the artery crosses the mandible 3 cm in front of the angle of the mandible.

Supraorbital artery – emerges from the orbit through the supraorbital notch or foramen to supply the scalp.

Superficial temporal artery – a terminal branch of the external carotid within the parotid gland, it passes outwards behind the temporomandibular joint and then turns up anterior to the tragus of the ear.

The superficial temporal pulse is felt anterior to the tragus of the ear.

Occipital artery – arises from the external carotid in the neck opposite the facial artery (which passes upwards and *forwards*), it then runs upwards and *backwards* to the scalp.

Lymph nodes and lymphatics – there are a few lymph nodes in the parotid gland and posterior to the ear, but there are no nodes within the scalp (only lymphatic channels). All lymph from the head drains to cervical nodes.

Temporalis – from the side of the skull it passes deep to the zygomatic arch and becomes attached to the coronoid process of the mandible (**Fig. 2.1**) and the anterior of the ramus, almost as far down as the last molar tooth.

Masseter – from the zygomatic arch it runs downwards to the outer side of the ramus of the mandible (**Fig. 3.22**).

Lateral pterygoid – from the *lateral side of the lateral pterygoid plate* and adjacent part of the base of the skull, its fibres run *posteriorly* to attach to the neck of the mandible, the capsule of the temporomandibular joint and its interarticular disc.

Medial pterygoid – mainly from the *medial side of the lateral pterygoid plate* (not the medial pterygoid plate), it runs *downwards and posteriorly* to the inner side of the angle of the mandible.

Temporomandibular joint – lies between the mandibular fossa and articular tubercle of the squamous part of the temporal bone and the head of the mandible. Inside the capsule there is a fibrocartilaginous interarticular disc that divides the joint cavity in two. If you lay a fingertip just anterior to the tragus of the ear and open your mouth wide, you can feel that the head of the mandible has moved downwards and forwards. The lateral pterygoid muscle is responsible for this movement along with gravity, pulling the head of the mandible out of its notch on the disc below the mandibular fossa onto the articular tubercle in front of the fossa, and allowing the chin to drop down. The *lowest* fibres of temporalis are responsible for restoring the normal position: they pull the coronoid process backwards because at their origin they lie *horizontally* before hooking down over the root of the zygomatic arch.

> In dislocation of the jaw the head of the mandible gets 'stuck' on the articular eminence and must be manually helped back into the fossa.

The powerful movement of closing the jaw is completed with contraction of the remaining temporalis fibres and masseter in particular. In less wide opening, the head of the mandible simply rotates slightly, without being pulled out of its fossa. Accessory muscles of mastication (in the floor of the mouth and attached to the hyoid bone, such as the mylohyoid and geniohyoid) assist the opening. The other mastication muscle (the medial pterygoid) also helps to *close* the mouth. Working in a coordinated way the pterygoids also produce the side-to-side grinding movements of chewing.

Inferior alveolar nerve – a branch of the mandibular nerve just inferior to the foramen ovale, it emerges between the two pterygoid muscles and runs down to enter the mandibular foramen with the companion vessels behind it (**Fig. 3.23**). It supplies all the lower teeth, the skin of the chin and the mucous membrane of the lower lip (for dental anaesthesia see p. 69). It gives off the nerve to the mylohyoid just before entering the foramen.

Lingual nerve – from the same origin as the inferior alveolar, it also emerges between the two pterygoids, but 1 cm anteriorly. It runs down and forwards to enter the floor of the mouth by passing under the lower border of the superior constrictor of the pharynx. It lies against the periosteum of the mandible (or on the origin of mylohyoid) just below and behind the third molar tooth, and enters the tongue to supply sensory fibres to the anterior part; it does not supply tongue *muscles*, which are innervated by the hypoglossal nerve (p. 68). When high up under the lateral pterygoid, the chorda tympani branch of the facial nerve joins the lingual nerve to provide taste fibres for the anterior two-thirds of the tongue and secretory fibres for the submandibular and sublingual glands via the (parasympathetic) submandibular ganglion, which is attached to the lingual nerve at the side of the tongue.

Buccal nerve – another mandibular nerve branch, it emerges through the lateral pterygoid to run down superficial to the buccinator to below the parotid duct; it supplies skin of the cheek as well as mucous membrane on the lateral oral cavity. In dissections of the infratemporal region (as in **Fig. 3.23**), note the three mandibular nerve branches running downwards: buccal, lingual and inferior alveolar, in that order from anterior to posterior, with the last two coming out between the two pterygoid muscles.

Auriculotemporal nerve – also from the mandibular nerve, has two roots that encircle the middle meningeal artery; the nerve then runs upwards, anterior to the ear, together with the superficial temporal

vessels (**Fig. 3.22**) to supply the face and scalp skin above and secretory nerve fibres to the parotid gland below (see above).

Posterior superior alveolar nerve – from the maxillary nerve to give two or more branches that run down the posterior wall of the maxilla and pierce the bone to supply the posterior upper teeth.

Maxillary artery – runs through or between the pterygoid muscles to pass through the pterygomaxillary fissure and enter the nose, where it is known as the sphenopalatine artery forming the main vessel of the nasal cavity (p. 70). Among the many branches

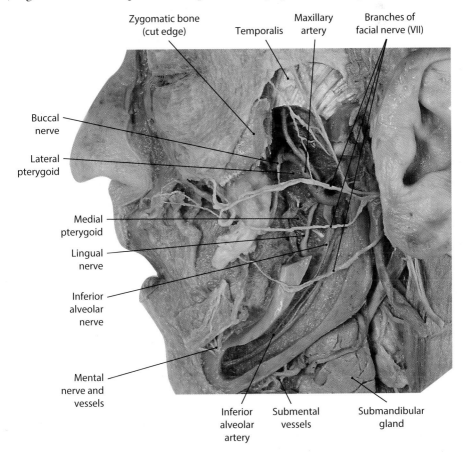

Fig. 3.23 Left infratemporal region, after removal of the parotid gland and part of the zygomatic arch and mandible. The facial nerve has been preserved.

are the middle meningeal artery (p. 36), which passes vertically *upwards* through the foramen spinosum, and the inferior alveolar artery, which runs *downwards* behind its companion nerve to enter the mandibular foramen.

Mouth

The mouth (oral cavity) is the start of the alimentary tract, with lips anteriorly at the front (containing the orbicularis oris), cheeks at the sides (containing the buccinator), the palate in the roof, the tongue and floor of the mouth below and the oropharyngeal isthmus posteriorly (the opening into the oral part of the pharynx – see Palate, below). The vestibule of the mouth is the space that separates the lips and cheeks from the teeth and gingivae (gums); the parotid ducts open into it opposite the second upper molar teeth, with numerous small mucous glands in the lips and cheeks. The mouth cavity is the part internal to the teeth and gums, with the hard and soft palates as its upper superior boundary and the tongue lying on its floor. Supporting the floor is the pair of mylohyoid muscles with the smaller geniohyoids lying just above them. The ducts of the submandibular and sublingual glands open into the cavity on the floor at the sides of the tongue base.

Sublingual gland – almond-shaped salivary gland that lies against the body of the mandible and makes a bulge in the mucous membrane over the floor of the mouth. Secretory fibres for this gland and the submandibular gland (in the neck, p. 88) come from the lingual nerve via the (parasympathetic) submandibular ganglion.

Tongue – a mass of skeletal muscle on each side of a midline fibrous septum, covered by a mucous membrane roughened by papillae and containing mainly mucous glands, with lymphoid follicles (lingual tonsil) posteriorly. There are also special nerve endings for taste (taste buds), found mainly towards the sides and back of the mucous membrane. The largest tongue muscle is the genioglossus, with bony attachment to the mandible, with the hyoglossus muscle passing from the hyoid bone more posteriorly. Other muscles of the tongue are smaller and join the tongue posteriorly to the palate and the styloid process above. All the tongue muscles are innervated by the hypoglossal nerve of their own side (**Fig. 3.38A**) (except for the palatoglossus attaching to the palate and innervated by the vagus nerve).

> In the rare hypoglossal nerve paralysis, the protruded tongue deviates towards the side of the lesion, because of the unopposed action of the muscles of the opposite side.

The mucous membrane of the anterior two-thirds of the tongue is innervated by the lingual nerve for ordinary sensations, like touch and temperature, but with fibres from the facial nerve's chorda tympani branch (which joins the lingual nerve below the foramen ovale) for the taste buds of this part. The posterior third is innervated by the glossopharyngeal nerve for both ordinary sensations and taste, with a small part of the front of the vallecula (p. 93) being supplied by the internal laryngeal branch of the vagus.

Gingivae – commonly called the gums, these are attached to the alveolar margins of the jaws and surround the necks of the teeth; they consist of dense fibrous tissue covered with mucous membrane.

Teeth – composed of a special mineralised tissue, dentine, with a central pulp cavity that contains vessels and nerves. Each tooth has an upper part or crown covered by enamel (the hardest of all tissues, thus the most opaque to X-rays), a neck surrounded by the gum and a root covered by cementum and anchored in the tooth socket by fibrous tissue, the periodontal ligament (periodontium).

Normal adult dentition consists of 32 teeth, 16 upper and 16 lower, eight in each half of each jaw, numbered and named from the midline laterally (listed here with approximate date of eruption in years): 1, central incisor (7 yr); 2, lateral incisor (8 yr); 3, canine (11 yr); 4, first premolar (9 yr); 5, second premolar (10 yr); 6, first molar (6 yr); 7, second molar (12 yr); and 8, third molar (18 yr or in later years of maturity, hence often called the 'wisdom tooth'). The deciduous dentition of the child ('milk teeth') consists of 20 teeth, five in each half jaw, lettered and named from the midline laterally (listed here with approximate date of eruption in months): A, central incisor (6 m); B, lateral incisor (8 m); C, canine (18 m), D, first molar (12 m); and E, second molar (24 m). Note that the deciduous molars are replaced by the permanent premolars, since the permanent molars have no precursors in the deciduous dentition.

To work on the teeth of the lower jaw, due to the density of the bone, dentists commonly need to produce an inferior alveolar and lingual nerve block by injecting anaesthetic solution through the inside of the cheek, so that it percolates around the nerves where they are labelled in **Fig. 3.23**, just above the mandibular foramen, and diffuses into them (the needle must not penetrate the nerves themselves). The teeth of the upper jaw can be anaesthetised by local injection into the mucous membrane that overlies the appropriate part of the jaw, because the bone of the maxilla is less dense and more porous than that of the mandible, so allowing the anaesthetic to penetrate into the bone and reach the roots of the teeth where the nerves enter them.

Palate – consists of the horizontal, bony hard palate (**Figs. 2.1C, 2.2B**), formed by parts of the maxillae and palatine bones and covered by a tough mucous membrane (mucoperiosteum) separating the oral cavity below from the nasal cavity above, and of the muscular soft palate (**Fig. 3.24**), which hangs down from the posterior edge of the hard palate (like a mobile curtain) to separate the nasopharynx above from the oropharynx below. One pair of soft palate muscles (the palatoglossus) runs to the side of the tongue to form the palatoglossal arch, which is the dividing line between the oral cavity and oropharynx; the palatine tonsils (p. 94) lie just behind this arch. A similar pair (the palatopharyngeus) run down into the pharynx (p. 93), while two other muscle pairs, the tensor veli palatini (tensor palati) and levator veli palatini (levator palati), pass superiorly from the palate to tense and raise it during swallowing, so helping to close off the nasopharynx and direct food and drink downwards. The lower border of the soft palate is not straight, but has a central downwards projection, the uvula, with its own pair of tiny muscles. All the muscles are innervated by pharyngeal branches of the vagus (p. 89), except for the tensor, which is innervated by a branch of the mandibular nerve via the nerve to the medial pterygoid muscle.

Saying 'Ah' with the mouth open raises the soft palate and enables more of the posterior pharyngeal wall to be seen.

Nose and paranasal sinuses

The nose, which is the start of the respiratory tract and where the organ of olfaction (smell) is located, consists of the external nose and the nasal cavity.

Conditions such as the common cold and hay fever cause increased secretion and swelling of the mucous membrane, and hence obstruction to the flow of air.

Draining into the cavity are the four pairs of paranasal air sinuses, named from the bones in which they lie; they are of uncertain function, but they add some resonance to the voice and by their shapes they may help to orientate the orbits so that the eyes can provide binocular vision.

External nose – the part that sticks out on the face. It is bony only in its upper part (the pair of nasal bones); the rest is cartilaginous. The openings are the nostrils (external nares).

Nasal septum – divides the nasal cavity into right and left halves. It is formed by the vomer posteriorly and part of the ethmoid bone centrally, with the rest being cartilaginous (**Fig. 3.4A**). The septum is rarely exactly in the midline, so that a slightly 'deviated septum' is a normal occurrence without clinical significance. Only if it is grossly deviated may it cause problems by obstructing one or more of the sinus openings.

> The lower anterior part of the septum is the common site for nose-bleed (epistaxis).

Nasal cavity – on either side of the nasal septum (**Fig. 3.24**), the roof of each half is only 1–2 mm wide, although the floor (the upper surface of the hard palate) is more than 1 cm wide. The lateral wall is the most complicated feature; its skeleton is made up of parts of the maxilla, the palatine and

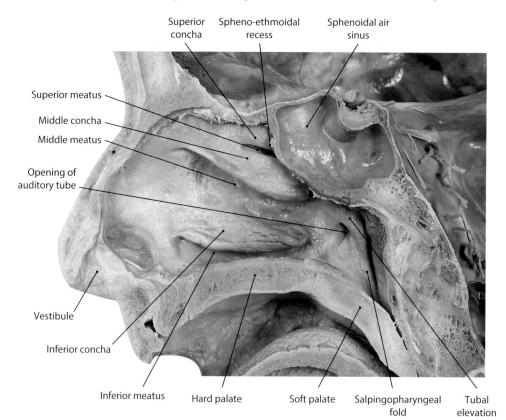

Fig. 3.24 Lateral wall of the right half of the nasal cavity.

ethmoid bones and the inferior nasal concha (the superior and middle nasal conchae are part of the ethmoid bone).

Superior, middle and inferior nasal conchae – form scroll-like projections from the lateral wall (**Fig. 3.24**), these are still sometimes called by their old names, the turbinate bones. They increase the surface area of the nasal mucous membrane and so help to warm inspired air. Immediately posterior to the *superior* concha is the spheno-ethmoidal recess, into which drain the sphenoidal sinus and posterior ethmoidal air cells. Posterior to the *middle* concha is the sphenopalatine foramen, through which the sphenopalatine artery enters the nose. About 1 cm posterior to the *inferior* concha is the opening of the auditory tube (in the nasopharynx).

Superior meatus – the space under the superior concha, into which drain the posterior ethmoidal air cells.

Middle meatus – under the middle concha, it features a swelling, the ethmoidal bulla (due to ethmoidal air cells), at the upper boundary of a curved groove, the semilunar hiatus, into which drain anterior and middle ethmoidal air cells, the maxillary sinus and the frontonasal duct (from the frontal sinus).

Inferior meatus – under the inferior concha, into which drains the nasolacrimal duct.

Blood supply – mainly by the sphenopalatine artery (the termination of the maxillary), with anastomoses with the anterior ethmoidal (internal carotid) and facial (external carotid) branches, in particular on the lower anterior part of the septum. There are corresponding veins.

Nerve supply – most of the nasal cavity (including the sinuses) is lined by respiratory mucous membrane (pseudostratified, with cilia), with sensory supplies by branches of the ophthalmic and maxillary nerves (trigeminal). Only a small area of the roof, the uppermost part of the septum and over the superior concha, is olfactory, with receptors for smell supplied by filaments of the olfactory nerve, which run through the foramina in the cribriform plate of the ethmoid bone to enter the olfactory bulb on the under surface of the frontal lobe of the brain. Nasal glands receive secretory fibres from the (parasympathetic) pterygopalatine ganglion (the 'ganglion of hay fever'), which is attached to the maxillary nerve just below (inferior to) the base of the skull, behind the foramen rotundum.

Frontal sinus – in the frontal bone above the orbit (**Figs. 3.2, 3.25**), draining into the middle meatus via the frontonasal duct.

Ethmoidal sinus – in the ethmoid bone on the medial wall of the orbit and lateral wall of the nose (**Fig. 3.25**), and made up of a variable number of ethmoidal air cells, which drain into the middle meatus (including the semilunar hiatus) or the superior meatus.

Sphenoidal sinus – in the body of the sphenoid bone (**Fig. 3.24**). The adjacent pair normally do not communicate with one another; they may vary greatly in size, and one or both may be indented by the pituitary fossa. Each drains into the spheno-ethmoidal recess behind the superior concha.

Maxillary sinus – in the body of the maxilla (and sometimes known by its eponym, the maxillary antrum of Highmore) (**Fig. 3.25**), it drains into the semilunar hiatus of the middle meatus through an opening that is high up on its medial wall, not near its floor, so that efficient drainage depends on the

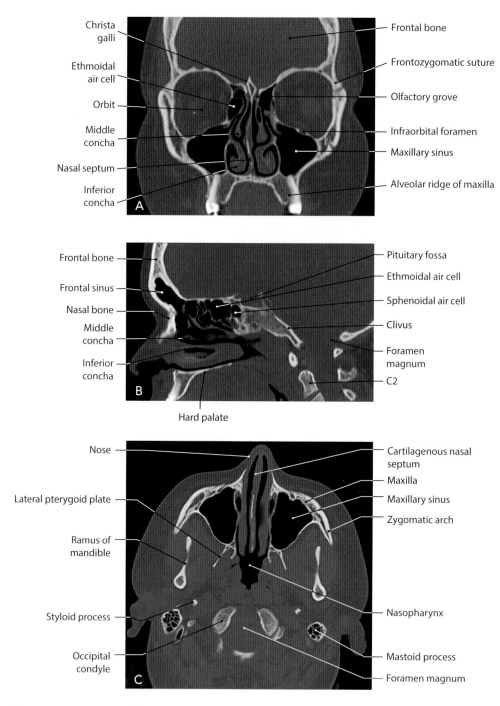

Fig. 3.25 CT images of the cranial air sinuses: (A) coronal view, (B) sagittal view, (C) axial view.

epithelial cilia (microscopic hairs), which beat to direct mucous secretion and debris upwards towards the opening.

Infection may spread from the nose or throat to any of the sinuses, but especially the maxillary, leading to sinusitis.

Eye and lacrimal apparatus

The eye (eyeball), the organ of vision, is almost a complete sphere, about 25 mm (1 inch) in diameter, lodged in the anterior half of the orbit (orbital cavity) of the skull and protected by the eyelids. Three layers make up the wall of the eye: the sclera, the choroid and the retina (from outside inwards); the retina contains the light receptors. However, anteriorly the sclera is replaced by, and is continuous with, the transparent cornea, which admits light into the eye. The optic nerve resides in the posterior half of the orbit, with most of the extraocular muscles that move the eye and other nerves and vessels all embedded in the orbital fat (**Fig. 3.29B**). The lacrimal apparatus starts with the lacrimal gland lying superiorly and laterally in the orbit, which secretes tears over the front of the eye, and is completed by the duct systems lying medially that dispose of these tears into the nose via the nasolacrimal duct.

Eyelids – each contains part of the orbicularis oculi muscle (p. 63), which closes the eye, and a plaque of dense fibrous tissue, the tarsal plate, which strengthens the protective capacity of the lid.

The facial nerve (VII) closes the eye (orbicularis oculi) but the oculomotor nerve (III) opens it.

The upper lid has an extra muscle to elevate it, the levator palpebrae superioris (**Figs. 3.26, 3.28**), unusual in that it

contains some smooth muscle fibres as well as skeletal fibres. The smooth muscle portion may have a separate designation as the superior tarsal muscle (of Müller). The gap between the lids when the eye is open is the palpebral fissure and located medially lie the puncta (openings) for the nasolacrimal duct. The edges of the lids contain the eyelashes and the tarsal (meibomian) glands, which are modified sebaceous glands.

Sclera – the 'white of the eye', the tough, fibrous outer layer (**Fig. 3.27**), to which are attached the extraocular muscles. The visible surface of the sclera is covered by a thin transparent membrane, the conjunctiva, which is continuous with the outer epithelial covering of the cornea and which also lines the inner surface of the eyelids.

'Something in the eye', like a speck of dust, readily irritates the conjunctiva, giving rise to conjunctivitis with enlarged and easily seen blood vessels.

Cornea – the transparent bulge at the front of the eye, continuous with the sclera at the sclerocorneal junction (limbus), and through which the iris and pupil can be seen.

Foreign bodies that damage the cornea may lead to loss of transparency with the formation of opacities and so interfere with vision.

Choroid – the thin and pigmented vascular layer that lies internal to the sclera (**Fig. 3.27**). The front part of the choroid is the ciliary body, which contains smooth muscle. From it is suspended the lens (whose shape can be altered by ciliary muscle to focus – accommodation); the part of the ciliary body anterior to the

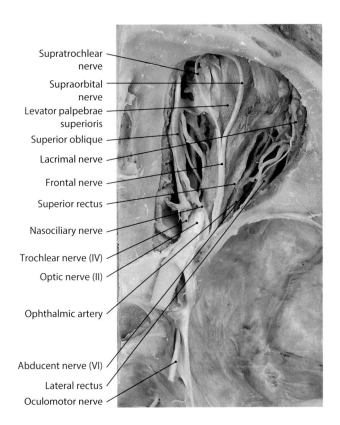

Supratrochlear nerve

Supraorbital nerve

Levator palpebrae superioris

Superior oblique

Lacrimal nerve

Frontal nerve

Superior rectus

Nasociliary nerve

Trochlear nerve (IV)

Optic nerve (II)

Ophthalmic artery

Abducent nerve (VI)

Lateral rectus

Oculomotor nerve

Fig. 3.26 Dissection of the right orbit, from above.

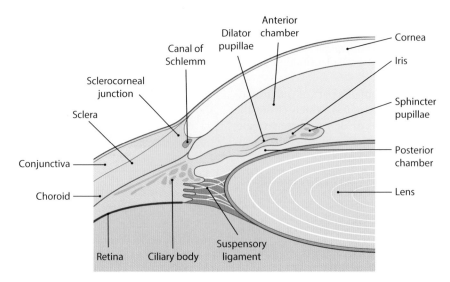

Anterior chamber

Dilator pupillae

Canal of Schlemm

Sclerocorneal junction

Sclera

Conjunctiva

Choroid

Retina   Ciliary body

Suspensory ligament

Cornea

Iris

Sphincter pupillae

Posterior chamber

Lens

Fig. 3.27 A section through the eye in the region of the sclerocorneal junction.

lens forms the pigmented iris, which gives the eye its colour and whose central opening is the pupil. Part of the ciliary muscle forms the sphincter pupillae, for constricting the pupil, and there are a few radial dilator pupillae fibres behind the sphincter fibres. The choroid, ciliary body and iris are sometimes collectively known as the uveal tract (from the Latin for grape, having the colour of a black grape).

The area between the cornea and the iris is the anterior chamber and that between the iris and the lens is the posterior chamber. Both chambers are continuous with one another through the pupil and contain a fluid, the aqueous humour, which is derived from blood vessels in the ciliary body and continuously circulates from the posterior chamber into the anterior chamber.

> Interference with the drainage of aqueous humour leads to an increase in intraocular pressure (glaucoma), which can eventually cause blindness due to retinal degeneration.

Here it is absorbed into a small channel, the canal of Schlemm (sinus venosus sclerae), at the iridocorneal angle, from where it drains away into ciliary veins.

Retina – the innermost layer, it contains the rods and cones, which are the light receptors. At the posterior pole of the eye is a particularly sensitive part of the retina, the macula lutea, where the clarity and sharpness of vision (visual acuity) are greatest.

> Macular degeneration is the common cause of loss of central vision in the elderly.

A little to the medial (nasal) side of the macula is the optic disc, devoid of rods and cones and therefore a blind spot, where nerve fibres leave the retina to pass back into the optic nerve.

> Detachment of the retina or retinal haemorrhage causes blind spots over the affected area.

From the optic disc branches of the central artery of the retina fan out and corresponding veins converge on to it. These vessels and the surface of the retina can be

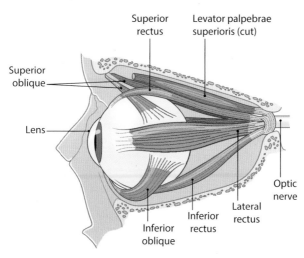

Fig. 3.28 Extraocular muscles of the left eye (the lateral rectus obscures the view of the medial rectus).

observed through an ophthalmoscope, a procedure commonly called examining the fundus of the eye.

> Study of the optic disc can give the clinician an indication of raised pressure within the cranial cavity as the CSF extends around the optic nerve enclosed in a dural sleeve, which is attached to the sclera. The fundus of the eye is the only place where blood vessels can be visualised during life. Clinicians make use of this when monitoring patients with conditions that can damage blood vessels such as hypertension or diabetes mellitus.

All the region internal to the retina (and behind the lens and ciliary body) is filled with a clear, gelatinous fluid, the vitreous body (vitreous humour); this has no connection with the aqueous humour; it helps to maintain the globular shape of the eye.

Extraocular muscles – four rectus muscles (superior and inferior, medial and lateral) and two oblique muscles (superior and inferior) (**Figs. 3.26, 3.28, 3.29B**). All except the inferior oblique arise from the posterior of the orbit and run forwards; the inferior oblique arises from the orbital floor anteriorly, near the nasolacrimal canal, to run posteriorly and laterally. These muscles are attached to the sclera in such a way that the muscles responsible for turning the eye *inwards* are the medial, superior and inferior recti, and those for turning it *outwards* are the lateral rectus and the superior and inferior obliques. Turning the eye *upwards* depends on the superior rectus and inferior oblique and *downwards* on the inferior rectus and superior oblique.

Motor nerve innervation – lateral rectus by the abducent nerve, superior oblique by the trochlear nerve and the other four by

the oculomotor nerve, which also innervates the skeletal fibres of the levator of the upper lid (the smooth muscle part receives sympathetic fibres).

The ciliary muscle and sphincter pupillae are innervated by parasympathetic fibres of the oculomotor nerve via the short ciliary branches of the ciliary ganglion, which lies on the lateral side of the optic nerve near the back of the orbit. Sympathetic fibres, which enter the orbit with the ophthalmic artery, cause dilation of the pupil.

Sensory nerve supplies – the cornea, an important part of the surface of the whole body, is innervated by the long and short ciliary nerves, which arise respectively from the ophthalmic branch of the trigeminal nerve and from the oculomotor nerve via the (parasympathetic) ciliary ganglion. They provide the afferent fibres for the corneal (blink) reflex; there are connections in the brainstem with neurons of the facial nerve that supply the orbicularis oculi, thus causing the protective closure of the eye.

Visual pathway – light impulses that fall on the rods and cones pass back in the optic nerve to the optic chiasma (**Fig. 3.29**), on the under surface of the brain just anterior to the stalk of the pituitary gland. At the chiasma, fibres from the nasal (medial) side of both retinas cross over, so that the optic tracts, which run posteriorly from the chiasma, contain fibres from the *temporal side* of the retina of one eye and from the *nasal side* of the retina of the *opposite* eye.

> Should the pituitary gland enlarge it can press upwards, damaging the fibres crossing in the chiasma with a classic peripheral visual loss (tunnel vision).

Each optic tract runs back round the side of the brainstem to reach a group of cells on the under surface of the thalamus,

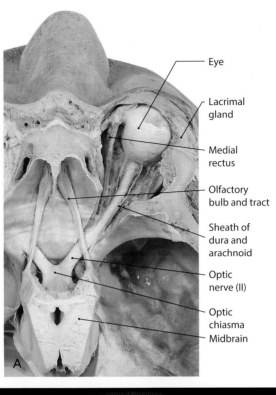

Eye

Lacrimal gland

Medial rectus

Olfactory bulb and tract

Sheath of dura and arachnoid

Optic nerve (II)

Optic chiasma

Midbrain

A

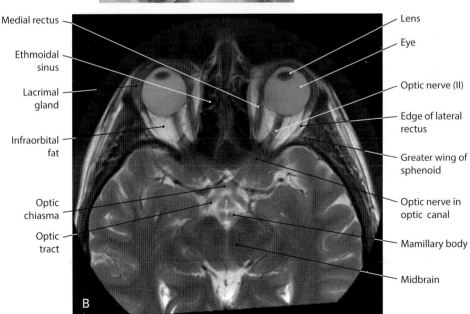

Medial rectus

Ethmoidal sinus

Lacrimal gland

Infraorbital fat

Optic chiasma

Optic tract

Lens

Eye

Optic nerve (II)

Edge of lateral rectus

Greater wing of sphenoid

Optic nerve in optic canal

Mamillary body

Midbrain

B

Fig. 3.29 Right orbit and optic nerve: (A) in a horizontal section of the head, (B) comparable axial MR image.

the lateral geniculate body, where the retinal fibres end by synapsing with cells whose fibres form the optic radiation, which passes to the visual area of the cerebral cortex, mostly on the medial surface of the occipital lobe.

Light reflexes – the general light reflex (e.g. blinking and turning away from a sudden bright light) involves connections in the brainstem and spinal cord so that the head and perhaps other parts of the body can respond.

The pupillary light reflexes depend on connections between retinal fibres in the optic nerve and certain neurons of the oculomotor nucleus; because of fibre cross overs in the optic chiasma and between the oculomotor nuclei of both sides, shining a light into one eye causes constriction of the pupils of both eyes. The final part of the pathway is via the (parasympathetic) ciliary ganglion, which lies near the back of the orbit on the lateral side of the optic nerve.

The accommodation–convergence reflex, sometimes called the near reflex, which enables the lens to focus for near vision and the eyes to converge slightly, as for reading, involves certain areas of the cerebral cortex as well as of the brainstem.

Lacrimal apparatus – concerned with the secretion and disposal of tears, which keep the visible part of the eye and the conjunctiva moist.

Lacrimal gland – in the upper outer corner of the orbit (**Fig. 3.30**), with about a dozen small ducts constantly discharging a small amount of secretion onto the surface of the eye. At the medial end of each eyelid is a tiny opening (lacrimal punctum) into a lacrimal canaliculus, which leads into the lacrimal sac situated in the lacrimal groove at the front of the orbit.

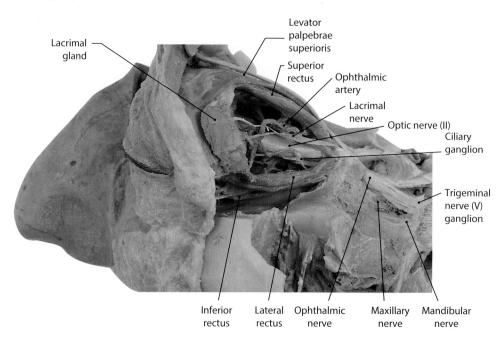

Fig. 3.30 Dissection of the left orbit, from the left, with the lateral rectus displaced downwards to show the ciliary ganglion.

The sac continues down as the naso-lacrimal duct, which opens into the inferior meatus of the nose (hence the 'snuffly nose' when crying, although excess tears also escape onto the face). The secretory nerve supply involves branches of the facial, maxillary and ophthalmic nerves and the (parasympathetic) pterygopalatine ganglion (p. 10).

Ear

The ear, the organ of hearing and balance, has three parts, named the external, middle and internal ear. All three are concerned with hearing, but only the internal ear with balance.

External ear – consists of the auricle (pinna), which projects from the side of the head, and the external acoustic meatus (ear canal). The auricle and the outer part of the meatus have a cartilaginous framework, but the deeper part of the meatus is part of the temporal bone. Special glands in the skin lining the meatus secrete wax (cerumen), whose purpose is to trap particles before they reach the eardrum (see below).

> The commonest cause of deafness is excess wax, which prevents the tympanic membrane from vibrating. Infections of meatal skin are very painful because the skin adheres very tightly to the underlying cartilage and bone.

Middle ear – a small air-filled cavity within the temporal bone, separated from the external acoustic meatus by the tympanic membrane (eardrum, **Figs. 3.31–3.33**). The cavity is bridged by three tiny bones, the auditory ossicles (malleus, incus and stapes, meaning hammer, anvil and stirrup, named from their shapes). It communicates anteriorly with the nasopharynx (p. 93) by the very narrow (1 mm or less) auditory tube (Eustachian tube). This is formed partly by the temporal bone and partly by cartilage, which can be moved slightly by small muscles attached

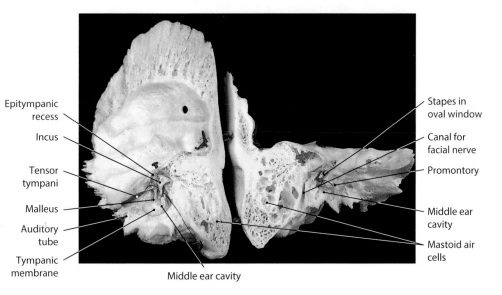

Epitympanic recess
Incus
Tensor tympani
Malleus
Auditory tube
Tympanic membrane
Middle ear cavity
Stapes in oval window
Canal for facial nerve
Promontory
Middle ear cavity
Mastoid air cells

Fig. 3.31 Bisected right temporal bone, to show the middle ear cavity. The fine threads over the promontory represent the tympanic plexus (glossopharyngeal nerve), which supplies the mucous membrane lining the middle ear cavity.

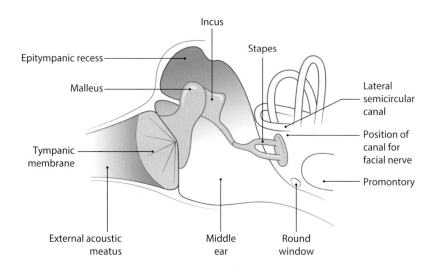

Fig. 3.32 The right middle ear.

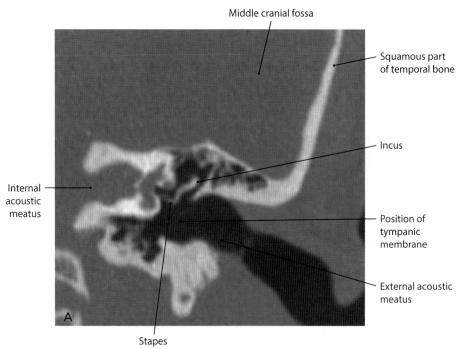

Fig. 3.33 CT images (magnified) of the ear anatomy: (A) coronal view of incus and stapes.
(Continued)

to it, in particular the tensor palati (tensor veli palatini); this increases the diameter of the tube when swallowing and helps to equalise the air pressure between the nasopharynx and middle ear cavity. Posteriorly, the cavity communicates with the sponge-like mastoid air cells, which reside within the mastoid process.

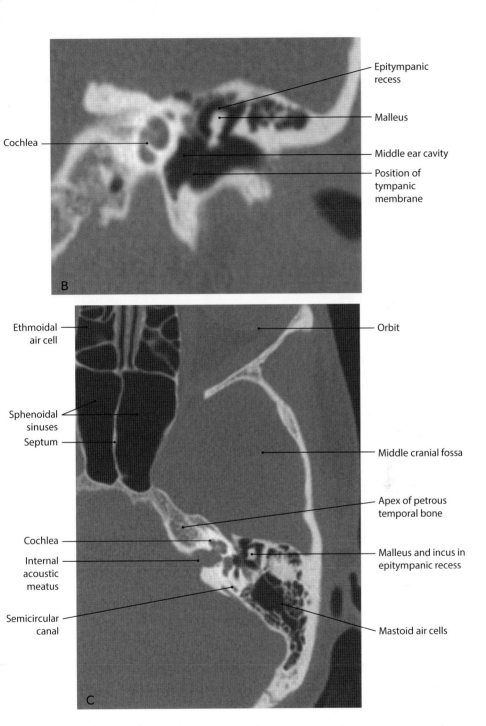

Fig. 3.33 *(Continued)* CT images (magnified) of the ear anatomy: (B) coronal view of malleus and cochlea, (C) axial view of cochlea and mastoid air cells.

Air within this cavity is required for the normal process of hearing.

Infections of the middle ear (otitis media) may cause rupture of the tympanic membrane (perforation of the eardrum) and may also invade the mastoid air cells (mastoiditis).

Internal ear – a complicated structure within the temporal bone that is concerned with hearing and balance. As explained below, it has bony and membranous parts (**Fig. 3.34**); to avoid confusion it is essential to remember what makes up these various parts and, in particular, to distinguish between those called *canals* (which are bony) and those called *ducts* (which are membranous).

The irregular-shaped space within the temporal bone comprising the internal ear is the osseous (bony) labyrinth. From front to back its parts are the cochlear canal (cochlea), the vestibule and the three semicircular canals (each at right angles to the other).

These bony spaces are occupied by a similarly shaped, thin fibrous sac, the membranous labyrinth. From front to back its parts are the cochlear duct (which occupies the bony cochlear canal), the utricle and saccule (which occupy the bony vestibule) and the semicircular ducts (which occupy the bony semicircular canals) and smaller ducts that connect these membranous structures to each other.

All the parts of the membranous labyrinth are filled with a fluid, the endolymph; outside the membranous labyrinth is another fluid, the perilymph, which separates the membranous labyrinth from the surrounding bony labyrinth. The two fluids do not communicate with one another.

Hearing – sound waves that cause the tympanic membrane to vibrate are conducted across the middle ear cavity by the malleus, incus and stapes. The movement of the stapes, against a membrane that fills a small opening (the oval window) in the cochlear canal, causes movement of the perilymph, which in turn causes movement of the endolymph within the cochlear duct. This, in its turn, stimulates the specialised auditory (hair) cells of the cochlear duct to send impulses into the brain via the cochlear nerve – the auditory part of the vestibulocochlear (eighth cranial) nerve. By various brainstem connections, the impulses are

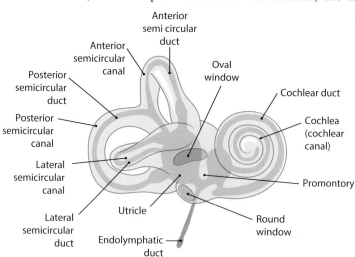

Fig. 3.34 The right osseous labyrinth with the membranous labrynth within.

conveyed to the auditory area of the cerebral cortex.

> A common cause of conductive deafness in the elderly is otosclerosis, where the stapes becomes fixed and cannot transmit vibrations to the inner ear.

Note that the stimulation of the special nerve receptors for hearing is by a rather indirect pathway: first, by vibration of the tympanic membrane, then through the chain of auditory ossicles, which modify the energy of the vibrations so that fluid can be vibrated, then to the perilymph, then to the endolymph and only then to the nerve receptors. It follows that disturbance of any part of this pathway could lead to impairment of hearing – ultimately deafness. Of the two types of deafness, conductive deafness is due to impairment of the conduction of vibrations in the external or middle ear (e.g. by wax in the external ear affecting the tympanic membrane or by middle ear disease preventing movement of the ossicles); sensorineural deafness is due to conditions that affect the internal ear or eighth nerve.

Balance – the vestibular nerve, the balance part of the vestibulocochlear nerve, supplies special nerve receptors (also hair cells) in the utricle, saccule and semicircular ducts that are stimulated by the movement of endolymph within these parts of the membranous labyrinth (which constitute the vestibular system). The body can make adjustments to its position according to these vestibular stimuli. In susceptible people, certain types of movement (as in travel by car, ship or plane) cause disturbances of vestibular function, which stimulate the vomiting centre in the brainstem - motion sickness. It is usually sudden changes in the position of the head that cause the movement of endolymph, and hence the feeling of dizziness (vertigo).

Neck and vertebral column

The skeleton of the neck is the cervical part of the vertebral column and the thoracic and lumbar parts of the vertebral column (p. 16) form the back of the thorax and abdomen, respectively (**Fig. 2.3B**). Significant muscles anterior to and lateral to the neck are mentioned below. Posterior to the neck and the thoracic and lumbar regions, there is on each side of the midline a large longitudinal mass of muscle, the erector spinae, the collective name for three groups of muscles located posterior to the spinal column.

Erector spinae – extend from the sacrum to the skull and form the bulge on each side of the line of the vertebral spines (**Figs. 3.35, 4.3, 6.5**). Each consists of large numbers of muscle bundles of varying lengths, with multiple attachments to vertebral spines, laminae and transverse processes and to the adjacent parts of ribs and sacrum, given different names depending on position and attachment. Collectively they make up this great extensor muscle of the vertebral column. It is one of the few muscles to be innervated segmentally by the *posterior rami* of spinal nerves. Multifidus, a deep component in the lumbar region, is also able to rotate and bend the spine laterally.

Sternocleidomastoid – prominent landmark (**Figs. 3.21, 3.36**) running obliquely upwards from the manubrium of the sternum and adjacent part of the clavicle to the mastoid process of the temporal bone. The part of the neck anterior to it, up to the midline, is the anterior triangle; the part posterior to it, as far as trapezius, is the posterior triangle. The muscle overlies much of the carotid vessels and the internal jugular vein (**Figs. 3.37, 3.38A**). Acting singly, it tilts the face upwards and to the opposite side; acting with its opposite fellow, the pair protrude the neck (as in peering over

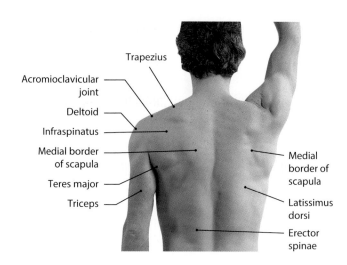

Fig. 3.35 Surface features of the trunk, from behind.

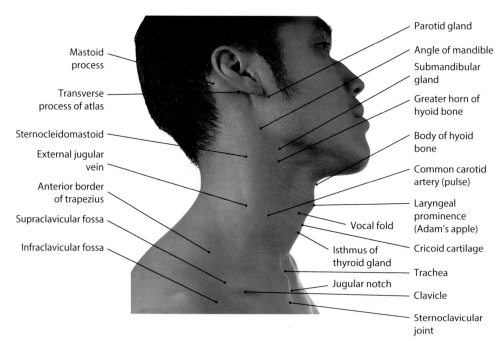

Fig. 3.36 Surface features of the right side of the neck.

someone's shoulder). They are innervated by the spinal part of the accessory nerve.

Cervical plexus – cutaneous branches fan out from the posterior edge of sternocleidomastoid: great auricular and lesser occipital nerves upwards, transverse cervical nerve forwards (**Fig. 3.22**) and branches of the supraclavicular nerve downwards (**Fig. 3.37**). By far the most important branch is the phrenic nerve (see below).

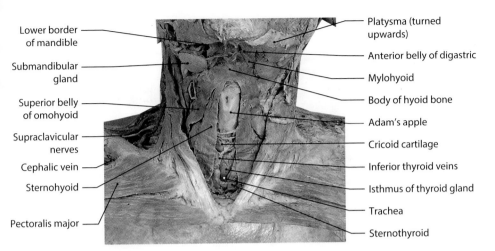

Lower border of mandible

Submandibular gland

Superior belly of omohyoid

Supraclavicular nerves

Cephalic vein

Sternohyoid

Pectoralis major

Platysma (turned upwards)

Anterior belly of digastric

Mylohyoid

Body of hyoid bone

Adam's apple

Cricoid cartilage

Inferior thyroid veins

Isthmus of thyroid gland

Trachea

Sternothyroid

Fig. 3.37 Superficial dissection of the neck, from the front.

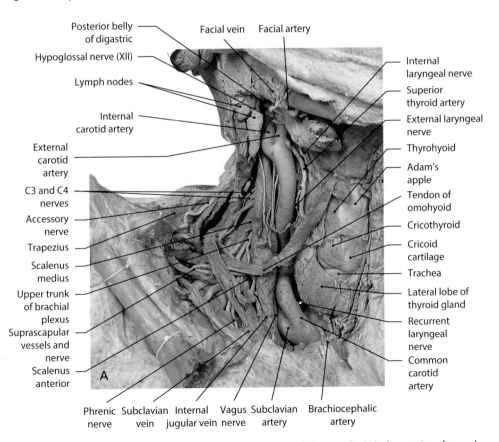

Posterior belly of digastric

Facial vein   Facial artery

Hypoglossal nerve (XII)

Lymph nodes

Internal carotid artery

External carotid artery

C3 and C4 nerves

Accessory nerve

Trapezius

Scalenus medius

Upper trunk of brachial plexus

Suprascapular vessels and nerve

Scalenus anterior

Internal laryngeal nerve

Superior thyroid artery

External laryngeal nerve

Thyrohyoid

Adam's apple

Tendon of omohyoid

Cricothyroid

Cricoid cartilage

Trachea

Lateral lobe of thyroid gland

Recurrent laryngeal nerve

Common carotid artery

A

Phrenic nerve   Subclavian vein   Internal jugular vein   Vagus nerve   Subclavian artery   Brachiocephalic artery

Fig. 3.38 Great vessels and nerves of the right side of the neck: (A) dissection from the front and the right, after removal of the sternocleidomastoid and with part of the clavicle turned down.   (Continued)

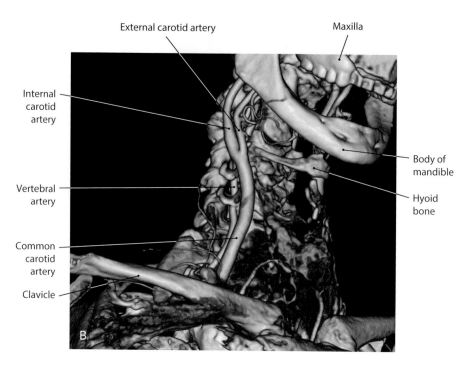

External carotid artery

Maxilla

Internal carotid artery

Body of mandible

Vertebral artery

Hyoid bone

Common carotid artery

Clavicle

B

Fig. 3.38 *(Continued)* Great vessels and nerves of the right side of the neck: (B) 3-D reconstruction from axial CT scans of the neck to show the arteries in relation to bones.

Hyoid bone – the body and greater horns are palpable below (inferior to) the mandible (**Figs. 3.36–3.38**), on a horizontal level with the C3 vertebra. It is connected inferiorly to the thyroid cartilage by the superior horn and the thyrohyoid membrane, which is pierced by the internal laryngeal nerve (from the superior laryngeal branch of the vagus) and the superior laryngeal artery (from the superior thyroid).

Laryngeal prominence (Adam's apple) – in the middle of the anterior of the neck (**Figs. 3.36–3.38A**), and more prominent in males than in females, especially post puberty, because the two laminae (plates) of the thyroid cartilage that form the Adam's apple (at the level of C4 and C5 vertebrae, as part of the larynx, p. 91) join at a more acute angle in adolescent and adult males. Posteriorly on each lamina are upward and downward projections, the superior and inferior horns; the inferior horns form the cricothyroid joints with the cricoid cartilage. The vocal folds within the larynx lie at a level midway between the laryngeal prominence and the lower border of the thyroid cartilage.

The whole larynx and hence the Adam's apple move upwards during swallowing.

Cricoid cartilage – shaped like a signet ring, with a narrow anterior arch and a broad posterior lamina, both of which give attachment to the cricothyroid membrane of the larynx. The arch is felt about 5 cm above the jugular notch of the manubrium of the sternum, at the horizontal level of the C6 vertebra, immediately anterior to the junction of the pharynx and oesophagus. From the cricoid artilage the trachea continues downwards *and backwards*, disappearing into the thorax behind the jugular notch through the thoracic inlet (see below).

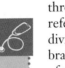

> Backward pressure on the cricoid cartilage can prevent the upward passage of vomit into the pharynx.

Common carotid artery – source of the carotid pulse (**Figs. 3.36, 3.38**), *vitally important in indicating circulation to the brain*.

> The carotid pulse is felt by pressing backwards in the angle between sternocleidomastoid and the thyroid cartilage (larynx).

Arising on the left from the arch of the aorta and on the right from the brachiocephalic trunk, each artery divides into internal and external carotid arteries at about the level of the upper border of the thyroid cartilage (C4 vertebra) (**Fig. 3.38**) just inferior to the posterior tip of the hyoid bone. **Note:** The carotid sheath is a fascia that encircles the common carotid, internal carotid, internal jugular vein and main stems of cranial nerves exiting the sigmoid and hypoglossal openings of the skull.

Internal carotid artery – passes vertically to the skull base. It enters the carotid canal running medially before passing anteriorly through the cavernous sinus (a course often referred to as the carotid syphon) before dividing into the anterior and middle cerebral arteries, which are major components of the arterial circle at the base of the brain (**Figs. 3.3, 3.13, 3.38B**).

External carotid artery – instantly identified from the common or internal carotids because it has numerous branches (**Figs. 3.38, 3.39**); the other two have no branches in the neck. The external carotid terminates by entering the parotid gland and dividing into the superficial temporal and maxillary arteries (**Figs. 3.22, 3.23**).

External jugular vein – prominent vessel that runs superficial to sternocleidomastoid and disappears behind the clavicle to join the subclavian vein (**Fig. 5.8**).

Scalenus anterior – small prevertebral muscle (**Figs. 3.38A, 5.4**) that runs from the transverse processes of C3–C6 vertebrae to the scalene tubercle of the first rib, where it separates the subclavian vein anteriorly from the subclavian artery posteriorly.

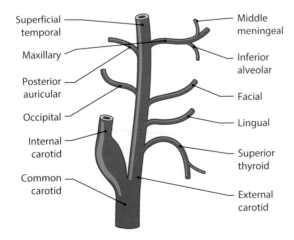

Superficial temporal

Maxillary

Posterior auricular

Occipital

Internal carotid

Common carotid

Middle meningeal

Inferior alveolar

Facial

Lingual

Superior thyroid

External carotid

Fig. 3.39 The carotid arteries and branches.

It is an important landmark in the lower neck; the phrenic nerve passes vertically downwards anterior to it and the roots of the brachial plexus emerge posterior to the subclavian artery.

Phrenic nerve – from C3, C4 and C5 (mainly C4) roots of the cervical plexus, it passes obliquely downwards over the scalenus anterior (**Figs. 3.38A, 5.4A**) to enter the thorax as *the main motor nerve to its own half of the diaphragm* (p. 140).

Brachial plexus – the roots, trunks, divisions and cords (p. 60) are each in a distinct position in the neck or axilla. The roots are in the neck between two of the prevertebral muscles (scalenus anterior and scalenus medius). The trunks (upper, middle and lower) are low down in the posterior triangle of the neck; the upper trunk gives rise to the suprascapular nerve (**Figs. 3.38A, 5.4A**), which supplies the supraspinatus and infraspinatus muscles of the shoulder. The divisions, which have no branches but vary greatly in length, lie posterior to the clavicle and form the lateral, medial and posterior cords in the axilla (p. 109).

Cervical lymph nodes – superficial nodes, which lie mainly along the external jugular vein, inferior to the mandible and behind the ear, and deep nodes along the internal jugular vein, including jugulodigastric (tonsillar) nodes below the angle of the mandible. Head and neck structures drain to these nodes, which in turn pass lymph to the right lymphatic duct or thoracic duct (on the left).

Palpation for cervical lymph nodes is an essential part of clinical examination.

Submandibular gland – salivary gland lying in the angle between the inner surface of the body of the mandible and the outer surface of mylohyoid (**Figs. 3.37, 3.38A**) with a small deep part that hooks deeply around the posterior border of that muscle.

The gland is palpable as a slight swelling 2.5 cm long about halfway along and inferior to the lower border of the mandible.

The submandibular duct, 2 cm long, runs forwards on the hyoglossus muscle at the lower part of the side of the tongue superior to the lingual artery and with the lingual nerve (with the submandibular ganglion attached to it) hooking inferior to the duct and the hypoglossal nerve above. The duct opens into the floor of the mouth beside the frenulum of the tongue.

Internal jugular vein – main vein of the head and neck, continuous with the sigmoid sinus in the skull through the jugular foramen (**Fig. 5.8**). It runs down on the lateral side of the internal and common carotid arteries (**Fig. 3.38A**) to join the subclavian vein deep to the sternoclavicular joint and form the brachiocephalic vein. It receives the inferior petrosal sinus and the pharyngeal, lingual, facial and superior and middle thyroid veins, in that order from above downwards. On the left, the thoracic duct (p. 134) joins the left side of the angle between the internal jugular and subclavian veins.

Right lymphatic duct – a short lymph vessel formed by channels that drain the right side of the head and neck, right upper limb and right side of the thorax, it joins the right side of the angle between the internal jugular and subclavian veins (similar to the thoracic duct on the left side).

Glossopharyngeal nerve – the smallest of the last four cranial nerves, it only innervates one muscle (the stylopharyngeus)

It gives sensory fibres to the back of the tongue and part of the pharynx, and has a highly important carotid branch, only found with meticulous dissection that runs down to the start of the internal carotid artery to supply specialised receptors in its wall and surrounding tissue. It conveys information on blood pressure and the carbon dioxide content of the blood to centres in the brainstem, and thus takes part in the reflex control of the heart rate.

Vagus nerve – runs straight down between the internal jugular vein and the internal and common carotid arteries (**Fig. 3.38A**) to enter the thorax. Among its branches in the neck are the pharyngeal branches and the superior laryngeal nerve, which divides into the internal laryngeal nerve (sensory to the larynx above the vocal folds), which passes downwards and forwards just below the greater horn of the hyoid bone to enter the larynx through the thyrohyoid membrane (**Figs. 3.38A, 3.40**), and the external laryngeal nerve (motor to the cricothyroid, the only laryngeal muscle visible on the outside of the larynx), which runs down behind the superior thyroid artery (**Fig. 3.38A**). There are also cervical cardiac branches that run down to the cardiac plexus (as well as thoracic cardiac branches).

Recurrent laryngeal nerve – from the vagus, but arising in the lowest part of the neck on the right (recurring/hooking under the right subclavian artery) and from within

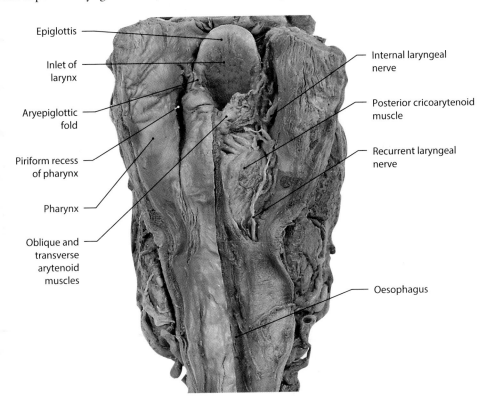

Epiglottis

Inlet of larynx

Aryepiglottic fold

Piriform recess of pharynx

Pharynx

Oblique and transverse arytenoid muscles

Internal laryngeal nerve

Posterior cricoarytenoid muscle

Recurrent laryngeal nerve

Oesophagus

Fig. 3.40 Larynx, pharynx and oesophagus, from behind. The pharynx and oesophagus have been incised in the midline and turned forwards; the mucous membrane has been dissected away on the right side.

the thorax on the left (recurring/hooking under the arch of the aorta, **Fig. 5.5**).

> The recurrent laryngeal nerves are among the most important in the body, since by their supply of the vocal fold muscles they control the size of the airway.

The nerves run cranially in the groove between trachea and oesophagus, to enter the pharynx and larynx (**Fig. 3.40**), passing behind the cricothyroid joint and supplying all the intrinsic laryngeal muscles (except the cricothyroid, supplied by the external laryngeal nerve) and the mucous membrane below the vocal folds.

Accessory nerve (spinal part) – runs down and backwards through the sternocleidomastoid to trapezius, which it enters about 5 cm above the clavicle (**Fig. 3.38A**). The nerve innervates both muscles.

Hypoglossal nerve – curls forwards just above the tip of the greater horn of the hyoid bone (**Fig. 3.38A**) to run into the tongue and supply its muscles.

Sympathetic trunk – lies posterior to the internal or common carotid arteries (but outside the carotid sheath), giving off from its three ganglia various branches to blood vessels, other cervical structures and also cardiac branches.

Vertebral artery – arising from the subclavian artery, it enters the foramen in the transverse process of the C6 vertebra and runs up through the same foramen in the succeeding vertebrae, eventually emerging from that of the atlas and then curling over the posterior arch of the atlas to enter the skull through the foramen magnum and unite with its fellow to form the basilar artery (**Figs. 3.13, 3.38B**).

Thyroid and parathyroid glands

Thyroid gland – consists of a small central isthmus anterior to tracheal rings 2 to 4 and on each side a lateral lobe, overlapped by the thin infrahyoid ('strap') muscles and sternocleidomastoid, and lying anterior to the common carotid artery, hugging the sides of the lower larynx and upper trachea (**Figs. 3.37, 3.38A, 5.4A**).

> The gland is usually only visible or palpable when enlarged (then called a goitre).

The gland's upper pole extends up to near the top of the lamina of the thyroid cartilage, and the lower pole down to tracheal rings 5 or 6. Being attached by connective tissue to the larynx, the gland *moves with swallowing*.

> The gland is best palpated with the examiner behind the patient, so that both hands can be brought forwards to feel the sides and front of the neck.

The gland usually has two arteries and three veins. The superior thyroid artery comes down from the start of the external carotid to the upper pole, and the inferior thyroid artery, from the thyrocervical trunk, arches up behind the lower pole. The recurrent laryngeal nerve (see above) may be in front of or behind this artery.

> This nerve is the most important structure related to the thyroid gland because it may be injured during thyroid surgery.

Superior and middle thyroid veins drain to the internal jugular, and one or more inferior thyroid veins enter the left brachiocephalic vein by running straight down anterior to the trachea (where they may be a hazard in tracheotomy).

The gland's iodine-containing secretion, thyroxine, is a general metabolic stimulant. Occasionally, a pyramidal lobe extending upwards towards the floor of the mouth can be found attached to the isthmus. This reflects the development of the gland from an outgrowth from the floor of the primitive oral cavity. This variation is not in itself pathological, but can contain pathology or a bleeding hazard when performing an emergency cricothyrotomy.

Parathyroid glands – usually two on each side, these are very small pea-like structures lying in contact with, or even within, the lower part of the back of the lateral lobe of the thyroid gland. All are supplied by the inferior thyroid arteries. Their endocrine secretion, calcitonin, helps to control blood calcium.

Larynx

The larynx (voice box) has a framework of cartilages and membranes (**Figs. 3.40–3.43**). The rather pyramidal-shaped arytenoid cartilages, with a vocal and a muscular process at their bases, sit on top of the (posterior) lamina of the cricoid cartilage to make the cricoarytenoid joints, while the inferior horns of the thyroid cartilage make the cricothyroid joints with the sides of the cricoid cartilage. The epiglottic cartilage is covered by mucous membrane to form the epiglottis, and lies anteriorly in the laryngeal inlet from the pharynx. The aryepiglottic folds of mucous membrane and muscle

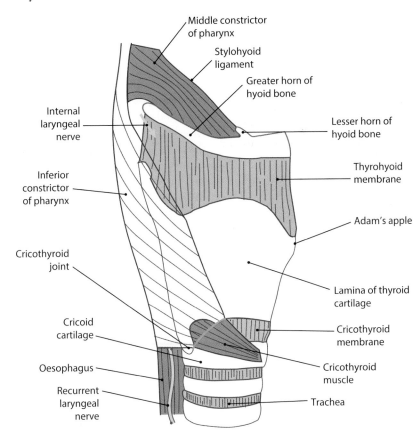

Fig. 3.41 The right side of the external surface of the larynx.

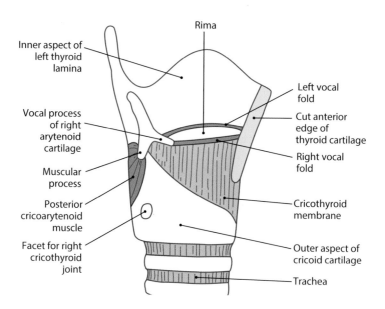

Rima

Inner aspect of left thyroid lamina

Vocal process of right arytenoid cartilage

Muscular process

Posterior cricoarytenoid muscle

Facet for right cricothyroid joint

Left vocal fold

Cut anterior edge of thyroid cartilage

Right vocal fold

Cricothyroid membrane

Outer aspect of cricoid cartilage

Trachea

Fig. 3.42 The vocal folds of the larynx, from the right, with the right lamina of the thyroid cartilage removed. The left arytenoid cartilage is obscured by the right one.

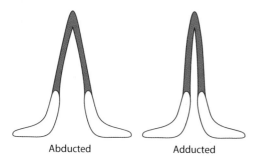

Abducted   Adducted

Fig. 3.43 The vocal folds in abducted and adducted positions.

form the lateral boundaries of this inlet, with the arytenoid cartilages and interarytenoid muscles posteriorly. The cavity of the larynx between the inlet and vocal folds (see below) is the vestibule of the larynx. At the cricoid cartilage (level of the C6 vertebra) the larynx becomes continuous with the trachea. Because of the attachment of some pharyngeal muscles (see below) to the larynx, the larynx moves upwards when swallowing.

Cricothyroid membrane – the most important of the membranes of the larynx. Attached all round the upper margin of the ring-like cricoid cartilage, it stretches up (like the lower part of a round tent) to be attached anteriorly to the midline junction of the thyroid laminae, midway between the laryngeal prominence and the lower borders of the laminae, and posteriorly to the vocal processes of the arytenoid cartilages (**Fig. 3.42**). These attachments alter the round shape to a V-shape, with the apex anteriorly. This upper free margin of the membrane is covered by mucous membrane and forms, on each side, the anterior 60% of the vocal fold or vocal cord; the posterior 40% is the vocal process of the arytenoid cartilage (**3.43**). The up-rush of air past these folds causes them to vibrate, hence the production of sounds. Slight rotational movements at the cricoarytenoid joints, but more importantly gliding movements up and down the sloping sides of the cricoid lamina (moving the arytenoids farther apart or closer together), alter the size of the rima of the glottis (the gap between the folds through which the air passes, **Fig. 3.43**) and so help to modify the sounds produced. The vestibular folds lie just above (superior to) the vocal folds; they are separate structures that do not move like the vocal folds, so they are often called the false vocal folds.

Posterior cricoarytenoid muscle – runs from the back of the cricoid lamina to the muscular process of the arytenoid cartilage. It is the *only muscle that can abduct the vocal fold* (i.e. increase the size of the rima of the glottis).

> The most important muscle of the larynx, because it increases the size of the airway.

The other intrinsic muscles either adjust the tension in the vocal folds, adduct them or alter the shape of the laryngeal inlet.

Innervation – the motor nerve supply of the laryngeal muscles is the recurrent laryngeal nerve, except for the cricothyroid (innervated by the external laryngeal nerve). The sensory supply of the mucous membrane below the vocal folds is also by the recurrent laryngeal nerve, but above the folds is by the internal laryngeal nerve (so it is all from the vagus, but by different branches).

Pharynx

The pharynx is a muscular tube that extends from the base of the skull to the C6 vertebra, where it becomes the oesophagus (**Figs. 3.4A, 3.5**). The nasal part (nasopharynx) is part of the respiratory tract, and the opening of the auditory tube (p. 79) lies in the lateral wall and the pharyngeal tonsil in the posterior wall. The oral and laryngeal parts (oropharynx and laryngopharynx) are common to the respiratory and alimentary tracts.

> 'Sore throats' (pharyngitis) and infection of the tonsils (tonsillitis) are common causes of enlarged and painful cervical lymph nodes.

The oropharynx has the (palatine) tonsils just behind the palatoglossal folds (junction with the mouth) yet in front of the palatopharyngeal folds. At the base of the tongue, in front of the epiglottis, lie two shallow depressions known as valleculae. The laryngopharynx has the larynx with the laryngeal inlet projecting backwards into it, with the piriform recess lateral to the aryepiglottic folds at each side where foreign objects (e.g. fish bones) may lodge.

Muscles – mainly the three pairs of constrictor muscles, arranged like three tumblers stacked one inside the other, but with large gaps anteriorly – openings into the nose, mouth and larynx. The inferior constrictor arises from the side of the cricoid and thyroid cartilages, the middle constrictor from the horns of the hyoid bone (**Fig. 3.41**) and the superior constrictor comes from the inside of the mandible, pterygomandibular raphe and medial pterygoid plate. Their fibres run backwards and upwards to converge posteriorly onto the midline pharyngeal raphe, which is attached to the pharyngeal tubercle of the base of the skull.

Three other pairs of small muscles run down from above to blend with the constrictors – the stylopharyngeus (from the styloid process), palatopharyngeus (from the soft palate) and salpingopharyngeus (from the cartilaginous part of the auditory tube). These, but more importantly the inferior constrictors, raise the larynx during swallowing; the sternothyroid, the elasticity of the trachea and the upper attachment of the oesophagus to the back of the cricoid cartilage pull it down.

Innervation – mainly from the pharyngeal plexus, found posteriorly on the middle constrictor, formed by pharyngeal branches of the vagus (which provide motor and sensory fibres) and glossopharyngeal nerves (which provide sensory fibres only). Note that stylopharyngeus has its motor supply from a separate glossopharyngeal nerve branch. The sensory supply to the mucosa of the nasopharynx (like the back of the nose) is mostly by the maxillary branches of the trigeminal nerves.

In swallowing (deglutition), the tongue is raised (a voluntary action) towards the hard palate and forces the food bolus posteriorly from the oral cavity into the oral part of the pharynx, while the soft palate is raised to block off the nasopharynx. The rest of the swallowing process is involuntary; sequential contraction of the pharyngeal constrictors carries on into the oesophagus and throughout its whole length to the stomach.

Tonsils – masses of lymphoid tissue (properly called the palatine tonsils), which lie in the oropharynx between the palatoglossal and palatopharyngeal arches (once collectively known as 'the pillars of the fauces'). The mucous membrane on the pharyngeal surface contains numerous downgrowths or crypts, which may become the site of infection, especially in the young. With the pharyngeal tonsil at the back of the nasopharynx and the lingual tonsil in the base of the tongue, there is thus a protective ring of lymphoid tissue at the start of the alimentary and respiratory tracts (Waldeyer's tonsillar ring).

Thoracic inlet – this is the term given to where structures of the root of the neck pass in/out of the thoracic cavity and marks the lowest border of the neck (**Fig. 3.44**). It is bounded anteriorly by the superior edge of the manubrium and laterally by the medial (inner) edge of the first rib and the T1 vertebra posteriorly. Dividing the inlet into right and left sides, the trachea lies anterior to the oesophagus, which in turn lies on the T1 vertebral body. On each side, the main structures passing through are the common carotid, subclavian and vertebral arteries, the brachiocephalic veins, the phrenic and vagus nerves descending into the chest, the sympathetic chain and

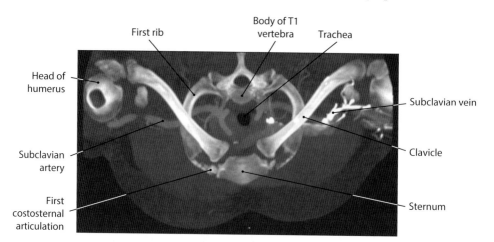

Fig. 3.44 CT reconstruction of the thoracic inlet from above.

posteriorly the T1 spinal nerve root passing upwards. On the left there is the recurrent laryngeal nerve and the thoracic duct passing into the root of the neck.

Summary

- Injury to the side of the head may rupture the *middle meningeal artery*, causing a dangerous build-up of pressure on the cerebral cortex (extradural or epidural haemorrhage).
- The most important tracts within the brain and spinal cord are the *corticospinal* (motor), *gracile* and *cuneate* (touch) and *spinothalamic* (pain).
- Arterial disease (haemorrhage and thrombosis) affecting the internal capsule is the common cause of *stroke* (hemiplegia).
- The *visual pathway* includes the retina, optic nerve, optic chiasma, optic tract, lateral geniculate body, optic radiation and the calcarine area of the cerebral cortex.
- The *cornea* is innervated by ciliary branches of the ophthalmic branch of the trigeminal nerve.
- The *muscles of the face* are innervated by the facial nerve, but facial skin is innervated by the ophthalmic, maxillary and mandibular branches of the trigeminal nerve.
- The *muscles of mastication* are innervated by the mandibular branch of the trigeminal nerve.
- The *hyoid bone* lies at the level of C3 vertebra, the *thyroid cartilage* at C4 and C5 vertebrae and the *cricoid cartilage* opposite C6 vertebra.
- The *carotid pulse* is felt in the angle between sternocleidomastoid and the upper thyroid cartilage, the *facial pulse* 2.5 cm anterior to the angle of the mandible and the *superficial temporal pulse* anterior to the tragus of the ear.
- The *isthmus of the thyroid gland* lies anterior to tracheal rings 2 to 4, with the lateral lobes extending between the levels of C5 to T1 vertebrae. The gland is not obvious to the naked eye, unless enlarged.
- The most commonly palpable *cervical lymph nodes* are those in the angle between the mandible and sternocleidomastoid and between sternocleidomastoid and the clavicle.
- The most important muscle of the larynx is the *posterior cricoarytenoid* – the only one that can abduct the vocal fold.

Questions

Answers can be found in Appendix A, p. 243.

Question 1

The pituitary gland is considered to be a key gland controlling body functions. Which of the following statements gives the most accurate description of the gland?

(a) Located within the body of the sphenoid and the anterior lobe has fibres joining it directly with the hypothalamus.

(b) It lies posterior to the body of the sphenoid and there is a venous portal system that controls secretions from the posterior lobe.

(c) Located superiorly in a depression in the body of the sphenoid and has a venous portal system that carries the stimulus to control secretions of the anterior lobe.

(d) Located inferiorly to a depression in the body of the sphenoid and the secretory cells of the posterior lobe are directly connected to the hypothalamus.

(e) Related to the superior aspect of the body of the sphenoid, it lies in a dural pocket and the important growth hormone is secreted by the posterior lobe.

Question 2

Many structures of the head and neck are midline structures. Which statement below is the most accurate description of the anatomy seen in such a section?

(a) The corpus callosum lies inferior to the third ventricle.

(b) The anterior communicating artery crosses the midline posterior to the pituitary gland.

(c) The aqueduct joining the third and fourth ventricles lies posterior to the pons.

(d) The basilar artery is located on the anterior aspect of the pons and terminates level with the midbrain.

(e) The fourth ventricle lies posterior to the midbrain between it and the cerebral hemisphere responsible for vision.

Question 3

The cells that store conscious thoughts are located on the surface of the brain. Which statement below is the most accurate?

(a) Motor cells responsible for movement of the hand are located in the gyrus just anterior to the calcarine sulcus.

(b) Motor cells responsible for the movement of the tongue are located in the temporal lobe just inferior to the lateral sulcus.

(c) Sensory cells responsible for the conscious appreciation of pin pricks to the hand are located on the gyrus just anterior to the central sulcus.

(d) Sensory cells responsible for noting vision are located just anterior to the parieto-occipital sulcus.

(e) Speech is controlled by cells located in the frontal lobe just above the anterior aspect of the lateral sulcus.

Question 4

Body functions are controlled by or through different parts of the central nervous system. Which statement below is the most accurate?

(a) Smooth movement of the limbs is coordinated through cells of the pre-central gyrus working with the basal ganglia and cerebellum.

(b) Smooth movement of the limbs is coordinated through cells of the post-central gyrus working closely with the cerebellum and basal ganglia.

(c) The respiratory centre is located in the medulla and responds to stimuli carried through the nucleus gracilis.

(d) The visual light reflex relies on connections between the optic nerves, internal capsule and the precentral gyrus.

(e) If the thalamus was damaged in a stroke, it would have no effect on the appreciation at a conscious level of touch, pain and temperature.

Question 5

Cranial nerves course from the brain to their target structure. Which statement below gives the most accurate description of the cranial nerve being described?

(a) This nerve commences at the junction of the medulla and pons and passes anteriorly into a dural pocket before dividing into three branches, one of which passes through the foramen ovale to innervate the muscles of mastication.

(b) This nerve commences at the junction of the medulla and the pons and passes anteriorly to run through the floor of the cavernous sinus to reach the facial sheet of muscles.

(c) This nerve commences at the posterior aspect of the midbrain and passes anteriorly around the midbrain to cross the edge of the tentorium cerebelli before passing in the medial wall of the cavernous sinus to reach a single muscle of the eye.

(d) This nerve commences from the lateral aspect of the medulla anterior to the olive and passes superiorly to the jugular foramen before passing to innervate the muscle sternocleidomastoid.

(e) This nerve commences on the anterior aspect of the pons and passes anteriorly to a dural pocket before dividing into three branches, one of which passes through the superior oblique fissure.

Question 6

Like the brain the spinal cord is divided into recognisable parts with different functions. Which statement below is most accurate?

(a) The main tracts carrying motor fibres down the cord are the lateral corticospinal tracts that cross in the brainstem.

(b) The main tracts carrying pain and temperature are uncrossed at spinal level and lie posteriorly as the gracile and cuneate tracts.

(c) The main spinothalamic tracts are crossed at spinal level and are located posteriorly in the cord either side of midline.

(d) The main tracts carrying touch are uncrossed in the cord and lie anterolaterally, rising to the nucleus cuneatus and gracilis.

(e) The main tracts carrying fibres that help coordinate muscular movement pass from the posterior horn cells to the cerebellum and are the anterior and lateral spinothalamic tracts.

Question 7

The teeth have an interesting history developmentally. Of the statements below, which one is accurate?

(a) With regard to the permanent dentition, the first central incisor normally erupts at 6 months of life.

(b) With regard to the permanent dentition, the canine teeth erupt first at 7 years of life.

(c) With regard to the deciduous dentition, the canine tooth normally starts to erupt at 8 months of life.

(d) With regard to the permanent dentition, the first molar tooth normally replaces the first deciduous molar tooth at 12 years of life.

(e) With regard to the deciduous dentition, the first molar tooth usually erupts at 12 months.

Question 8

Modern clinical anatomy involves viewing cross sections, so knowing what structures are normally related to other structures at a level is important to understand images. Which statement below most accurately reflects relations to cervical vertebrae?

(a) The hyoid bone lies anterior to the larynx at the level of C2.

(b) The bifurcation of the common carotid artery occurs just inferior to the hyoid bone at the level of the upper border of C4.

(c) The isthmus of the thyroid gland is located anterior to the cricoid at the level of C6.

(d) The vocal cords are level with the upper border of C3.

(e) The back of the oral cavity is level with the anterior arch of the atlas C2.

Question 9

A 23-year-old man suffers severe head trauma in a car crash. Weeks after he recovers from the immediate effects of a concussion, it is noted that he is constantly thirsty and urinates frequently. Urinalysis reveals that his urine is very dilute. Which intracranial structure has most likely been damaged in this patient to cause these symptoms?

(a) The arterial circle (of Willis).

(b) The pituitary stalk.

(c) The flax cerebri.

(d) The cavernous sinus.

(e) The pons.

Question 10

Following a severe sinus infection, a 55-year-old man experiences headaches, exophthalmos (bulging eyes) and a decrease in his vision. Physical examination reveals that his right eye is adducted (deviated medially). Which of the following is the most likely diagnosis?

(a) Cavernous sinus thrombosis.

(b) Aneurysm of the middle cerebral artery.

(c) Erosion through the cribriform plate of the ethmoid bone.

(d) Migraine headache.

(e) Tumour in the temporal lobe of the brain.

Question 11

A 22-year-old man sustains head trauma during a motorcycle accident and is unresponsive at the scene. He is rushed to the nearest Emergency Department where a doctor observes that the pupils of both the patient's eyes are dilated and do not constrict when a light is projected into them. With these and other findings, the physician declares the patient dead. Which of the following is the most likely explanation for the absence of pupillary reflexes to light?

(a) One or both internal carotid arteries are blocked.

(b) One or both superior cervical sympathetic ganglia have been compromised.

(c) One or both ciliary ganglia have been traumatised.

(d) The oculomotor nuclei are no longer functioning.

(e) Cranial nerve IV and/or cranial nerve VI have been lesioned.

Question 12

A 4-year-old girl is suffering from an upper respiratory tract infection. Her mother takes her to the local clinic. The examining physician notes that the child has diminished hearing, which is of recent origin. The physician inserts an otoscope into the child's external acoustic meatus to visualise the tympanic membrane (eardrum). This examination reveals fluid in the tympanic cavity (middle ear cavity). Which of the following is the most likely explanation for diminished hearing in this young patient?

(a) Cranial nerve VII is compressed.

(b) The endolymph is under pressure and cannot stimulate hair cells properly.

(c) The tympanic membrane cannot vibrate freely.

(d) The stapes cannot move unimpeded.

(e) Fluid in the tympanic cavity is putting pressure on the oval window.

Question 13

A 35-year-old woman has a severe allergic reaction to a bee sting and tissues in her pharynx swell rapidly and severely. In the Emergency Department it is decided that swelling will soon cause an obstruction to her airway and an emergency cricothyrotomy is performed. During this procedure there is copious bleeding that is difficult to control. Which of the following is the most likely cause of this bleeding?

(a) The superior thyroid artery was inadvertently cut.

(b) The inferior thyroid artery was inadvertently cut.

(c) An inferior thyroid vein was cut.

(d) The isthmus of the thyroid gland was incised.

(e) A pyramidal lobe was incised.

Question 14

While eating fish, a 55-year-old man experiences "something stuck in his throat". This is quite irritating and he reports to a local clinic seeking help with his condition. Which of following is the most likely location for a foreign object to become lodged?

(a) Piriform recess.

(b) Between the palatoglossal arch and the palatopharyngeal arch.

(c) The vestibule of the larynx.

(d) Between the vestibular (false vocal) folds.

(e) In the nasopharynx.

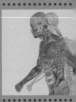

Introduction

The upper limb accounts for 5% of the body weight. The movements of the clavicle and scapula, humerus, radius, ulna and wrist have one collective purpose – to put the hand into the desired position for whatever it is required to do. Since the limb is essentially suspended from the trunk of the body mainly by muscles and not by a large joint, it has great freedom of movement.

The small sternoclavicular joint is the only bony connection between the upper limb and the axial skeleton (**Figs. 4.1, 4.4A, 5.3**). All other connections are *muscular*, mainly pectoralis major anteriorly, serratus anterior laterally and trapezius and latissimus dorsi posteriorly (**Figs. 4.2, 4.3**), accounting for the great mobility of the shoulder girdle compared with the hip girdle (p. 22). Small gliding and rotatory movements take place at the clavicular joints to accompany scapular movements against the chest wall.

Shoulder, axilla and arm

Shoulder (glenohumeral) joint position is maintained lateral to the side of the trunk by the clavicle, giving it freedom to be the most mobile of all body joints.

Bony prominences – the clavicle (**Figs. 4.1, 4.4A, 5.3**) is palpable throughout its length and can be traced from the sternoclavicular joint to its lateral end, where it makes the acromioclavicular joint with the acromion, which is at the lateral end of the spine of the scapula. The acromion lies at a slightly lower level than the clavicle; on palpation there is a small 'step down' from clavicle to acromion. The tip of the coracoid process of the scapula is just deep to the anterior border of the deltoid and can be felt by pressing laterally in the deltopectoral groove (see below) about 1 cm inferior to the clavicle.

Sternoclavicular joint – between the bulbous medial end of the clavicle and the manubrium of the sternum, the capsule encloses two joint cavities because a fibrocartilaginous disc separates the two bones. Adjacent to the joint is the costoclavicular ligament, which passes from the first rib and costal cartilage to the inferior surface of the clavicle, and is important as the fulcrum about which movements of the clavicle take place.

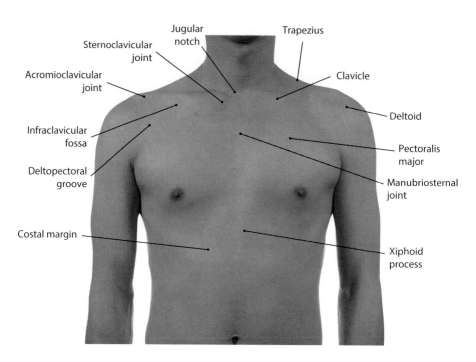

Fig. 4.1 Surface features of the upper trunk and upper limb, from the front (for the back view see Fig. 3.35).

Acromioclavicular joint – between the flattened lateral end of the clavicle and the acromion of the spine of the scapula (**Fig. 4.4**). There is a capsule, but the main factor keeping the bones in place is the coracoclavicular ligament, which runs from the coracoid process of the scapula to the inferior surface of the clavicle near its lateral end and consists of two parts, the conoid and trapezoid ligaments. These are strong and highly important in maintaining the integrity of the joint.

> In dislocation, they are torn and the 'step down' from clavicle to acromion is markedly increased. Clinically this is 'shoulder separation'.

Pectoralis major – from the medial half of the clavicle (clavicular head), upper 6(7) costal cartilages and sternum (sternal head)

it converges on to the lateral lip of the intertubercular groove of the humerus (**Fig. 4.2**). It is a powerful flexor, adductor and medial rotator of the shoulder joint and innervated by the medial and lateral pectoral nerves.

Pectoralis minor – small and lying deep to pectoralis major, passing from ribs 3, 4 and 5 to the coracoid process of the scapula (**Fig. 4.2**). It helps to fix the scapula to the anterior chest wall. It is important as a landmark in the axilla (see below).

Serratus anterior – from the upper eight ribs anterolaterally (**Fig. 4.2**) fibres converge along the length of the medial border of the scapula, but half of them are concentrated on the inferior angle to assist in lateral rotation of the scapula (see Shoulder joint (movements), p. 108). It is innervated by the long thoracic nerve.

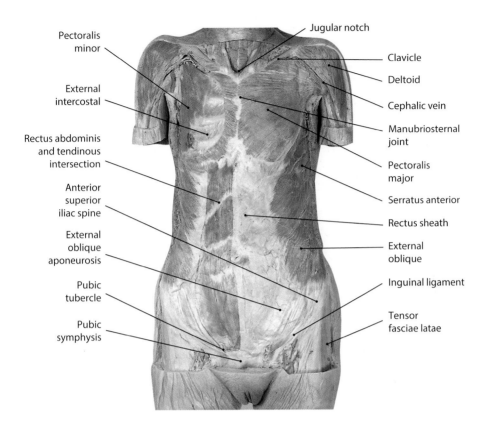

Fig. 4.2 Superficial dissection of the trunk, shoulder region and inguinal region, from the front.

The long thoracic nerve may be injured during operations in the axilla causing paralysis of the serratus anterior, which results in 'winging' of the scapula.

shrugs (elevates) the shoulder. Working as a whole it also rotates the scapula laterally (see Shoulder joint (movements), p. 108). It is innervated by the spinal part of the accessory nerve (p. 90).

Trapezius – from a wide medial attachment to the occipital region of the skull and the spines of all the cervical and thoracic vertebrae, the fibres pass laterally to converge on the lateral third of the clavicle, the inner edge of the acromion and the spine of the scapula (**Fig. 4.3**). By its upper fibres descending from the occiput and upper cervical spine to the clavicle and acromion, it is the main muscle that

Latissimus dorsi – arising from the spines of the lower six thoracic vertebrae, lumbar fascia (attaching to the spines of all lumbar vertebrae) and the posterior part of the iliac crest (**Fig. 4.3**), the fibres pass cranially and laterally, converging on a narrow tendon that curls around teres major to attach in the floor of the intertubercular groove of the humerus. It is a powerful adductor, extensor and medial rotator of the humerus, innervated by the thoracodorsal nerve.

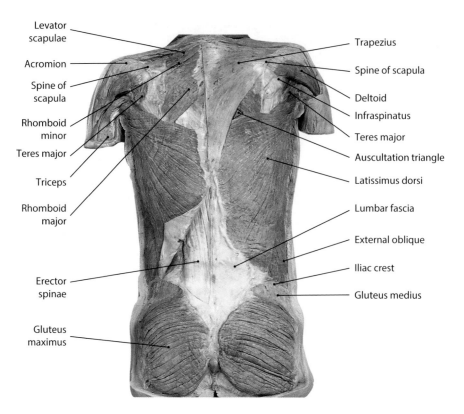

Fig. 4.3 Superficial dissection of the trunk, shoulder region and gluteal region, from behind.

Triangle of auscultation – formed by the adjacent borders of the trapezius, latissimus dorsi and medial scapula (**Fig. 4.3**). It is where there is the least tissue between the skin and the rib cage, making it the best location on the back to place a stethoscope and listen to (auscultate) breath sounds.

Teres major – from the inferior angle of the scapula (**Fig. 4.3**), it passes *anterior to* the long head of triceps to attach to the medial lip of the intertubercular groove of the humerus. It will form the lower boundary of the axilla posteriorly along with the latissimus dorsi tendon curling around anterior to it. It is an extensor, adductor and medial rotator of the humerus innervated by the lower subscapular nerve.

Rotator cuff muscles – a group of four muscles (see below) that fuse with the capsule of the glenohumeral (shoulder) joint and embrace the head of the humerus, designed and function to ensure that the head remains in contact with the glenoid cavity of the scapula (**Fig. 4.5**).

Subscapularis – from the subscapular fossa of the anterior (deep surface) of the scapula it reaches the lesser tubercle of the humerus to lie anterior to the glenohumeral joint (**Fig. 4.5C**). Apart from stabilising this joint, it is a medial rotator of the humerus, innervated by the upper and lower subscapular nerves.

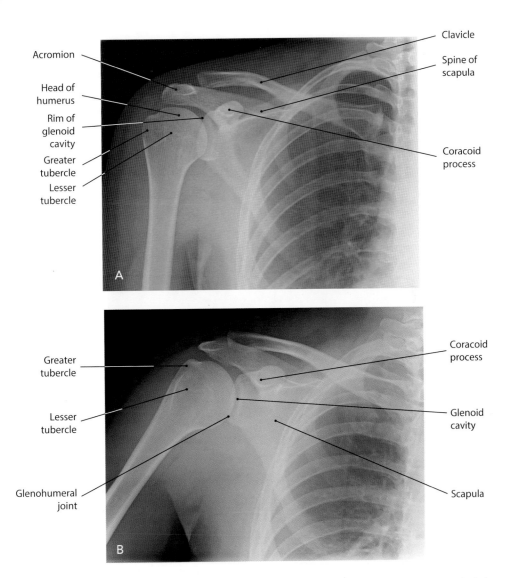

Acromion

Head of
humerus

Rim of
glenoid
cavity

Greater
tubercle

Lesser
tubercle

Clavicle

Spine of
scapula

Coracoid
process

A

Greater
tubercle

Lesser
tubercle

Glenohumeral
joint

Coracoid
process

Glenoid
cavity

Scapula

B

Fig. 4.4 Radiographs of the right shoulder: (A) posteroanterior view, (B) slightly abducted anteroposterior view; note the resultant elevation of the acromion and attached clavicle.

Supraspinatus – from the supraspinous fossa of the scapula it runs laterally superior to the shoulder joint to the upper facet of the greater tubercle of the humerus (**Figs. 4.5A & B**). Apart from stabilising the shoulder joint, it initiates the first 10° of abduction (as seen in **Fig. 4.4B**) and then acts with the deltoid to abduct the arm further. It is innervated by the supras-capular nerve.

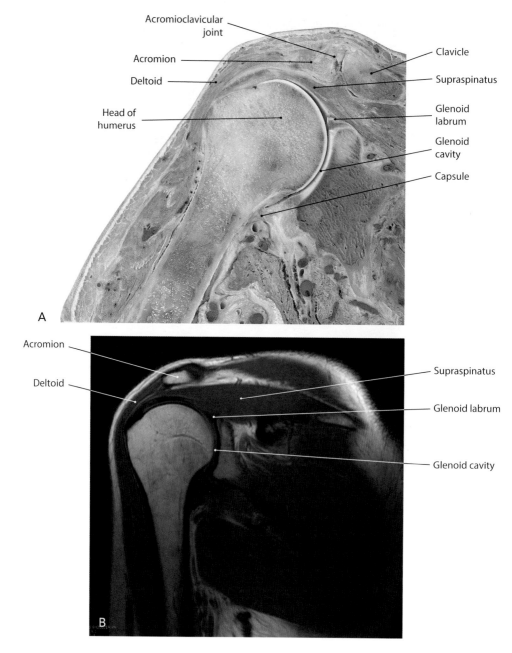

Fig. 4.5 Right shoulder joint: (A) coronal section, (B) coronal MR image. *(Continued)*

Infraspinatus – from the infraspinous fossa (**Figs. 4.3, 4.5C**) it runs laterally to the middle facet on the posterior aspect of the greater tubercle of the humerus. Apart from stabilising the shoulder joint, it is a lateral rotator of the humerus, innervated by the suprascapular nerve.

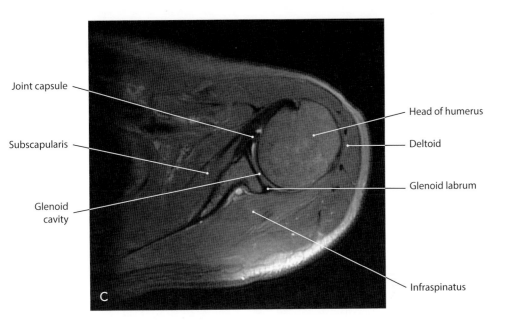

Joint capsule

Subscapularis

Glenoid cavity

Head of humerus

Deltoid

Glenoid labrum

Infraspinatus

C

Fig. 4.5 *(Continued)* Right shoulder joint: (C) axial MR image.

Teres minor – from the lateral border of the scapula, just above teres major, it passes *posterior to* the long head of triceps to the lower facet on the posterior aspect of the greater tubercle of the humerus. Apart from stabilising the shoulder joint, it is a lateral rotator of the humerus, innervated by the axillary nerve.

Deltoid – forms the most lateral mass of the shoulder, covering the greater tubercle of the humerus (**Figs. 4.2, 4.3, 4.5**). It runs from proximally the lateral third of the clavicle, the acromion and spine of the scapula to distally halfway down the lateral side of the shaft of the humerus. It is the most important abductor of the shoulder joint; its anterior fibres also assist in medial rotation and flexion of the humerus and the posterior fibres in lateral rotation and extension. It is innervated by the axillary nerve.

Deltopectoral groove – the gap between the deltoid (attached to the *lateral third* of the clavicle) and pectoralis major (attached to the *medial half* of the clavicle), in which lies the cephalic vein passing proximally to reach the subclavian vein without being compressed by the muscles (**Fig. 4.2**).

Shoulder (glenohumeral) joint – between the glenoid cavity of the scapula and the head of the humerus (**Figs. 4.4, 4.5**). The glenoid cavity is slightly deepened at the periphery by the fibrocartilaginous glenoid labrum.

> The stability of the shoulder depends on its surrounding muscles and not on its bony structure. As a result, it is the most mobile joint in the body and the most frequently dislocated.

The tendon of the long head of biceps runs over the top of the head of the humerus within the joint cavity and passes out of the joint capsule, surrounded by a tubular sleeve of synovial membrane to lie in the intertubercular (bicipital) groove of the humerus.

The capsule is very lax, to allow for the wide range of movement. There are some thin bands within the capsule (referred to as glenohumeral ligaments) which surgeons 'tighten' when treating recurrent shoulder dislocations. The lowest part of its attachment to the humerus is to the medial side of the surgical neck; elsewhere, it surrounds the anatomical neck. The rotator cuff muscles compensate for the laxness of the capsule. The coraco-acromial ligament forms a fibrous arch superior to the joint; between it and the supraspinatus tendon is the subacromial bursa (sometimes called the subdeltoid, since it projects laterally beyond the acromion deep to deltoid).

> In laypersons' jargon, 'bursitis' is typically inflammation of this bursa.

Normally this bursa does not communicate with the joint cavity, but if the supraspinatus tendon is torn there will then be a direct communication between the two cavities.

The principal muscles that produce movements at the shoulder joint are:

- **Abduction** – supraspinatus (to 10°), deltoid (beyond 10°).
- **Adduction** – pectoralis major, latissimus dorsi and teres major.
- **Flexion** – pectoralis major (sternal part especially when the arm is extended), deltoid (anterior part) and biceps.
- **Extension** – latissimus dorsi, teres major, deltoid (posterior part) and pectoralis major (clavicular part, especially when the arm is flexed).
- **Lateral rotation** – infraspinatus, teres minor and deltoid (posterior fibres).
- **Medial rotation** – pectoralis major, subscapularis, latissimus dorsi, teres major and deltoid (anterior fibres).

The amount of abduction possible at the shoulder joint itself (produced by the supraspinatus and deltoid working together) is about 120°. Abduction to 180° (straight up beside the head) requires movement at the joint to be supplemented by rotation of the scapula, tilting the glenoid cavity upwards. This is produced by trapezius upper fibres pulling the clavicle and acromion upwards, the middle group of fibres pulling the acromion and spine medially and the lower fibres pulling down on the medial point of the scapular spine to create lateral rotation of the scapula. This is aided by the lower part of serratus anterior (pulling on the inferior angle of the scapula).

> Cutting the accessory nerve in the neck (in operations to remove cervical lymph nodes) paralyses trapezius and limits abduction of the shoulder to around 90°. Similarly, cutting the long thoracic nerve (e.g. during axillary lymph node clearance) also limits abduction.

Note that the supraspinatus passes right over the centre of the top of the joint and is an abductor, not a rotator, despite belonging to the group called 'rotator cuff'.

Axilla – commonly called the armpit, whose anterior wall is formed by pectoralis major and minor and the posterior wall by subscapularis superiorly and with latissimus dorsi inferiorly, curling around teres major at the lower border. The medial wall is the rib cage covered by serratus anterior and the lateral wall is the bicipital groove where the pectoralis major and latissimus dorsi converge. The main contents are the axillary vessels, cords of the brachial plexus and their branches, lymph nodes and fat (**Fig. 4.6**).

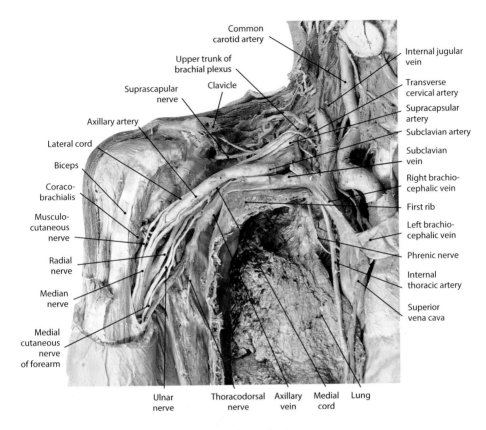

Fig. 4.6 Right axilla and root of the neck, from the front.

Axillary artery – continuation of the subclavian artery at the outer border of the first rib, and becoming the brachial artery in the arm at the lower border of teres major. The axillary vein lies medial to the artery. The vessels lie deep to pectoralis minor – the guide to the artery and the surrounding cords of the brachial plexus.

Cords of the brachial plexus – arranged around the axillary artery and named according to their positions – lateral, medial and posterior (**Fig. 3.18**). To assist in identifying the major branches of the cords, note the capital-M pattern made by the ulnar nerve, the two roots of the median nerve and the musculocutaneous nerve. (For other parts of the plexus, see pp. 60 and 88. For the distributions of dermatomes and cutaneous nerves, see **Figs. 3.17** and **4.12**.)

It is of note that many variations of the components of the brachial plexus have been described, which can hinder correct identification of its components, but these variations normally have no clinical significance, unless they form tight bands constricting a major axillary vessel.

Lateral cord – gives rise to the musculocutaneous nerve, lateral root of the median nerve and lateral pectoral nerve.

Medial cord – gives rise to the ulnar nerve, medial root of the median nerve, medial pectoral nerve and the medial cutaneous nerves of arm and forearm.

Posterior cord – gives rise to the radial nerve, axillary nerve, subscapular nerves and thoracodorsal nerve.

Musculocutaneous nerve – most lateral of the large branches, it pierces the coraco-brachialis, a feature that identifies it from all other branches of the plexus. It supplies biceps, coracobrachialis and brachialis (all of the flexors in the arm), and then becomes the lateral cutaneous nerve of the forearm. In some individuals this nerve consists of a small branch to coracobrachialis only and a more substantial branch arising more dis-tally to biceps and brachialis.

Median nerve – formed by its two roots, which unite anterior to the axillary artery, it runs down the arm anterior to the brachial artery, overlapped by the bicipital aponeu-rosis, into the cubital fossa lying medial to the artery. There are no muscular branches in the arm.

Ulnar nerve – largest branch of the medial cord, it runs medial to the axillary artery and just *posterior to* the medial cutaneous nerve of the forearm. Halfway down the arm the ulnar nerve passes into the posterior com-partment to continue its downwards course superficial to triceps; at the elbow it lies posterior to the medial epicondyle of the humerus, where it is palpable and most vul-nerable to damage. There are no muscular branches in the arm.

Medial cutaneous nerve of the arm – small, lying medial to the axillary vein.

Medial cutaneous nerve of the forearm – almost as large as the ulnar nerve, but lying anterior to it (as might be expected since it is heading for skin) and not to be confused with it.

Radial nerve – largest nerve of the brachial plexus, from the posterior cord, posterior to the axillary artery; anterior to the wide tendon of latissimus dorsi on the lower posterior axillary wall. It is the nerve of the extensor muscles in the arm and forearm (including brachioradialis).

> Radial nerve injury from fracture of the humerus does not usually paralyse triceps because the branches that supply it arise high in the axilla above the level of injury.

It curls around posterior to the humerus in the radial groove, between the medial and lateral heads of triceps, to emerge laterally deep to brachioradialis to innervate it and all the extensors in the forearm. It divides into a relatively unimportant superficial cutaneous branch and the highly important deep radial nerve, which carries the motor supply to all the forearm extensor muscles. The deep radial nerve runs between the two heads of the supinator and emerges distally as the posterior interosseous nerve.

> Radial nerve paralysis (e.g. from fracture of the shaft of the humerus) causes 'wrist drop' because the wrist extensors are paralysed.

Remember, therefore, that the radial nerve, which comes from the *posterior* cord of the brachial plexus, is the nerve that sup-plies the muscles of the *posterior* aspect of the *arm and forearm.*

Axillary nerve – large nerve arising high up from the posterior cord, it runs down-wards and laterally to disappear posteriorly between the tendons of subscapularis and teres major and the humerus, to innervate the deltoid (and teres minor) and, clinically important, a small overlying patch of skin inferior to the acromion.

Axillary lymph nodes – up to about 50 nodes scattered in the axillary fat and mainly located near the axillary vessels and their branches. They are divided into groups (anterior or pectoral group, posterior and lateral), all draining to a central group, which in turn drain to an apical group in the axillary apex.

> The axillary lymph nodes are commonly invaded by cancerous spread (metastases) from the breast – one of the commonest sites for cancer in females.

Apart from receiving lymph from the upper limb, they are of supreme clinical importance because most of the lymphatic drainage from the breast passes to these nodes.

Biceps – the prominent muscle on the anterior of the arm, with a long head originating from the supraglenoid tubercle within the shoulder joint, and a short head arising from the coracoid process with coracobrachialis. At the elbow its tendon is attached to the *posterior* of the tuberosity of the radius. It is not only a flexor of the elbow joint (and a weak flexor of the shoulder), but also (with the elbow flexed and forearm pronated) the most powerful supinator of the forearm (p. 120). There is a thin expansion (bicipital aponeurosis) of the tendon, which passes superficially and medially to lie between the antecubital veins, commonly used for venepuncture, and the deeper located brachial artery and median nerve. It is innervated by the musculocutaneous nerve.

Brachialis – deep to biceps, from the anterior of the distal humerus to the anterior of the coronoid process and tuberosity of the ulna. It is a powerful flexor of the elbow joint innervated by the musculocutaneous nerve.

Coracobrachialis – from the coracoid process of the scapula (with the short head of biceps) passing halfway down the medial side of the humerus. Very weak flexor of the shoulder joint and notable because the musculocutaneous nerve runs through and innervates it – a useful identifying feature.

Triceps – extensor of the elbow (with the long head also weakly extending the shoulder), the largest muscle on the posterior of the arm, with heads of origin from the scapula inferior to the glenoid cavity (long head), the upper part of the posterior of the humerus (lateral head) and the rest of the posterior of the humerus (medial head). All unite in a tendon inserted into the posterior of the olecranon of the ulna. It is innervated by the radial nerve.

Anconeus – a very small triangular muscle from the posterior surface of the lateral humeral epicondyle passing distally to the posterior surface of the ulna. Innervated by the radial nerve, it has a role in stabilising the elbow joint.

Brachial artery – runs down the arm just deep to the medial border of biceps. In the upper (proximal) part of the arm the brachial pulse can be felt by pressing *laterally, not backwards*, because at this level the artery lies *medial* to the humerus, not in front of it.

> This is the artery that is compressed for recording blood pressure; the stethoscope used for listening to the pulsation sounds is placed over the *lower* end of the artery (Fig. 4.7) in the antecubital fossa (see below) medial to the biceps tendon, just above where it divides into the radial and ulnar arteries.

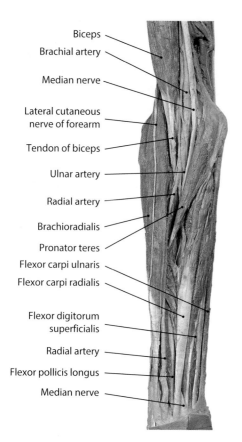

Biceps
Brachial artery
Median nerve
Lateral cutaneous
nerve of forearm
Tendon of biceps
Ulnar artery
Radial artery
Brachioradialis
Pronator teres
Flexor carpi ulnaris
Flexor carpi radialis
Flexor digitorum
superficialis
Radial artery
Flexor pollicis longus
Median nerve

Fig. 4.7 Superficial dissection of the right cubital fossa and forearm.

Elbow, forearm and hand

The power and the range of upper limb activity are enormous, extending from the relatively crude movements of wielding a hammer to the most delicate brush strokes of the artist or the steady manipulations of the neurosurgeon. The coordination of motor and sensory activities in the hand is matched only by those of the eye. The twisting movements of the forearm that turn over the hand and the unique rotatory movement at the base of the thumb, allowing it to be carried towards the palm of the hand to give a firm grip, have given a degree of manual dexterity that has contributed to

the human species becoming the world' most dominant animal.

Additional terms are required to describe the twisting of the forearm. To understand these, flex your elbow to a right angle and look at the palm of the hand (supine position), then turn the hand over so that you are looking at the dorsum of the hand (placing it in the prone position). This is the movement of *pronation*, where the lower end of the radius (the lateral bone of the forearm) rotates round the lower end of the ulna (the medial bone of the forearm), carrying the hand with it. Now turn the hand over so that you are looking at the palm (supine) again; this is the movement of *supination* For many common actions, like holding a glass, the forearm and hand are used in the mid-prone position, midway between full pronation and full supination. The ligaments of the radioulnar joints and the fibrous interosseous membrane stretching between the radius and ulna keep the two bones together during these movements.

Bony prominences – at the elbow the medial and lateral epicondyles of the humerus are easily palpable at the sides, and posteriorly is the olecranon of the ulna and the whole length of the subcutaneous posterior border of the ulna (**Fig. 2.6**). The medial epicondyle gives origin to several flexor muscles and forms the common flexor tendon; similarly, the common extensor tendon attaches to the lateral epicondyle.

> Any of these bony prominences are easily hit against objects and a resultant fracture of the more prominent medial epicondyle can damage the ulnar nerve, which lies in close contact.

With the elbow straight (extended), the head of the radius can be felt on the posterior aspect of the elbow (at the bottom of a small depression lateral to the olecranon), where it articulates with the capitulum of the humerus.

At the sides of the wrist, the styloid process of the radius extends 1 cm distal to the styloid process of the ulna.

> In the common fracture of the lower end of the radius (Colles' fracture) the two styloid processes come to lie at the same level because the lower broken end is forced upwards/posteriorly.

Near the distal skin crease (anteriorly) at the wrist on the radial side is the tubercle of the scaphoid, and on the ulnar side is the pisiform bone with the tendon of flexor carpi ulnaris running into it. On the dorsum of the hand, all the metacarpals are palpable; in a clenched fist, the heads of the metacarpals form the knuckles. In the thumb and fingers, all the phalanges are easily felt.

The hand is mostly attached to the radius, which bears the brunt of upward pressure applied to the hand. When the hand is in the anatomical position with the palm facing forwards, the forearm is in the position of supination. When the forearm is pronated, the head of the ulna makes a prominent bulge; note that this bulge is the anterior surface of the head of the ulna (confirm this on an articulated skeleton). Muscles named with the word 'carpi' (meaning 'of the carpus' or wrist), such as flexor carpi radialis and extensor carpi radialis, are usually attached to the bases of metacarpals and are designed to move the wrist, while those with the word 'digitorum' (of the digits) have longer tendons that run beyond the wrist to phalanges of the fingers and so can move the fingers as well as the wrist. The thumb (pollex) has its own muscles, indicated by 'pollicis.'

Cubital fossa – a descriptive triangular region anterior to the elbow, bounded by pronator teres medially, brachioradialis laterally and above by a line that joins the humeral epicondyles (**Fig. 4.7**). Brachialis and supinator form the floor. It contains, from lateral to medial, the tendon of biceps, the brachial artery and the median nerve. The radial nerve is deep to brachioradialis on the lateral side and so is not visible unless the muscle is displaced laterally, where the nerve can be seen dividing into its superficial (cutaneous) and deep (posterior interosseous) branches.

Pronator teres – arising proximally from the common flexor origin, the muscle crosses the forearm obliquely to be attached distally halfway down the lateral side of the radius. It has a small deep head from the coronoid process of ulna, and the median nerve, by which it is innervated, passes distally between the two heads.

Brachioradialis – from the lateral side of the humerus proximal to the lateral epicondyle, the muscle runs distally to the lower end of the radius just proximal to the styloid process. In the commonly used mid-prone position of the forearm, it helps to maintain the required angle of elbow flexion. It is the only flexor innervated by the radial nerve.

Supinator – a deep muscle that arises partly from the supinator crest on the posterior of the ulna, it passes laterally to wrap around the posterior of the proximal end of the radius, thus helping to 'unwind' the pronated radius. It is innervated by the deep radial nerve, which runs through the muscle to become the posterior interosseous nerve.

Brachial artery – in the cubital fossa, the artery is located with the elbow extended by palpating on the medial side of the biceps tendon (the median nerve lies medial to the artery); the artery is not quite in the centre of the fossa, but a little towards the medial side deep to the bicipital aponeurosis.

It is commonly noted that the brachial artery can divide proximal to the cubital fossa into the radial and ulnar arteries, and occasionally the ulnar branch may lie superficial to the bicipital aponeurosis.

Superficial veins – commonly make an H or M pattern anterior to the cubital fossa (**Fig. 4.8**). The cephalic vein on the lateral side and the basilic vein on the medial side both begin from the dorsal venous network on the dorsum of the hand.

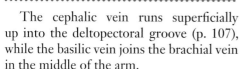

Any of these veins is frequently used for intravenous injections and to collect blood for tests.

The cephalic vein runs superficially up into the deltopectoral groove (p. 107), while the basilic vein joins the brachial vein in the middle of the arm.

Elbow joint – between the trochlea and capitulum of the distal humerus, the trochlear notch of the ulna and the head of the radius (**Figs. 4.9, 4.10**). The capsule is reinforced by medial and lateral ligaments, with the annular ligament holding the head of the radius in contact with the ulna (see proximal radioulnar joint, below).

The principal muscles that produce flexion and extension movements at the hinge-like elbow joint are:

- **Flexion** – brachialis, biceps and brachioradialis.
- **Extension** – triceps.

Pronation and supination are not movements of the elbow joint but occur at the radioulnar joints (see p. 119).

Radial artery – runs deep to brachioradialis and, distally, lies subcutaneously at the wrist, where it is the common site for feeling the pulse (**Fig. 4.11**).

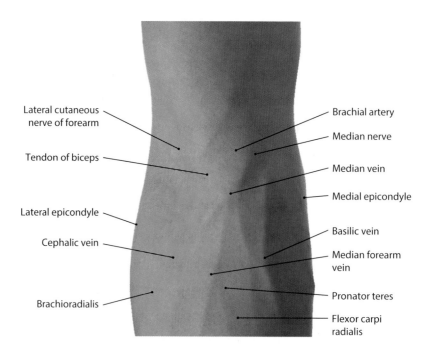

Fig. 4.8 Surface features of the right elbow region (cubital fossa), from the front.

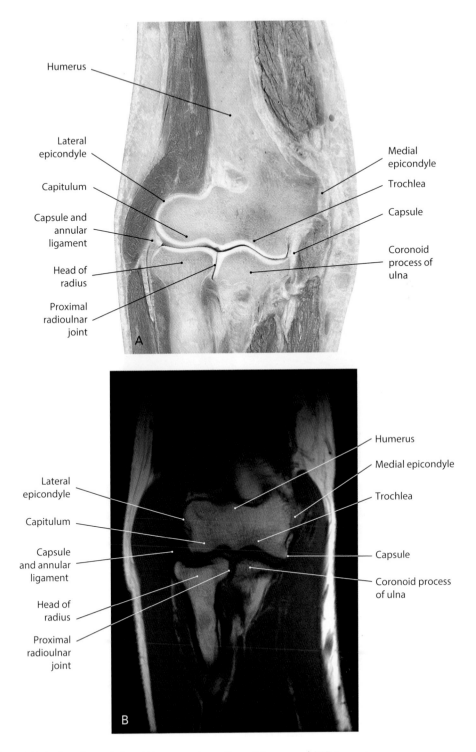

Fig. 4.9 Right elbow joint: (A) coronal section, (B) coronal MR image.

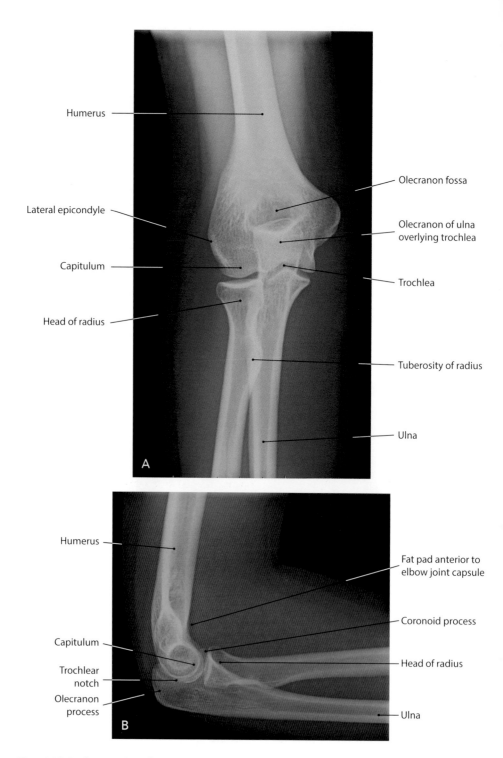

Fig. 4.10 Radiographs of the right elbow joint: (A) posteroanterior view, (B) lateral view.

The radial pulse is felt by pressing the artery against the distal end of the radius, on the radial (lateral) side of the tendon of flexor carpi radialis.

It then passes dorsally through the anatomical snuffbox (p. 119) and into the deep palm between the two heads of the first dorsal interosseous muscle, to become the deep palmar arch, usually uniting with the deep branch of the ulnar artery. This arch lies at a level 1 cm proximal to the superficial arch (see below) and is deep to the long flexor tendons.

Ulnar artery – usually smaller than the radial artery, it enters the hand lateral to the pisiform and superficial to the flexor retinaculum.

The ulnar pulse can usually be felt (though less easily than the radial pulse) on the radial side of the tendon of flexor carpi ulnaris, just before it becomes attached to the pisiform bone.

The artery continues into the palm as the superficial palmar arch (**Fig. 4.11**); it extends no farther into the hand than the level of the web of the outstretched thumb. It is usually J-shaped; only in one-third of hands is the arch completed by union with the superficial palmar branch of the radial artery. The arch lies deep to the palmar aponeurosis, superficial to the long flexor tendons, and its digital branches run up the sides of the fingers, joining with corresponding vessels from the deep arch.

Median nerve – runs deep to flexor digitorum superficialis and innervates most of the long flexor muscles of the wrist and fingers. At the wrist it lies on the *ulnar* side of the flexor carpi radialis tendon and superficial to the long flexor tendons, partly overlapped by the palmaris longus tendon (if present) (**Figs. 4.11, 4.13B**).

This subcutaneous position is the most common site for median nerve injury (e.g. cuts of the wrist by broken glass).

The median nerve may be injured in the carpal tunnel as a result of trauma or because of compression secondary to medical conditions such as rheumatoid arthritis. Such injury interferes with gripping and causes loss of sensation at the tips of the thumb and adjacent fingers.

The nerve enters the hand by running *deep* to the flexor retinaculum (carpal tunnel) of the wrist and then gives off the highly important muscular (recurrent) branch, which supplies the three small muscles of the base of the thumb (p. 121). It also innervates the lumbricals of the index and middle fingers. Other cutaneous branches supply palm and finger skin, including that of the pulps of the thumb, index and middle fingers – among the most important sensory areas in the body (**Fig. 4.12**).

Ulnar nerve – after passing posterior to the medial epicondyle of the humerus it runs distally between the long flexor muscles on the medial side of the forearm to enter the hand *superficial* to the flexor retinaculum (**Fig. 4.11**). It innervates flexor carpi ulnaris and the ulnar half of flexor digitorum profundus, and all the small muscles of the hand (except for the three at the base of the thumb and the first two lumbricals [innervated by the median nerve]), which are so important for intricate movements of the fingers (p. 121–124).

Injury to the ulnar nerve at the elbow gives rise to 'claw hand', due to the inability to extend the fingers, and interferes with sensation on the ulnar side of the hand.

Cutaneous branches supply skin of the ulnar side of the palm and dorsum of the little and ring fingers.

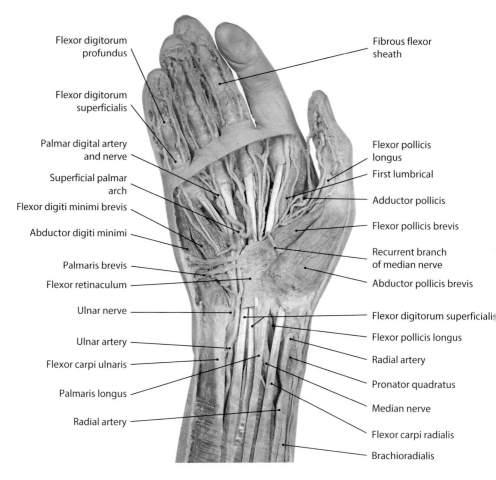

Fig. 4.11 Superficial dissection of the right lower forearm and palm of the hand.

Flexor tendons – the prominent superficial tendons anterior to the wrist are those of the flexor carpi radialis (reaching the bases of metacarpals 2 and 3) towards the radial side, palmaris longus (attaching to the palmar aponeurosis) almost in the midline (although this muscle is missing in about 13% of limbs), with those of flexor digitorum superficialis deep to it, and that of the flexor carpi ulnaris running to the pisiform bone on the ulnar side (**Figs. 4.11, 4.13**). At a deeper level (not palpable) are flexor pollicis longus and flexor digitorum profundus, whose lower ends pass anterior to the quadrangular-shaped pronator quadratus, which

occupies the lower quarter of the anterior o[f] the ulna and runs straight across to the dis[-] tal quarter of the radius. The pollicis longu[s] and profundus tendons are attached to the *base* of the *distal* phalanx of the respectiv[e] digits; the superficialis tendons split int[o] two to attach to the *sides* of the *middle* pha[-] lanx of each finger, thus allowing the pro[-] fundus tendons to pass through to the dista[l] phalanx (**Fig. 4.13A**).

Flexor retinaculum – tough fibrous tis[-] sue (**Figs. 4.11, 4.13**) (the size of a smal[l] postage stamp) passing from the pisifor[m] and hamate medially to the scaphoid an[d]

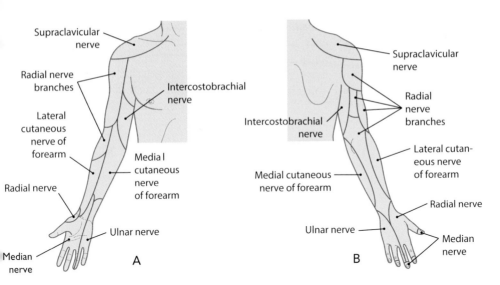

Fig. 4.12 Cutaneous nerves of the right upper limb: (A) front, (B) back.

trapezium laterally to form with them and other carpal bones the carpal tunnel (**Fig. 4.13B**), through which run the tendons to the thumb and fingers (along with their synovial sheaths) *and the median nerve.* The ulnar nerve and artery lie medial and superficial to the retinaculum.

Fibrous flexor sheaths – form on the palmar side of the phalanges of each digit. They prevent the flexor tendons from bowing anteriorly when the digits are flexed (**Fig. 4.11**).

Synovial sheaths – surround the tendons in the carpal tunnel and are situated within the fibrous sheaths of the fingers, to allow tendon movement with minimal friction.

Anatomical snuffbox – the hollow seen distal to the styloid process of the radius on the lateral side of the base of the thumb. Its lateral boundary is formed by abductor pollicis longus and extensor pollicis brevis, whereas the medial boundary is the tendon of extensor pollicis longus. The scaphoid bone and trapezium lie in its floor and the radial artery crosses it to pass to the dorsal aspect of the first web space.

> Following a fall on the outstretched wrist with no obvious fracture of the radius, pain on palpation of this fossa is indicative of a possible fracture of the scaphoid.

Extensor muscles and extensor retinaculum – occupy the posterior of the forearm and hand (**Fig. 4.14**). The tendons with synovial sheaths are kept in place on the dorsum of the wrist by the extensor retinaculum. At the level of the metacarpophalangeal joints the extensor digitorum tendons form triangular-shaped dorsal digital expansions, which wrap around the sides of the joints and receive the attachments of the interosseous and lumbrical muscles. The central parts of the tendons continue on to the bases of the middle and distal phalanges.

Proximal radioulnar joint – between the head of the radius and the radial notch of the ulna (**Figs. 4.9, 4.10**), held together by the annular ligament wrapping around the radial neck to allow the head of the radius to rotate, and shares the same capsule and joint cavity as the elbow joint.

Distal radioulnar joint – between the head of the ulna and the ulnar notch of the radius (**Fig. 4.15**), the bones are held together by the triangular fibrocartilaginous disc, which normally separates this joint from the wrist joint.

The principal muscles that produce movements at the proximal and distal radioulnar joints are:

- **Pronation** – pronator quadratus, pronator teres (and flexor carpi radialis).
- **Supination** – supinator, biceps (and extensor pollicis longus).

Wrist joint – between (proximally) the lower end of the radius and the disc of the distal radioulnar joint and (distally) three carpal bones – the scaphoid, lunate and triquetral (**Figs. 2.6, 4.15**). The capsule is reinforced by radial and ulnar ligaments.

The principal muscles that produce movements at the wrist joint are:

- **Flexion** – flexor carpi radialis, flexor carpi ulnaris, Palmaris longus (when present) and flexor digitorum superficialis and profundus.

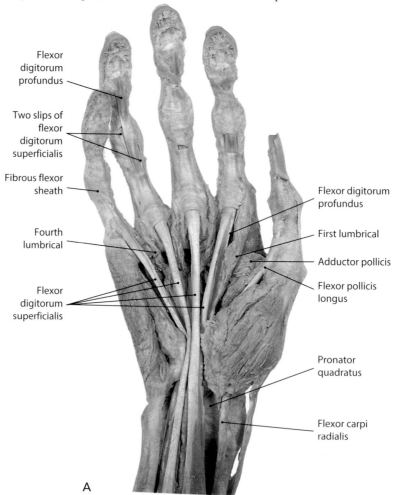

Flexor digitorum profundus

Two slips of flexor digitorum superficialis

Fibrous flexor sheath

Fourth lumbrical

Flexor digitorum superficialis

Flexor digitorum profundus

First lumbrical

Adductor pollicis

Flexor pollicis longus

Pronator quadratus

Flexor carpi radialis

A

Fig. 4.13 Flexor tendons of the right wrist and hand in the carpal tunnel visualised: (A) after removal of the flexor retinaculum and all vessels and nerves. *(Continued)*

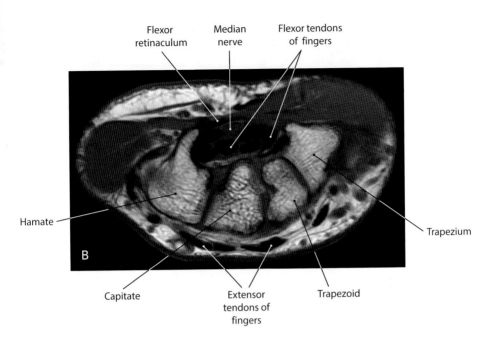

Fig. 4.13 *(Continued)* Flexor tendons of the right wrist and hand in the carpal tunnel visualised: (B) axial MR image.

- **Extension** – extensor carpi radialis longus and brevis, extensor carpi ulnaris and extensor digitorum.
- **Abduction** – flexor carpi radialis and extensor carpi radialis longus and brevis.
- **Adduction** – flexor carpi ulnaris and extensor carpi ulnaris.

The main movements are flexion and extension (which are accompanied by some movement between the two rows of carpal bones – the mid-carpal joint), with some degree of adduction and a lesser degree of abduction (because the styloid process of the radius extends lower than the styloid process of the ulna). Adduction allows the axis of a tool held in the hand to be lined up with the long axis of the forearm (as in using a screwdriver).

Small muscles of the hand – muscles of the thumb and fingers. The bulge on the palmar surface of the base of the thumb,

the thenar eminence, is due to flexor pollicis brevis (medially) and abductor pollicis brevis (laterally) superficial to opponens pollicis (**Fig. 4.11**). Arising mainly from the flexor retinaculum and trapezium, flexor and abductor pollicis brevis are inserted into the base of the proximal phalanx of the thumb, and are of great importance for opposition of the thumb (see below). They are normally innervated by the median nerve (see above), but flexor pollicis brevis is unique in being the muscle that has the most variable nerve supply of any in the body – median nerve or ulnar nerve, or both. Opponens pollicis inserts along the shaft of the first metacarpal bone and is important in rotating the thumb at the first carpometacarpal joint, so that it can oppose the pads of the other digits (opposition).

On the ulnar side of the hand, over the fifth metacarpal, is the hypothenar eminence, with similar muscles for the little finger (all supplied by the ulnar nerve).

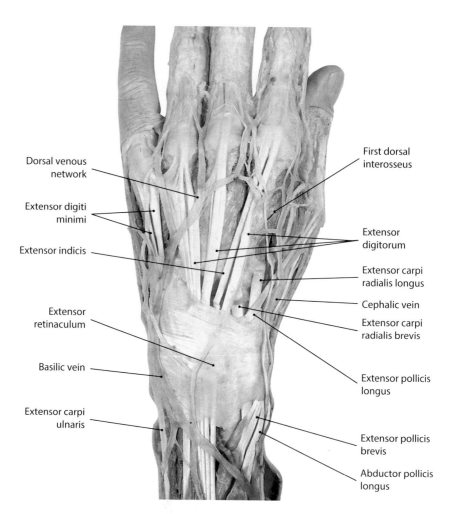

Dorsal venous network

Extensor digiti minimi

Extensor indicis

Extensor retinaculum

Basilic vein

Extensor carpi ulnaris

First dorsal interosseus

Extensor digitorum

Extensor carpi radialis longus

Cephalic vein

Extensor carpi radialis brevis

Extensor pollicis longus

Extensor pollicis brevis

Abductor pollicis longus

Fig. 4.14 Extensor (dorsal) surface of the left wrist and hand.

There are also interosseous muscles (four dorsal and three palmar) that arise from adjacent metacarpals and four lumbrical muscles that arise from the lateral side of the tendons of flexor digitorum profundus. All are attached to the dorsal digital expansions (see above), with the interosseous muscles also having attachments to the proximal phalanges; all are innervated by the ulnar nerve, except for the two lateral lumbrical muscles (innervated by the median nerve, as are the two tendons they attach to). For their actions, see below.

First carpometacarpal joint – between the trapezium and the base of the first metacarpal (**Fig. 4.15B**), it is of great importance. The *saddle-shaped* bone surfaces allow the movement of *opposition* of the thumb carrying the thumb across the palm towards the pads of the fingers. This is essential for a firm thumb grip (pulp to pulp opposition) and also allows for more delicate movements, like bringing together the tip of the flexed thumb with the tips of the flexed fingers. Since the first metacarpal lies at right angles to

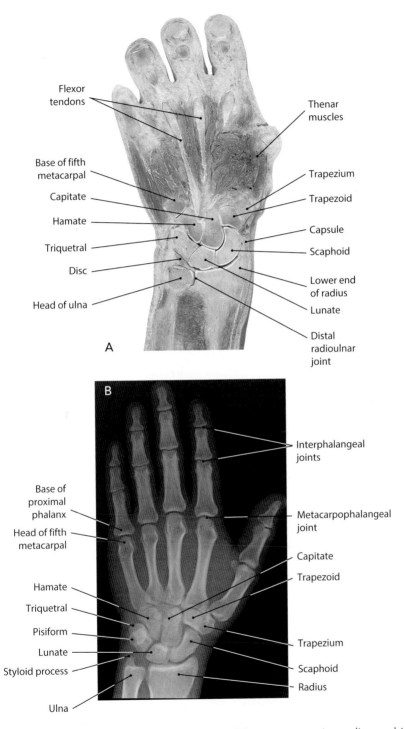

Flexor tendons

Thenar muscles

Base of fifth metacarpal

Capitate

Hamate

Triquetral

Disc

Head of ulna

Trapezium

Trapezoid

Capsule

Scaphoid

Lower end of radius

Lunate

Distal radioulnar joint

A

B

Interphalangeal joints

Base of proximal phalanx

Head of fifth metacarpal

Metacarpophalangeal joint

Capitate

Trapezoid

Hamate

Triquetral

Pisiform

Lunate

Styloid process

Trapezium

Scaphoid

Radius

Ulna

Fig. 4.15 Right wrist and hand: (A) coronal section, (B) anteroposterior radiographic view.

the others, flexion of the thumb means bending it parallel to the plane of the palm and extension implies stretching the 'web' of the thumb, but still in the plane of the palm. Abduction lifts the thumb away from the palm at right angles and adduction restores the normal anatomical position. Opposition involves a mixture of abduction, flexion and rotation.

Metacarpophalangeal and interphalangeal joints – all have a similar structure, with a small capsule reinforced on each side by a collateral ligament (**Fig. 4.15B**).

It is reasonable to assume that the flexor muscles on the anterior of the forearm and hand will produce flexion of the wrist and/or fingers, and that the extensor muscles on the posterior aspect will extend them. However, it is unexpected that (as far as finger movements are concerned) extensor digitorum can only produce extension of the metacarpophalangeal joints; it cannot by itself extend the interphalangeal joints. To extend these joints the assistance of the interosseous and lumbrical muscles is required; by pulling on the extensor expansions (although the exact mechanism by which they act is not clear) at the same time, these muscles help to flex the metacarpophalangeal joints. A less important action of the dorsal interosseous muscles is to fan the fingers out from one another (abduction, with the middle finger as the axis), and of the palmar interosseous muscles is to bring them together (adduction). These actions are usually remembered by the mnemonics DAB and PAD – **D**orsal **AB**duct and **P**almar **AD**duct. Since all these small muscles are innervated by the ulnar nerve (except for the two lateral lumbrical muscles – median nerve), the ulnar is the all-important nerve for intricate movements of the fingers, such as the upstroke in writing, playing the violin, etc. Contrast this with the median nerve, which supplies the small muscles of the thumb but also most of the long forearm flexors used for grosser digital movements, such as gripping a hammer. The lumbrical muscles are essential to ensure the normal digital sweep seen in action of the long digital flexors, ensuring flexion of the metacarpophalangeal joint first followed by that of the interphalangeal joints. Lack of lumbrical function results in clawing of the digit, with flexion of the interphalangeal joints first.

Summary

- The *shoulder joint* is the most mobile in the body and the one most frequently dislocated. Abduction (by supraspinatus and deltoid – suprascapular and axillary nerves, respectively) depends not only on movement at the joint itself, but is accompanied by rotation of the scapula on the chest wall, tilting the glenoid cavity upwards (by the action of trapezius and serratus anterior).
- At the *elbow joint* only flexion and extension can occur; the forearm movements of pronation (mainly by pronator teres and pronator quadratus – median nerve) and supination (mainly by biceps – musculocutaneous nerve – when the elbow is flexed) take place at the two radioulnar joints.
- Fine *finger* movements depend on the interossei and lumbricals, mainly supplied by the ulnar nerve. The small muscles of the thumb, essential for gripping, are supplied by the median nerve.

- The skin of the pulp of the thumb, index and middle fingers, so necessary for the appreciation of touch, is supplied by the *median nerve*. The skin of the ulnar edge of the hand and the little finger is supplied by the *ulnar nerve*.
- The *radial nerve*, from the posterior cord of the brachial plexus, supplies muscles on the posterior surface of the arm and forearm; its skin supply on the hand is negligible.
- *Blood pressure* is taken by occluding the brachial artery with an inflatable cuff placed round the arm above the elbow. The cuff is slowly released and blood pressure is measured in millimetres of mercury (mmHg). Systolic pressure is measured when blood audibly begins to pass through the artery and diastolic pressure is measured when it is no longer audible.
- The brachial artery is palpated on the anterior of the elbow (in the cubital fossa) medial to the tendon of biceps.
- The *radial pulse* is felt by pressing the radial artery against the distal end of the radius, lateral to the tendon of flexor carpi radialis.
- Injury to the *radial nerve* is commonest in the upper arm (from fracture of the mid shaft of humerus) and causes 'wrist drop' due to paralysis of the extensors of the wrist and fingers.
- Injury to the *ulnar nerve* is commonest at the elbow (where it is subcutaneous posterior to the medial epicondyle of the humerus) and causes 'claw hand' due to inability to extend the fingers, with anaesthesia (lack of sensation) on the ulnar side of the hand.
- Injury to the *median nerve* is commonest at the wrist, due to lacerations or raised pressure in the carpal tunnel (carpal tunnel syndrome), and interferes with opposition of the thumb, with anaesthesia (lack of sensation) over the pulps of the thumb and adjacent fingers.
- The segments of the spinal cord mainly concerned in supplying major limb muscles are: C5 – deltoid; C6 – biceps; C7 – triceps; C8 – wrist and finger flexors and extensors; T1 – small muscles of the hand.

Questions

Answers can be found in Appendix A, p. 245.

Question 1

The spinal nerve roots C5, C6, C7, C8 and T1 come together, dividing and joining to form a plexus connecting the lower neck to the nerves of the upper limb. Which of the statements below accurately describes the normal path taken by nerve fibres in the stated nerve to reach the destination nerve given?

(a) The anterior division of the C7 root joins the anterior division of the C8 and T1 roots to lie lateral to the subclavian artery before passing into the musculocutaneous nerve.

(b) The anterior division of the C8 root joins the posterior root of the C6 root to form the musculocutaneous nerve posterior to the subclavian artery.

(c) The anterior division of the C5 root joins the anterior division of the C8 root to lie medial to the subclavian artery in the ulnar nerve.

(d) The anterior division of the C8 root joins the anterior division of the T1 root to lie medial to the subclavian artery before passing anterior to this artery to form the median nerve.

(e) The anterior division of the C8 root joins the anterior division of the T1 root to lie lateral to the subclavian artery before passing anterior to this artery to form the musculocutaneous nerve.

Question 2

The glenohumeral (shoulder) joint appears to be capable of a great range of movement. Which of the statements below most accurately describes muscles involved with movements of this joint?

(a) In abduction, supraspinatus initiates the movement followed by deltoid.

(b) In abduction, deltoid is involved throughout aided by trapezius and the lower fibres of serratus anterior.

(c) In lateral rotation the movement is initiated by infraspinatus working with supraspinatus and deltoid.

(d) In adduction the movement is initiated by subscapularis aided by deltoid.

(e) In medial rotation the movement is initiated by subscapularis working with only the other muscles of the rotator cuff.

Question 3

The elbow joint is a hinge joint with muscles arranged appropriately to allow its movement. Which statement below most accurately describes muscle location and action at this important joint?

(a) Attaching to the medial epicondyle, this muscle attaches to the distal radius and is involved in flexion.

(b) Attaching to the supercondylar ridge laterally, this muscle attaches to the distal radius and is involved in flexion.

(c) Attaching to the distal humerus posteriorly, this muscle attaches to the coronoid process of the ulna and is involved in flexion.

(d) Attaching to the mid shaft of the humerus, this muscle with two heads passes distally to attach to the radial tuberosity and is involved in flexion.

(e) Attaching to the lateral epicondyle and the supinator crest of the ulna and passing distally to the posterior aspect of the mid-shaft to the ulna, this muscle is involved in supination.

Question 4

At the level of the wrist many structures are related to the flexor retinaculum, forming the carpal tunnel. Which statement most accurately describes the relationship?

(a) The ulnar artery passes medial to the long flexor tendons before passing through the tunnel medial to the median nerve.

(b) The radial artery passes lateral to the long flexor tendons across the scaphoid bone before passing through the tunnel lateral to the median nerve.

(c) The median nerve passes through the tunnel deep to the tendons of flexor digitorum superficialis but superficial to the tendons of flexor digitorum profundus.

(d) The median nerve passes just deep to palmaris longus superficial to the flexor retinaculum and to the ulnar artery, which passes through the tunnel.

(e) The median nerve passes into the carpal tunnel deep to the tendon of palmaris longus yet superficial to the long digital flexors while the radial artery passes superficial to the scaphoid bone posteriorly around the wrist and is not related to the tunnel.

(c) Median nerve.

(d) Radial nerve.

(e) Axillary nerve.

Question 5

Concerning movement of the thumb, which combination of muscles and nerves would be involved with the movement being described?

(a) All three thenar muscles innervated only by the ulnar nerve are involved in opposition of the thumb.

(b) To facilitate opposition of the thumb all of the thenar muscles innervated normally by the median nerve are involved along with the posteriorly located radial innervated forearm abductor.

(c) The median innervated first lumbrical is involved with flexor pollicis longus and brevis in the normal digital sweep of the thumb.

(d) The ulnar innervated first dorsal interosseous muscle is involved with abductor pollicis brevis in abduction of the thumb.

(e) The radial innervated abductor pollicis longus is the only muscle capable of abducting the thumb.

Question 6

A 20-year-old woman suffers severe trauma in a fall. Medical examination reveals that the deltoid muscle is flaccid and a small patch of skin inferior to the acromion is insensate (numb). A plain radiograph reveals a fracture of the surgical neck of the humerus. Which of the following has most likely been injured in this patient?

(a) Upper trunk of the brachial plexus.

(b) Middle trunk of the brachial plexus.

Question 7

A 25-year-old man suffers from frequent shoulder dislocations. His orthopaedic surgeon recommends surgery to stabilise the shoulder. Which of the following structure(s) is most likely to be shortened during this surgery?

(a) Coracoclavicular ligament.

(b) Capsule of the acromioclavicular joint.

(c) Acromioclavicular ligament.

(d) Glenohumeral ligaments.

(e) Serratus anterior muscle.

Question 8

A 20-year-old man is injured in a motorcycle crash. Physical examination reveals that he cannot extend his wrist or fingers. Radiographs reveal a fracture of the mid-shaft of his humerus. Which of the following injuries is most likely to account for his symptoms?

(a) Tear of the triceps brachii.

(b) Lesion of the median nerve.

(c) Laceration of the brachial artery.

(d) Lesion of the radial nerve.

(e) Avulsion of the long head of the biceps brachii tendon.

Question 9

A 23-year-old male medical student is bitten at the base of his thumb by a dog. Infection set in and spread into the radial bursa.

The tendon(s) of which of the following muscles is most likely affected?

(a) Flexor carpi radialis.

(b) Flexor pollicis longus.

(c) Flexor pollicis brevis.

(d) Flexor digitorum superficialis.

(e) Flexor digitorum profundus.

Question 10

A 20-year-old woman fell on her outstretched hand and immediately experienced severe wrist pain. Palpation of the anatomical snuffbox exacerbated the pain. A radiograph is most likely to reveal a fracture of which of the following?

(a) Styloid process of the ulna.

(b) Scaphoid bone.

(c) Distal radius (Colles' fracture).

(d) Capitate bone.

(e) First metacarpal bone.

Question 11

A 22-year-old man suffered a laceration of his hand while handling a knife. Physical examination reveals that he is able to extend the metacarpophalangeal joints of all his fingers of the injured hand. He cannot extend the interphalangeal (IP) joints of the fourth and fifth digits, and extension of the IP joints of the second and third digits is very weak. Which of the following nerves has most likely been injured?

(a) Deep branch of the ulnar nerve.

(b) Recurrent branch of the median nerve.

(c) Deep branch of the radial nerve.

(d) Superficial branch of the radial nerve.

(e) Median nerve in the carpal tunnel.

Question 12

A 57-year-old female typist presents with bilateral wrist pain that is exacerbated when she goes to extremes of flexion and extension at the wrist. She is diagnosed with carpal tunnel syndrome. Which of the following muscles are most likely to be weak in this patient?

(a) Thenar.

(b) Hypothenar.

(c) Palmar interossei.

(d) Dorsal interossei

(e) Third and fourth lumbricals.

Question 13

A 24-year-old man falls while rock climbing and reports pain in his left elbow. Physical examination and radiographs reveal a fracture of medical epicondyle of the humerus. The patient is not able to abduct or adduct the fingers of his left hand. Which of the following nerves is most likely injured?

(a) Musculocutaneous.

(b) Radial.

(c) Axillary.

(d) Median.

(e) Ulnar.

Question 14

A 62-year-old woman is diagnosed with arthritis in her right wrist. This painful condition is limiting her activities of daily living. Which of the following peripheral nerves is most likely conducting pain sensation from her wrist?

(a) Musculocutaneous.

(b) Axillary.

(c) Long thoracic.

(d) Median.

(e) Suprascapular.

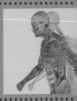
Introduction

The bony thoracic cage and its associated muscles form an airtight container that protects the heart and lungs, although the main purpose of the ribs is to assist with respiration. In normal quiet respiration, the principal muscle involved is the diaphragm, the muscular and tendinous partition separating the thorax and abdomen. Perhaps the most unexpected feature of the thorax is the height to which the right and left domes of the diaphragm rise; the capacity of the thorax is much smaller than would be imagined from looking at the outside and the width of the shoulders obscures the small size of the uppermost part.

The skeleton of the thorax (**Fig. 2.3**) is covered superficially by the muscles joining the upper limb to the chest wall (**Figs. 4.2, 4.3**), with the overlying breasts on the anterior chest wall. The intercostal spaces (between adjacent ribs and costal cartilages (p. 21) are numbered from the rib lying superior (cranial) to the space and filled in by three layers of thin intercostal muscles, with the main intercostal vessels and nerves running between the middle and inner layers along the *lower (caudal) border* of each rib (**Figs. 5.1, 5.2**).

> Needles or drainage tubes are inserted through the chest wall immediately above a rib, to keep away from the main intercostal vessels and nerves.

The diaphragm (**Fig. 5.2**), with the liver immediately inferior (caudal) to it, bulges upwards from the abdomen to a level (viewed from the front) as high as the fifth rib and costal cartilage on the right and the fifth intercostal space on the left (**Fig. 5.2**). The gap between the upper border of T1 vertebra, the two first ribs and costal cartilages, and the upper border of the manubrium of the sternum is known as the thoracic inlet (although sometimes also known as the thoracic outlet) (p. 94; **Fig. 3.44**).

The chest wall receives its blood supply via the pairs of intercostal vessels arising on the posterior thoracic wall, which anastomose anteriorly with the internal thoracic vessels on each side of midline. These descend just deep to the medial edge of the upper six costal cartilages before supplying

> Clinically the left internal thoracic artery in particular can be used as an arterial source for performing a coronary artery bypass.

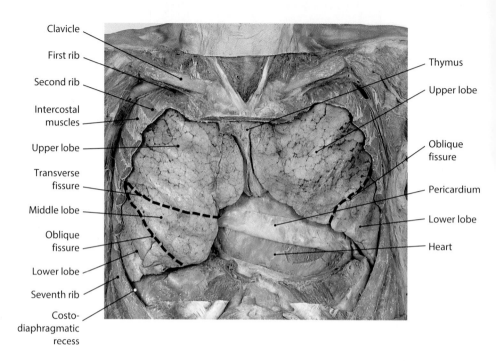

Clavicle
First rib
Second rib
Intercostal muscles
Upper lobe
Transverse fissure
Middle lobe
Oblique fissure
Lower lobe
Seventh rib
Costo-diaphragmatic recess

Thymus
Upper lobe
Oblique fissure
Pericardium
Lower lobe
Heart

Fig. 5.1 Thoracic contents, from the front, after removal of most of the sternum and ribs. The pericardium has been incised and turned upwards.

the anterior abdominal wall. The central region of the thoracic cavity is the mediastinum, which contains principally the heart and great vessels, while at each side is a lung (**Figs. 5.1, 5.2**) lying within the pleural membranes.

The pleura is a smooth mesothelial (simple squamous epithelium) membrane that adheres to the surface of the lung as the visceral pleura; it is continuous at the root of the lung with the parietal pleura, that part that lines the inside of the thoracic wall (costal pleura), continuous with pleura on the upper surface of the diaphragm (diaphragmatic pleura) and the surface of the mediastinum (mediastinal pleura). The pleural membrane as a whole thus forms a closed sac, the pleural cavity. However, over most of their surfaces the visceral and parietal layers are in contact with one another by the surface tension of

a thin layer of pleural fluid; the slight negative pressure within the pleural sac keeps the lung expanded.

> If the negative pressure in the pleural cavity is destroyed (e.g. by a penetrating wound of the chest wall), the lung collapses (pneumothorax). If breathing is compromised, a tube may need to be inserted.

> Pleurisy (inflammation of the pleura) may be intensely painful because the normally smooth adjacent surfaces become roughened and rub against one another, irritating the parietal pleura supplied by spinal nerves.

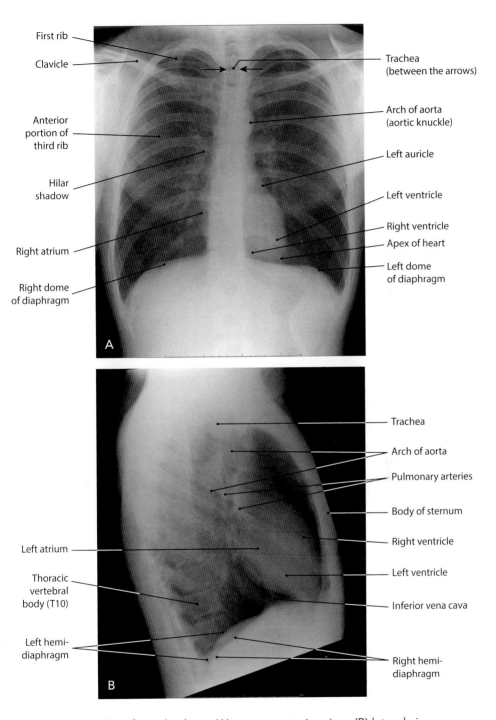

First rib

Clavicle

Anterior portion of third rib

Hilar shadow

Right atrium

Right dome of diaphragm

Trachea (between the arrows)

Arch of aorta (aortic knuckle)

Left auricle

Left ventricle

Right ventricle

Apex of heart

Left dome of diaphragm

A

Trachea

Arch of aorta

Pulmonary arteries

Body of sternum

Right ventricle

Left ventricle

Inferior vena cava

Left atrium

Thoracic vertebral body (T10)

Left hemi-diaphragm

Right hemi-diaphragm

B

Fig. 5.2 Radiographs of a male chest: (A) posteroanterior view, (B) lateral view.

Inflammation or cancer may cause fluid to collect in the pleural space (pleural effusion), compressing the lung and causing difficulty in breathing. It may be necessary to drain such fluid through a needle or drainage tube.

Manubriosternal joint (sternal angle of Louis) – a most important landmark anteriorly on the thorax (**Figs. 4.1, 5.3**). It lies about 5 cm caudal to the jugular notch and is almost always palpable, if not always visible. It indicates the level of the second costal cartilages and ribs on each side. The body of the sternum is opposite the middle four thoracic vertebrae (T5–T8).

The second costal cartilage is palpable at the sternal angle, allowing the second rib to be identified. The first rib is too high under the clavicle to be felt. The others can be identified anteriorly by counting downwards from the second. On a traditional chest radiograph the anterior aspect of the second rib lies superimposed on the posterior aspect of the 4th/5th ribs (**Figs. 5.2A, 5.15**).

Breasts

Each breast (mammary gland) lies on the anterior chest wall, largely anterior to (in front of) the muscle pectoralis major (**Figs. 4.2, 5.3**). Despite the variations in size of the non-lactating female breast (due to its fat content, not the amount of glandular tissue), the extent of the *base* of the breast is very constant: from near the midline to near the mid-axillary line, and from the second to the sixth rib. About 15 lactiferous ducts open on the nipple, which projects from the central pigmented area of skin, the areola.

The blood supply is from the internal thoracic and adjacent intercostal arteries. Since the breast is such a common site for cancer in the female, the lymph drainage is of *supreme clinical importance.*

Palpation of axillary lymph nodes is an important part of clinical examination. However, it is not reliable and ultrasound scanning of the axilla is now routine in cases of breast cancer. Enlargement of the axillary nodes occurs when there is infection or malignancy present in their drainage territory, for example in patients with breast cancer.

Most lymph drains to axillary nodes, especially to the pectoral group (p. 110) (which may become palpable and enlarged), but it may also pass through lymph channels that penetrate the chest wall to parasternal nodes within the thorax, beside the internal thoracic vessels (and therefore not palpable). The male breast normally remains very small and rudimentary but nevertheless can become cancerous.

Diaphragm

The diaphragm is the muscular and tendinous partition between the thorax and the abdomen (**Figs. 5.2, 5.15–5.17A**). Muscle fibres arise from the anterolateral aspect of the upper two lumbar vertebrae on the left (to form the left crus) and the upper three on the right (right crus, pleural crura; **Figs. 6.16A, 6.19**), from the tendinous bands passing laterally anterior to the upper attachments of psoas major and quadratus lumborum muscles (p. 162) and from the inner (deep) surfaces of the lower six ribs, with a few fibres from the xiphoid process of the sternum. All these fibres converge on the central tendon, which has the shape of a trefoil leaf, has no bony attachment and fuses

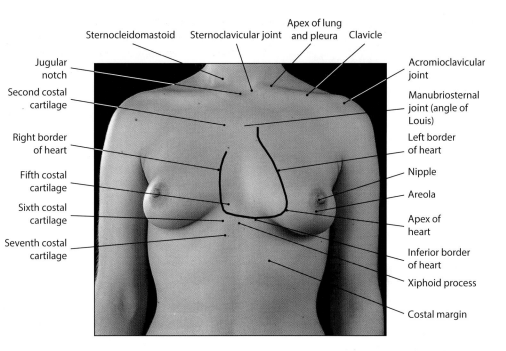

Fig. 5.3 Surface features of the front of the female thorax. The solid line indicates the borders of the heart.

above with the fibrous pericardium. Each half of the muscular part receives its motor nerve innervation from the phrenic nerve (passing caudally from the C3, C4 and C5 nerve roots). The diaphragm contains three main openings and several smaller ones for the passage of structures between the thorax and abdomen.

Aortic opening – not strictly *in* the diaphragm, but *behind* the union of the two crura, at the level of the T12 vertebra. Here the aorta, thoracic duct and perhaps the azygos vein (which may make its own hole in the right crus) all pass through.

> The main openings in the diaphragm are at vertebral levels T12 (aortic), T10 (oesophageal) and T8/9 (vena caval).

Oesophageal opening – lies in the *muscular* part, usually just to the *left* of the midline, but it is embraced by fibres of the *right* crus at the level of the T10 vertebra. Here the oesophagus, branches of the left gastric vessels and, importantly, the two vagal trunks pass into the abdomen.

Vena caval foramen – this lies in the *tendon*, at the level of the disc between T8 and T9 vertebrae, for the passage of the inferior vena cava with the right phrenic nerve to its right.

Smaller openings – in the crura, for the thoracic splanchnic (sympathetic) nerves. The sympathetic trunks pass posterior to the diaphragm, just anterior to psoas major, and the subcostal vessels and nerves also run in this location, but more laterally, anterior to quadratus lumborum.

Mediastinum

The mediastinum (**Figs. 5.2A, 5.4–5.6**) is the central region of the thoracic cavity (between the two pleural sacs). The superior mediastinum (**Fig. 5.5B**) is the part superior to the level of a line drawn from the manubriosternal joint anteriorly to the lower border of the body of the T4 vertebra posteriorly. The principal structures in it are: (1) the arch of the aorta with its branches (the brachiocephalic, left common carotid and left subclavian arteries); (2) the right and left brachiocephalic veins, lying anteriorly to the branches of the aorta and uniting to form the superior vena cava; (3) the phrenic and vagus nerves lying laterally; and (4) the trachea and oesophagus (and thoracic duct on the left) posterior to the aortic arch. Because of human variation and the state of respiration, the arch of the aorta might lie inferior to the manubrium.

The region lying posterior to the heart and inferior (caudal) to the level of the T4 vertebra is the posterior mediastinum (**Fig. 5.2B**), continuous with the superior mediastinum and containing principally the bifurcation of the trachea into the two main bronchi, the oesophagus with the plexus of vagus nerves around it, and the thoracic duct. The heart and its covering pericardium (see below) lie in the middle mediastinum, although this term is not often used. This leaves a narrow gap anterior to the heart and deep to the sternum, which is the anterior mediastinum. This may contain the lower part of the thymus and the internal thoracic vessels stuck just on the lateral edge of the sternum.

> Any infection of the mediastinum (mediastinitis) is highly dangerous because it is deeply seated and can spread widely in the connective tissue between the main structures

Trachea – begins in the neck as the continuation of the larynx at the level of the C6 vertebra. It is palpable superior to the jugular notch of the manubrium between the heads of sternocleidomastoid (**Figs. 3.37, 5.2A, 5.4A**), with the oesophagus behind it (but not palpable) (**Fig. 3.5**). The lumen is kept open as the airway by bands of cartilage in the front and side walls (but not the posterior wall, which contains the smooth muscle, where it is in contact with the oesophagus); although called tracheal rings, they are U-shaped and not completely circular. Overall the trachea is about 10 cm long and divides into the two main bronchi just inferior to the level of the manubriosternal joint (**Fig. 5.16**).

Oesophagus – begins in the neck as the continuation of the pharynx at the level of the C6 vertebra, then continues down anterior to the vertebral column through the superior and posterior mediastinum (**Figs. 5.5–5.7**), to pass through the oesophageal opening in the diaphragm, which is usually just to the left of the midline at the level of the T10 vertebra, giving it an overall length of about 25 cm.

Thoracic duct – begins as an upward continuation of the cisterna chyli, a sack-like dilatation under the *right* crus of the diaphragm at the level of the L1 vertebra in the abdomen, and ascends through the chest in the posterior mediastinum. Initially it passes superiorly through the diaphragm posterior to the right crus and anterior to the vertebral column to lie posterior to the oesophagus between the aorta and the azygos vein. Posterior to the trachea the duct turns as it ascends to the left of midline, passing through the thoracic inlet posterior to the left common carotid artery. In the root of the neck it starts to pass anteriorly to the confluence of the left internal jugular and subclavian veins (**Fig. 5.8**). It drains lymph from the whole body, except

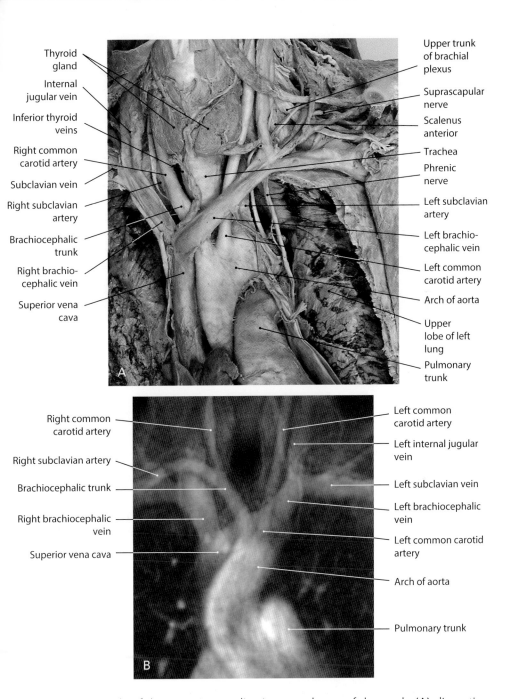

Thyroid gland

Internal jugular vein

Inferior thyroid veins

Right common carotid artery

Subclavian vein

Right subclavian artery

Brachiocephalic trunk

Right brachio-cephalic vein

Superior vena cava

Upper trunk of brachial plexus

Suprascapular nerve

Scalenus anterior

Trachea

Phrenic nerve

Left subclavian artery

Left brachio-cephalic vein

Left common carotid artery

Arch of aorta

Upper lobe of left lung

Pulmonary trunk

Right common carotid artery

Right subclavian artery

Brachiocephalic trunk

Right brachiocephalic vein

Superior vena cava

Left common carotid artery

Left internal jugular vein

Left subclavian vein

Left brachiocephalic vein

Left common carotid artery

Arch of aorta

Pulmonary trunk

Fig. 5.4 Great vessels of the superior mediastinum and root of the neck: (A) dissection from the front, (B) MR angiogram.

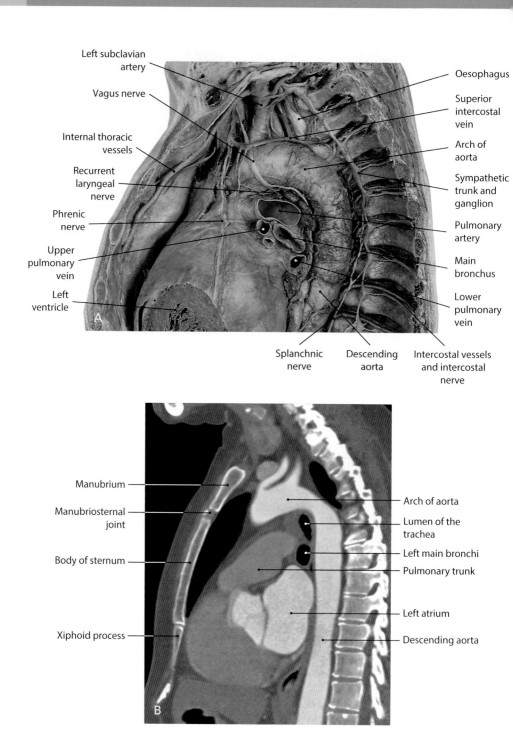

Left subclavian artery

Vagus nerve

Internal thoracic vessels

Recurrent laryngeal nerve

Phrenic nerve

Upper pulmonary vein

Left ventricle

Oesophagus

Superior intercostal vein

Arch of aorta

Sympathetic trunk and ganglion

Pulmonary artery

Main bronchus

Lower pulmonary vein

Splanchnic nerve

Descending aorta

Intercostal vessels and intercostal nerve

Manubrium

Manubriosternal joint

Body of sternum

Xiphoid process

Arch of aorta

Lumen of the trachea

Left main bronchi

Pulmonary trunk

Left atrium

Descending aorta

Fig. 5.5 Left side of the mediastinum: (A) dissection, (B) comparable sagittal CT section.

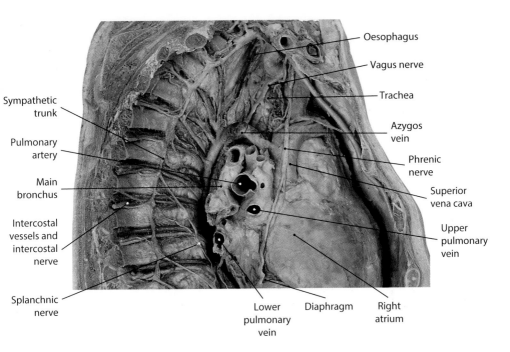

Fig. 5.6 Right side of the mediastinum.

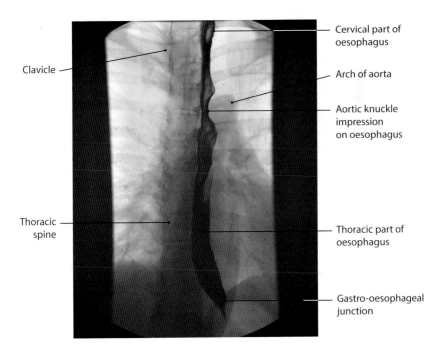

Fig. 5.7 Barium swallow demonstrating the course of the thoracic oesophagus. (Note: The patient is slightly rotated.)

for the three right-sided areas (head, neck and right upper limb) that drain to the right lymphatic duct (p. 88).

> Cancers of the GI tract may spread to a lymph node palpable between the heads of the left sternocleidomastoid muscle (Virchow's node).

Aorta – leaves the left ventricle of the heart, starting at the level of the aortic valve as the ascending aorta and giving off the left and right coronary arteries at this level. It ascends deep to the right side of the sternum before curving posteriorly (backwards) and to the left as the arch of the aorta (**Figs. 1.4, 5.4**). Superiorly it gives off its main branches: the brachiocephalic trunk (which divides into the right common carotid and right subclavian arteries), the left common carotid and finally the left subclavian arteries. The arch can pass cranially as

> The aortic arch gives the characteristic 'aortic knuckle' in posteroanterior radiographs of the chest (**Figs. 5.2A, 5.15**).

high as the midpoint of the manubrium; it then continues inferiorly (downwards) as the descending (thoracic) aorta (**Fig. 5.5**), which passes posterior to the diaphragm at the level of the T12 vertebra to become the abdominal aorta. Throughout its descent it gives pairs of intercostal arteries at each vertebral level as well as small branches to the bronchi and oesophagus.

Superior vena cava – lying on the right of the ascending aorta, it is formed superiorly by the union of the right and left brachiocephalic veins (**Figs. 5.4, 5.6, 5.8**) behind the lower border of the right first costal cartilage, and runs down to enter the right atrium of the heart at the level of the lower border of the right third costal cartilage.

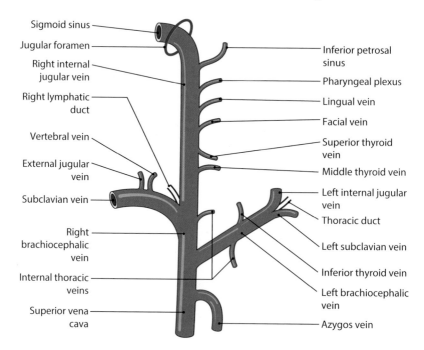

Fig. 5.8 The superior vena cava and tributaries.

Classically, at the level of the second costal cartilage (but can be below this), it receives the azygos vein that drains intercostal spaces and arches over the right lung root.

Brachiocephalic veins – each is formed by the union of the internal jugular and subclavian veins deep to the sternoclavicular joints. The left brachiocephalic vein thus runs from left to right deep to the upper half of the manubrium, crossing anterior to the three large branches from the aortic arch (**Fig. 5.4**).

Pulmonary trunk – starting as the outflow from the right ventricle of the heart and passing to lie to the left and slightly anterior to the ascending aorta, it runs superiorly and posteriorly to divide under the aortic arch (**Figs. 1.3, 1.4, 5.4, 5.17B**) into the right and left pulmonary arteries. The left pulmonary artery is joined to the arch by a fibrous cord, the ligamentum arteriosum, the remains of the embryonic ductus arteriosus that re-routed blood into the aorta because it could not easily pass through the then non-functioning lungs due to high vascular resistance. The ductus normally closes within hours after birth.

> A patent ductus arteriosus is the commonest congenital defect of the heart and great vessels. Normally it must be closed either surgically or using interventional radiological techniques.

Thymus – the source of production of T (for thymic) lymphocytes, it lies anterior to the great vessels and upper pericardium (**Fig. 5.1**) and usually extends into the root of the neck. It may appear to be a single structure, but in fact is two lobes closely applied to one another. It is maximal in size in childhood and thereafter regresses, but remains active throughout life. The function of thymic hormones is still being elucidated.

Sympathetic trunks – each enters the thorax by crossing the neck of the first rib and then runs vertically down through the thorax beside the vertebral column (**Figs. 5.5A, 5.6**), giving off from its ganglia various branches that join intercostal nerves or provide splanchnic nerves for thoracic and abdominal viscera and blood vessels. It is from all the thoracic and upper lumbar spinal nerves that the trunk receives its connections to the central nervous system. Two thoracic nerves (T1 and T2) pass cranially through the thoracic inlet to supply the head and neck; thoracic nerves 3 and 4 (T3 and T4) usually carry fibres destined for the upper limbs.

> Patients with excessive sweating in the upper limbs can have a sympathectomy. The T3 and T4 nerve connections are destroyed, but occasionally this can affect the T1 and T2 branches, resulting in a Horner's syndrome with anhydrosis (lack of sweating) of the face, a drooping eyelid and a small pupil on the affected side. Horner's syndrome can also arise as a result of cancers of the apex of the lung invading the sympathetic trunk or its branches.

Vagus nerves – descending from the neck (p. 89), the left vagus crosses to the left of the aortic arch (**Fig. 5.5A**) and the right vagus runs down the right side of the trachea (**Fig. 5.6**). Both give branches to the cardiac plexus (the left vagus also gives off the left recurrent laryngeal nerve, p. 89) before passing posterior to the lung roots to unite and form the oesophageal plexus around the lower oesophagus in the posterior mediastinum. From this plexus are formed the left and right vagal trunks, which pass through the oesophageal opening in the diaphragm to supply the foregut and midgut (notably stomach acid secretion) (p. 169). Related to the rotation of the gut during embryology, the left vagal trunk comes to lie anterior and the right trunk becomes posterior.

Phrenic nerves – *descending* from the neck (p. 88), the left phrenic nerve (**Figs. 5.4A, 5.5A**) runs caudally over the left side of the arch of the aorta and the pericardium overlying the left ventricle to pierce the *muscular* part of the diaphragm. The right phrenic nerve (**Fig. 5.6**) runs caudally beside the superior vena cava and the pericardium overlying the right atrium to pass through the right side of the vena caval foramen in the tendon of the diaphragm. Both phrenic nerves spread out on the abdominal surface of the diaphragm as the motor supply to the muscle fibres of their respective halves. Although the peripheral part of the diaphragm receives fibres from lower intercostal nerves, these are afferent only; the only motor supply is from the phrenic nerves. The phrenic nerves also have a large afferent area of supply: diaphragm, mediastinal and diaphragmatic pleura, pericardium and subdiaphragmatic peritoneum (hence referred pain from these areas is commonly to the C4 dermatome just superior to the shoulder; **Fig. 3.17**).

Heart

The heart (**Figs. 1.3, 5.9–5.15**) is the muscular pump of the cardiovascular system. It has four chambers – right and left atria, and right and left ventricles (**Figs. 5.9, 5.10**). The pulmonary circulation (which involves the right-sided chambers of the heart) is the part of the cardiovascular system that conveys blood to the lungs and brings it back to the left side of the heart. This is distinct from the systemic circulation (which involves the left-sided chambers of the heart) that takes blood to the rest of the body and returns it to the right side of the heart. The (hepatic) portal venous system is the part of the systemic circulation concerned with taking blood from the digestive tract (and the spleen) to the liver, so that the absorbed products of digestion can be delivered directly to the liver for chemical processing.

The heart lies within a tough fibrous sac, the fibrous pericardium, lined internally by a serous mesothelial membrane known as the pericardium, which, like the pleura, has a parietal layer lining it and a visceral layer adhering to the heart and adjacent parts of the great vessels.

Cardiac tamponade arises when fluid collects in the pericardium as a result of inflammation, malignancy or trauma. It is an emergency situation as the fibrous pericardium is non-elastic and the heart becomes compressed and cannot function normally.

Chambers and great vessels – the right atrium (**Fig. 5.9**) receives venous blood mainly from the superior vena cava and the inferior vena cava, but also from the coronary sinus (see below), the main vein of the heart itself and some other small veins. The internal wall is largely smooth, although there is a rough walled part separated from the smooth wall by a ridge, the crista terminalis, marked externally as a groove, the sulcus terminalis. The rough wall ridges are known as the musculi pectinate and extend out from the crista into the right atrial appendage and represent the primitive atrium of the heart. Internally, on the smooth wall just above the inferior vena cava beside the opening of the coronary sinus, is a shallow depression, the fossa ovalis (**Fig. 1.3**), lying on the interatrial septum, representing the remnants of the foramen ovale (a right to left interatrial shunt in foetal life). The blood passes from the atrium through the tricuspid valve

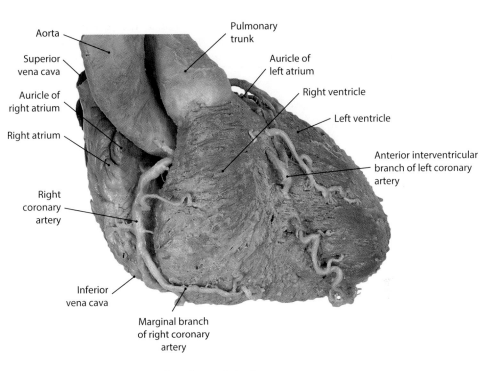

Aorta

Superior
vena cava

Auricle of
right atrium

Right atrium

Right
coronary
artery

Inferior
vena cava

Marginal branch
of right coronary
artery

Pulmonary
trunk

Auricle of
left atrium

Right ventricle

Left ventricle

Anterior interventricular
branch of left coronary
artery

Fig. 5.9 Anterior (sternocostal) surface of the heart.

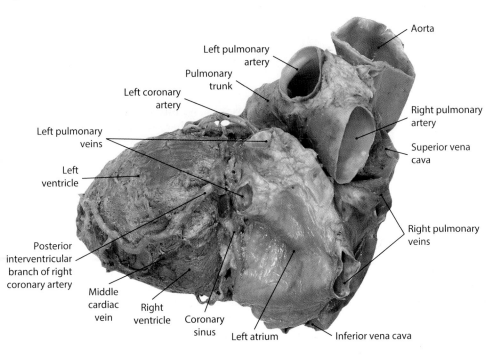

Left pulmonary
artery

Pulmonary
trunk

Left coronary
artery

Left pulmonary
veins

Left
ventricle

Posterior
interventricular
branch of right
coronary artery

Middle
cardiac
vein

Right
ventricle

Coronary
sinus

Left atrium

Aorta

Right pulmonary
artery

Superior vena
cava

Right pulmonary
veins

Inferior vena cava

Fig. 5.10 Heart, from the left and behind.

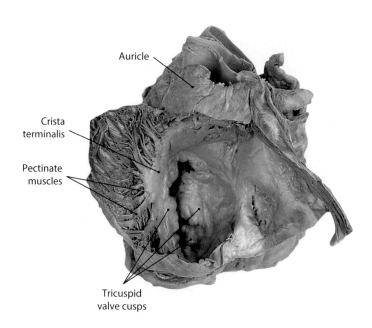

Fig. 5.11 Interior of the right atrium, opened up from the right to show the tricuspid valve.

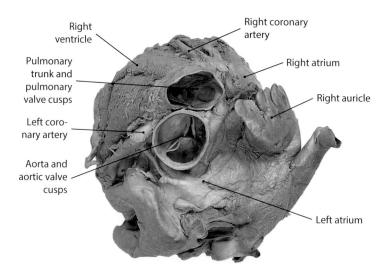

Fig. 5.12 Aortic and pulmonary valves, from above.

(**Fig. 5.11**) into the right ventricle, then through the pulmonary valve (**Fig. 5.12**) into the pulmonary trunk, and so to the right and left pulmonary arteries, conveying deoxygenated blood from the right ventricle to the lungs.

From the lungs, oxygenated blood is carried by the pulmonary veins (usually two on each side) to the left atrium (**Figs. 5.12, 5.14B**) and then passes through the (bicuspid) mitral valve into the left ventricle (**Fig. 5.13**), from where

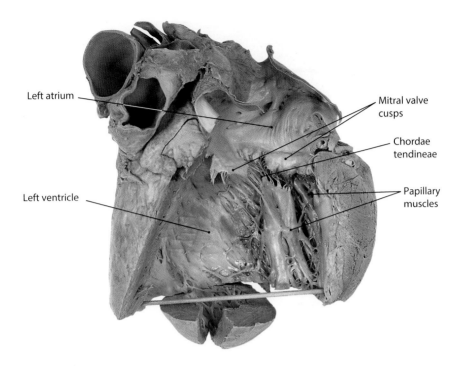

Left atrium

Mitral valve cusps

Chordae tendineae

Left ventricle

Papillary muscles

Fig. 5.13 Left atrium and left ventricle, opened up from the left.

it leaves through the aortic valve to enter the aorta, the body's largest vessel. The wall of the left ventricle is thicker (almost four times) than that of the right ventricle (**Fig. 5.14**) because the pressure of blood in the systemic circulation is much greater than that in the pulmonary circulation.

Fibrous chordae tendineae (**Fig. 5.13**) attach the margins of the cusps of the mitral and tricuspid valves to the papillary muscles that project from the ventricular walls. They prevent the cusps from being 'blown back' into the atria when the ventricles contract, so ensuring that the blood passes out through the aortic and pulmonary valves and does not regurgitate back into the atria. It is essential that the papillary muscles contract at the very start of ventricular contraction or the valve may fail to close and leak blood back into the atria.

The aortic and pulmonary valves are each composed of three semilunar leaflets (previously called cusps): the aortic valve has one anterior leaflet, where the ostium for the right coronary artery is located, and two posterior leaflets, the left one containing the ostium for the left coronary artery; the pulmonary valve has two anterior leaflets and one posterior leaflet. Alternatively, these six leaflets have been described as the aorta having a left leaflet associated with the ostia for the left coronary, a right leaflet with the ostia for the right coronary artery and a posterior leaflet (sometimes called the non-coronary leaflet), and the pulmonary valve having left, right and anterior leaflets. The difference is accounted for by the orientation of the specimen being studied. At the level of these valves the arterial wall is dilated to form a sinus. Closure of these valves relies on blood flowing backwards

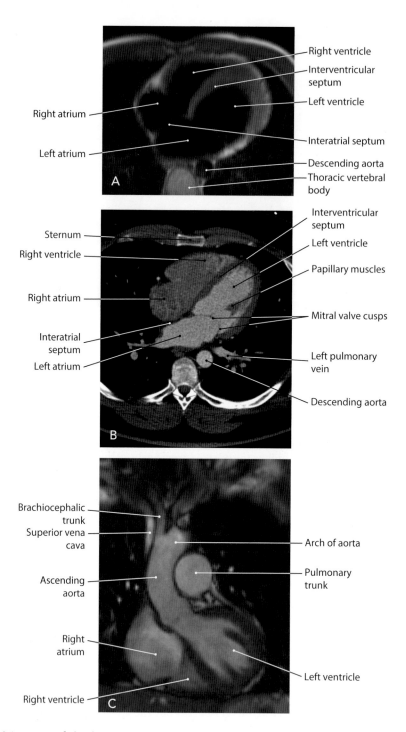

Fig. 5.14 Images of the heart: (A) Axial MR image (blood is black), (B) axial MR image (blood is light grey), (C) coronal MR image (blood is light grey).

at the end of systole towards the heart, filling the sinus and so pushing the valve leaflets together. The force for this retrograde flow is the elastic recoil of the aorta and pulmonary trunk. The four main

> The commonest valvular diseases of the heart are mitral stenosis (narrowing of the mitral valve) and aortic incompetence (improper closure leading to backflow through the aortic valve).

heart valves are all attached to a valve ring, otherwise known as the cardiac skeleton, to which the atria attach on one side and the ventricles on the other.

Note that the pulmonary trunk and pulmonary arteries contain deoxygenated blood, whereas the pulmonary veins contain oxygenated blood; the vessels are named, like all other blood vessels, from the direction of blood flow within them (to or from the heart), not from the state of oxygenation of their contained blood. Note also that the left and right atria do not normally communicate with one another, being separated by the interatrial septum, nor do the left and right ventricles intercommunicate, being separated by the interventricular septum. The systemic and pulmonary circulations thus remain separate unless there is a pathological opening.

> In many congenital heart diseases the septa are not properly developed, so the circulations become mixed and require surgical correction.

The heart does not 'hang straight down' from the great vessels superiorly, with the right chambers on the right and the left chambers on the left, but projects forwards (anteriorly) and is rotated

to the left. Thus, most of the anterior or sternocostal surface (**Figs. 5.9, 5.14**) is formed by the right ventricle, with the pulmonary trunk leaving its superior end; the right atrium is to the right of the right ventricle, and the left ventricle is to the left of, but mostly posterior to, the right ventricle (**Fig. 5.14**). The lower left extremity of the left ventricle forms the apex of the heart, located deep to the fifth intercostal space in the left mid-clavicular line. The aorta leaves the superior part of the left ventricle to the right of the pulmonary trunk and slightly posterior to the pulmonary trunk (**Fig. 5.9**). Thus, the order of the three great vessels superior to the heart from right to left is: superior vena cava, aorta, pulmonary trunk. The left atrium lies posteriorly and so forms the posterior surface or base of the heart; only the auricle of the left atrium is seen to the left of the pulmonary trunk when looking at the anterior surface.

Borders – it is important to appreciate the borders of the heart, as seen when looking from the front (visualised in a standard chest radiograph; **Figs. 5.2A, 5.15**), and to visualise them in relation to the surface of the thorax (**Fig. 5.3**).

> Radiography of the chest to ascertain whether the heart borders and lung fields are normal is one of the most important of all clinical procedures. Cardiac enlargement is recognised on a radiograph when the greatest diameter of the cardiac shadow is greater than 50% of the maximum diameter of the thoracic cavity.

The right border is formed by the right atrium, which runs from the third costal cartilage to the sixth costal cartilage at the right border of the sternum. The inferior

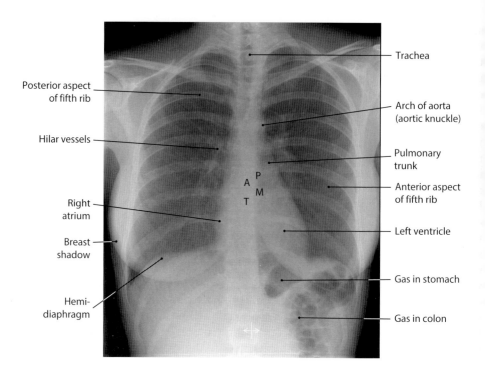

Fig. 5.15 Posteroanterior radiograph of a female chest. The standard 'straight radiograph of the chest', with heart valve locations superimposed. A, aortic; P, pulmonary; M, mitral; T, tricuspid.

border is formed mostly by the right ventricle, with the left ventricle (apex) at the left edge, and runs from the right sixth costal cartilage to the left fifth intercostal space, normally the mid-clavicular line; this is where the apex beat can be felt on the chest wall when the patient is leaning forward. The left border is formed by the left ventricle, with the left auricle at the superior end, and runs from the apex to the left third costal cartilage at the lateral border of the sternum. Radiographically, the pulmonary trunk can be seen lying superior to the left auricle. Higher still, the arch of the aorta can be seen passing posteriorly to produce a prominent bulge called the aortic knuckle.

Sound reverberates through the heart and chest wall in such a way that the positions on the chest wall where the sounds of

the heart valves are best heard with a stethoscope are not directly over the valves, but along the line of blood flow ('downstream'). Generally, the sounds of the pulmonary valve are best heard over the left second or third intercostal space at the sternal margin, those of the aortic valve over the second right intercostal space at the costal margin, those of the mitral valve at the apex of the heart, and those of the tricuspid valve over the lower right part of the sternum, fifth intercostal space or, equally well, at the same level just to the left of the sternum (**Fig. 5.15**).

Conducting system – the impulse for cardiac contraction begins in a small specialised area of pale heart muscle cells, the sinoatrial (SA) node, located superiorly in the right atrium just beside the entry of the superior vena cava (**Fig. 5.9**) where the superior end of the sulcus terminalis meets the atrial appendage. From there the impulse spreads through the cardiac muscle of the atria and reaches a specialised area of large pale muscle cells, the atrioventricular (AV) node, located in the lower part of the interatrial septum. The conduction continues through specialised myocardial cells, known as Purkinje fibres, from the AV node into the interventricular septum as the AV bundle of His, passing through the fibrous cushion before splitting into the left and right bundles and passing on the respective sides of the interventricular septum. These pass to the apex of the heart from where the wave of depolarisation that causes muscle contraction spreads across the ventricular walls. Within each ventricle several branches have been described passing from the main bundles. These have been referred to as moderator bands and they ensure that the wave of depolarisation is widely distributed, especially to the papillary muscles, so they contract at exactly the same time as the apex. However, only the one seen in the right ventricle is commonly referred to as the moderator band (or septomarginal trabeculum). These specialised tissues form the conducting or conduction system of the heart.

> Persistent ventricular arrhythmias may be treated by targeted ablation of parts of the conducting system using radio frequency waves delivered through a catheter passed through the venous system into the heart.

Blood supply – by two coronary arteries that arise from the ascending aorta just above the aortic valve (**Fig. 5.9**). The right coronary artery runs downwards in the right AV groove, giving off a large marginal branch, usually near the lower border of the heart, and a posterior interventricular branch on the inferior (diaphragmatic) surface. The left coronary artery, after a short course *posterior to* the pulmonary trunk,

> Disease of the coronary vessels, leading to narrowing and so to a reduced blood supply to cardiac muscle (ischaemic heart disease), is the commonest cause of sudden death in the UK.

> The anterior interventricular coronary artery is the one most frequently affected by disease and, because it is on the anterior aspect of the heart, it is easy to approach surgically for bypass operations.

continues in the left AV groove as the circumflex branch, after giving off the anterior interventricular branch (sometimes called by clinicians the left anterior descending artery or LAD), that runs in the anterior interventricular groove. The circumflex branch will also give a left marginal branch and a variable number of branches to the left ventricle. Again, the driving force for this blood flow is elastic recoil of the aorta. Importantly, this propels blood through the myocardium during diastole when vascular resistance is lowest. This phenomenon is diastolic perfusion.

> In about 30% of patients the posterior interventricular artery arises from the circumflex branch of the left. In these circumstances the left coronary artery is dominant and some refer to such a vessel as 'the widow maker', as occlusion of the main stem usually results in patient death.

The veins of the heart mostly run with the arteries (although they have different names) and mostly drain into the *coronary sinus*, which is situated in the AV groove on the posterior aspect of the heart (**Fig. 5.10**). The sinus opens into the lower part of the right atrium, near the opening of the inferior vena cava. Unlike the arteries, the veins of the heart are curiously unaffected by disease.

Nerve supply – by numerous sympathetic and parasympathetic (vagal) fibres, forming the cardiac plexus inferior to the arch of the aorta and at the bifurcation of the trachea. Increased vagal activity slows the heart rate and sympathetic activity increases it. Pain

> The pain of ischaemic heart disease is commonly felt behind the sternum, but is often referred to the neck or left upper limb. The patient may initially interpret it as indigestion.

fibres run with the sympathetic nerves and, because other parts of the same nerves supply other structures, such as blood vessels in the arm and neck, pain due to heart disease may appear to come from elsewhere, especially the left upper limb and side of the neck (referred pain, p. 60).

Lungs and pleura

The paired lungs are the principal organs of the respiratory system, where the exchange of gases (oxygen and carbon dioxide) takes place between air and blood. The other parts of the respiratory system (respiratory tract), consisting of the nose and paranasal sinuses, pharynx, larynx, trachea and main bronchi, are simply conducting pathways with no gaseous exchange. The trachea, the bronchi and the branches of the bronchi are often collectively called the 'bronchial tree'.

> Cancer of the lung invariably means cancer of one of the larger bronchi, hence the more correct technical term bronchial carcinoma.

By repeated divisions the bronchi become progressively smaller and eventually form the bronchioles, from which the air sacs (alveoli) bud off to form the sponge-like mass of aerated tissue where the exchange of gases (oxygen and carbon dioxide) takes place between the air in the air sacs and the red blood cells in the capillaries of the thin alveolar walls.

Lobes – the trachea divides into two main (primary) bronchi supplying each lung, which divide appropriately into the lobar (secondary) bronchi to supply each lobe. The left lung has upper and lower lobes, separated by an oblique fissure, but the right lung has upper, middle and lower lobes, separated by oblique and transverse (horizontal) fissures (**Figs. 5.1, 5.16, 5.17**). The secondary bronchi in the right lung to the middle and lower lobes branch from a common stem known as the bronchus intermedius. The visceral pleura, which covers the outer surface of the lobes, dips down into the fissures. The next division of each secondary bronchi, the (tertiary) bronchi, create the bronchopulmonary segments. Each segment is a functionally independent segment of lung supplied by a third order bronchus and has its own pulmonary artery and pulmonary vein. Each segment is separated from its neighbour by a fascial plane and as such can be surgically separated from the rest of the lung. The right lung usually has 10 segments and the left eight segments.

Surface markings – the surface marking of the oblique fissure of both lungs is on a line from the spine of the T3 vertebra posteriorly (T4 vertebral body) round to the sixth costal cartilage anteriorly, and is

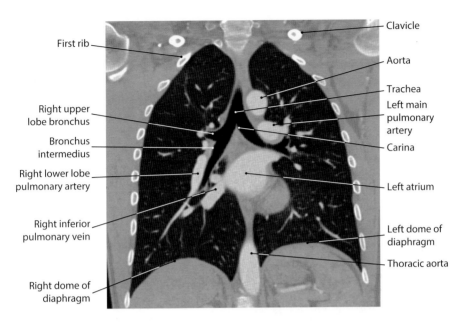

Fig. 5.16 Coronal CT chest image (lung setting) through the carina. (Note: Intermediate bronchus equals the bronchus to the right middle and lower lobes.)

approximately level with the medial border of the scapula when the arm is abducted to 180° (**Fig. 3.35**). The surface marking of the transverse fissure of the right lung is on a line drawn horizontally from the right fourth costal cartilage to where it meets the line of the oblique fissure.

> When listening with the stetho-scope on the front of the chest, it is mainly breath sounds in the upper lobes (and middle right lobe) that are heard; when listening on the back it is mainly the lower lobe sounds that are heard.

The lower parts of the lower lobes do not completely fill the pleural cavities, even with the deepest respiration. From the sixth costal cartilage level on the anterior chest, the lower level of the pleura extends posteriorly to the tenth rib in the mid-axillary line and the twelfth rib at the lateral border of the erector spinae (**Fig. 5.2B**), but the lower limit of the lung only extends to the level of the eighth rib in the mid-axillary line and the tenth rib at the lateral border of the erector spinae. The part of the pleural cavity without any lung (at the periphery of the diaphragm) is the costodiaphragmatic recess of the pleura and is where fluid accumulates in an upright patient (**Fig. 6.10**).

Hilum – the hilum of each lung (where the great vessels and main bronchus enter or leave it to form the lung root; **Figs. 5.5, 5.6, 5.16, 5.17B**) lies posterior to the costal cartilages 3 and 4 (level with T5, T6 and T7 vertebrae). Remember the numbers 3, 4, 5, 6 and 7: 3 and 4 for costal cartilages and 5, 6 and 7 for vertebrae. The main bronchus is the most posterior structure in each lung root and the lower pulmonary vein the lowest structure. The upper pulmonary vein lies anterior to the pulmonary artery, which in turn is anterior to the main bronchus. Remember the sequence vein, artery, bronchus from

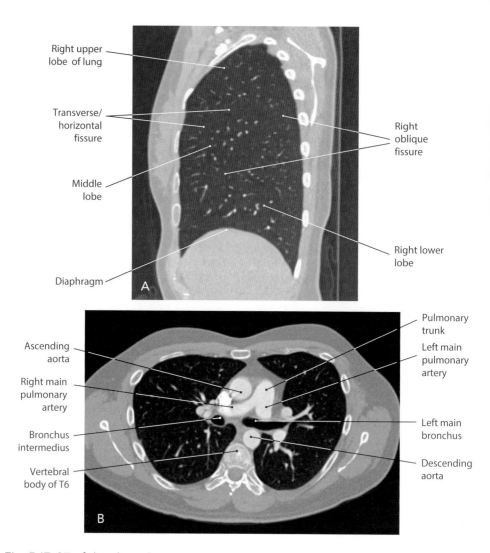

Fig. 5.17 CT of the chest (lung setting): (A) parasagittal section through the right lung. (B) axial view.

anterior to posterior (compare with vein, artery, ureter in the hilum of the kidney).

> The right main bronchus is more vertical than the left main bronchus, so inhaled foreign bodies (such as extracted teeth and peanuts) are more likely to enter the right main bronchus than the more 'horizontal' left one.

Pleura – the two pleural membranes (parietal and visceral) come together in the midline of the sternum between the levels of the second to fourth costal cartilages. The pleura and lung on the right side continue down to the level of the sixth costal cartilage, but on the left the presence of the heart causes an indentation (cardiac notch) in the lung and overlying pleura.

On each side, the apex of the pleura (cervical pleura) and lung extends for about 3 cm above the medial third of the clavicle (**Fig. 5.3**) in the thoracic inlet (**Fig. 3.44**).

> Stab wounds of the lower neck may injure the pleura and lung. When examining clinically it is important, therefore, to carry out percussion and auscultation above the clavicle in order to examine the apex of the lungs.

Blood supply – although the pulmonary arteries and veins concerned with oxygenation of blood are the largest vessels in the lung, the lung tissue itself is supplied by its own very small vessels, the bronchial arteries (direct branches of the aorta level with the fifth and sixth thoracic vertebrae) and veins.

> Blood clots, known as pulmonary emboli, commonly from deep venous thrombosis in the lower limbs (p. 230), may become impacted in the pulmonary circulation; if large they can cause sudden death.

Nerve supply – the smooth muscle of the blood vessels and bronchi of the lungs are supplied by various autonomic nerves that also provide the important pathways for the cough reflex, enabling the bronchial tree to be cleared of excess mucus and other debris. The visceral pleura is insensitive but the parietal pleura is supplied by spinal nerves such as the intercostal and the phrenic nerves, which are able to localise pain precisely.

> Spasm of smooth muscle in the bronchial walls is one of the features of asthma, with constriction of bronchi and particular difficulty with expiration.

> Pleural pain is experienced as a sharp, stabbing sensation, worse on inspiration as the parietal pleura is stretched.

Summary

- The *bony thorax* consists of the 12 thoracic vertebrae, 12 pairs of ribs and costal cartilages, and the three parts of the sternum – manubrium, body and xiphoid process.
- The most important landmark on the surface of the thorax is the *manubriosternal joint*, palpable about 5 cm inferior to the jugular notch at the level of the second costal cartilages and ribs. By counting down from these cartilages and ribs the surface markings of the heart, pleura and lungs can be identified.
- The *manubrium* of the sternum lies opposite the middle four thoracic vertebrae (T5–T8).
- The *apex beat* of the heart (left ventricle) is normally in the left fifth intercostal space about 9 cm from the midline; the *left border* of the heart (left ventricle with left atrial appendage lying superiorly) extends from the apex to the left third costal cartilage; *right border* (right atrium) from the right third to sixth costal cartilages; and the *inferior border* (mostly right ventricle) from the right sixth costal cartilage to the apex (left fifth intercostal space).

Continued

Continued

- The base of the heart is its posterior surface (left atrium), not the top end where large vessels are attached.
- The order of the *great vessels* superior to the heart from right to left is: superior vena cava, aorta, pulmonary trunk.
- The right and left *coronary arteries* arise from the ascending aorta just above the anterior and left posterior aortic valve leaflets, respectively.
- The arch of the *aorta* rises as high as the midpoint of the manubrium, and from right to left gives origin to the brachiocephalic, left common carotid and left subclavian arteries.
- The *tricuspid valve* lies between the right atrium and right ventricle, with the *pulmonary valve* between the right ventricle and pulmonary trunk; the *mitral valve* is between the left atrium and left ventricle, with the *aortic valve* between the left ventricle and ascending aorta.
- The *hilum* of the lung is on a level with the third and fourth costal cartilages and the order of the principal structures from front to back in the hilum is: vein, artery, bronchus.
- Posteriorly, the back of the *pleura* extends as low as the twelfth rib at the lateral border of the erector spinae, but the lung extends only as low as the tenth rib; the empty part of the pleural cavity is the costodiaphragmatic recess.
- The *trachea* divides into the two main primary bronchi just inferior to the level of the manubriosternal joint.
- The *oesophagus* runs down through the thorax immediately anterior to the vertebral column, with the thoracic duct passing upwards at first posterior to the right margin of the oesophagus and then crossing to the left to enter the neck posterior to the left common carotid before passing into the junction of the left internal jugular and subclavian veins.

Questions

Answers can be found in Appendix A, p. 246.

Question 1

There are two pleural membranes, visceral and parietal, separated normally by a very small volume of fluid for lubrication. Which statement below is also an accurate description relating to pleura?

(a) Normally the lowest part of the left pleural cavity is at the level of the tenth thoracic vertebra, due to the presence of the heart, and would be dull to percussion due to the presence of the liver.

(b) If percussing the anterior chest wall on the right between the fourth rib and the sixth rib, one is percussing the right middle lobe of the lung.

(c) If percussing the posterior aspect of the left side of the chest over the second intercostal space, you would be percussing the lower lobe of the left lung.

(d) Pathology contained within the middle lobe of the lung will cause pain that is easily located as it is innervated by the intercostal nerves that lie in direct contact with it.

(e) Pain due to pathology contained within the middle lobe is carried to higher centres through the closely related right phrenic nerve.

Question 2

Which statement below accurately describes heart valve anatomy?

(a) The aortic valve cusps are attached via cordae tendinae to papillary muscles, which are necessary to ensure proper closing of the valve.

(b) The pulmonary valve is located anterior to the aortic valve and the right coronary artery ostia lies in the right anterior cusp of this valve.

(c) The orientation of the tricuspid valve is such that valve sounds can be heard best on either the right side or left side of the sternum at the level of the third intercostal space.

(d) The orientation of the heart is such that the mitral valve sounds are best heard in the fifth intercostal space mid-clavicular line to the left of midline.

(e) The three cusps of the tricuspid valve are positioned superior on the valve ring (cushion) to the cusps of the pulmonary valve.

Question 3

Which of the statements below best describes the normal course of the given coronary artery?

(a) The left coronary artery arises from the left posterior cusp of the aortic valve and passes anterior to the pulmonary trunk to run down the anterior wall of the interventricular septum.

(b) The left coronary artery lies posterior to the pulmonary trunk where it bifurcates to form the circumflex and anterior interventricular branches.

(c) The right coronary artery lies posterior to the pulmonary trunk before bifurcating and descending in the AV groove between the right atrium and ventricle.

(d) The right coronary artery arises from the anterior cusp of the aortic valve before passing into the AV groove between the left atrium and ventricle.

(e) The left coronary artery arises from the right posterior cusp of the aortic valve and passes posterior to the pulmonary trunk in the AV groove between the left atrium and ventricle.

Question 4

The fissures of the lungs divide the lungs into lobes and are projected onto the chest wall. In quiet respiration, which statement below most accurately describes their normal projection?

(a) The transverse fissure follows the left fourth costal cartilage and rib around the chest to meet the oblique fissure in the mid-axillary line.

(b) The oblique fissure on the left follows the line joining the sixth thoracic vertebral spine posteriorly to the seventh costal cartilage anteriorly.

(c) The oblique fissure on the right follows the line joining the second thoracic vertebral spine posteriorly to the fifth costal cartilage anteriorly.

(d) The transverse fissure on the right follows a line joining the fourth thoracic vertebral spine posteriorly to the fourth costal cartilage anteriorly.

(e) The oblique fissure on the left passes along a line joining the fourth thoracic vertebral body posteriorly to the sixth costal cartilage anteriorly.

Question 5

An elderly man develops right middle lobe pneumonia. The resulting consolidation of the lung is recognised clinically by a dull percussion note. Where on the chest wall will this best be detected?

(a) Anteriorly, below the level of the fourth costal cartilage.

(b) Anteriorly, above the level of the fourth costal cartilage.

(c) In the mid-axillary line above the level of the fourth costal cartilage.

(d) Posteriorly, below the level of the sixth vertebral spine.

(e) Posteriorly, above the level of the sixth vertebral spine.

Question 6

Repeated severe vomiting can lead to rupture of the oesophagus in the thorax with leakage of food and subsequent infection. Which part of the thoracic cavity will initially be affected?

(a) Superior mediastinum.

(b) Anterior mediastinum.

(c) Posterior mediastinum.

(d) Costodiaphragmatic recess.

(e) Costophrenic angle.

Question 7

An 87-year-old woman had a complete removal of a breast (mastectomy) and the adjacent axillary lymph node to remove a cancerous tumour. She says that since the surgery she has had difficulty raising her arm above horizontal to brush her hair. Injury to which of the following structures is the most likely cause of this patient's longstanding problem?

(a) Suprascapular nerve.

(b) Axillary nerve.

(c) Long thoracic nerve.

(d) Pectoralis major muscle.

(e) Pectoralis minor muscle.

Question 8

A 52-year-old woman is diagnosed with breast cancer. The team providing her health care is concerned about the possible spread of malignant cells via lymphatic pathways. Which the following lymph nodes are most likely to become involved in the spread of the pathology?

(a) Inguinal lymph nodes.

(b) Parasternal lymph nodes.

(c) Axillary lymph nodes.

(d) Epitrochlear lymph nodes.

(e) Cysterna chyli.

Question 9

A 49-year-old man presents with ptosis (drooping) of the right eyelid. Physical examination reveals that the pupil of the right eye is constricted. It is also noted that there is no sweating on the right side of his face. Radiological examination reveals a tumour near the apex of his right lung. Which of the following structures has most likely been compromised by the tumour?

(a) Thoracic duct.

(b) Right vagus nerve.

(c) Right phrenic nerve.

(d) Right sympathetic trunk.

(e) Right subclavian artery.

Question 10

A 50-year-old man presents to his doctor complaining of shortness of breath (dyspnoea), which has become increasingly worse in the last weeks. On physical examination a murmur is detected when the stethoscope is placed over the apex of the patient's heart. Which of the following structures is most likely involved in this patient's clinical presentation?

(a) Tricuspid valve.

(b) Pulmonary valve.

(c) Mitral valve.

(d) Aortic valve.

(e) Ascending aorta.

Question 11

A 54-year-old man is admitted to the clinic with difficulty breathing (dyspnoea). Radiological examination reveals a tumour invading the surface of the lung anterior to the hilum. Which of the following nerves is most likely compressed, leading to the symptom in this patient?

(a) Vagus.

(b) Phrenic.

(c) Intercostal.

(d) Recurrent laryngeal.

(e) Greater thoracic splanchnic.

Question 12

A 68-year-old woman with a long history of smoking cigarettes complains of recent hoarseness. Laryngoscopy reveals a flaccid left vocal fold. Which of the following structures is most likely to be compromised?

(a) Left recurrent laryngeal nerve.

(b) Right recurrent laryngeal nerve.

(c) Left vagus nerve.

(d) Left phrenic nerve.

(e) Left sympathetic trunk.

Question 13

A 56-year-old man is scheduled to undergo a coronary bypass operation. The coronary artery of primary concern is the vessel that supplies much of the left ventricle and right and left bundle branches of the cardiac conducting system. Which of the following arteries is the surgeon most concerned with?

(a) Circumflex.

(b) Anterior interventricular.

(c) Posterior interventricular.

(d) Right marginal.

(e) Artery to the SA node.

Question 14

A 58-year-old woman is admitted to the Emergency Department with severe chest pain. Electrocardiography and radiological examination provide evidence of a significant myocardial infarction (heart attack) and accumulation of fluid within the pericardial cavity (cardiac tamponade). Emergency aspiration of the fluid (pericardiocentesis) is performed. Based on the surface anatomy, which of the following locations might be the safest for the needle to be inserted in this procedure?

(a) Triangle of auscultation.

(b) Left sixth intercostal space just lateral to the sternum.

(c) Right third intercostal space 2 cm lateral to the sternum.

(d) Right seventh intercostal space in the mid-axillary line.

(e) Left fifth intercostal space in the mid-clavicular line.

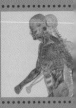

Introduction

The abdomen or abdominal cavity (in popular parlance the 'tummy') is the part of the trunk below the diaphragm that separates it from the thoracic cavity. Abdominal pain is a common reason to visit the doctor. The abdomen is also the site where excess fat is deposited. While most of the digestive system lies within the abdomen, the oesophagus is mostly in the thorax and the digestive system also extends below the pelvic brim in the lowest part (p. 190) into the pelvic cavity or pelvis. The upper abdomen also contains the kidneys, adrenal glands and spleen. Because of the way the diaphragm bulges upwards into the thorax, the abdominal cavity is larger than might be expected when looking at the outside of the trunk, but lower down it is less capacious than might be expected because of the way the lumbar region of the vertebral column projects forwards in the middle of the posterior abdominal wall. Muscles form the rest of the posterior wall, as they do the anterolateral wall.

> The possibility of disease or injury affecting so many organs makes abdominal surgery one of the more common reasons for admission to hospital.

The peritoneum is a smooth serosal membrane that lines the abdominal and pelvic walls and forms supporting folds for certain abdominal organs. The layer of peritoneum that lines the abdominal and pelvic walls is the parietal peritoneum, whereas that covering abdominal and pelvic viscera is the visceral peritoneum. Some organs, such as the kidneys, ureters, adrenal glands and pancreas, are plastered onto the posterior abdominal wall behind parietal peritoneum (i.e. they are retroperitoneal), whereas the stomach and much of the small and large intestines are suspended by folds (mesentery) of peritoneum (i.e. they are intraperitoneal). This shiny, lubricated membrane allows free movement between the mobile viscera that can change their size and shape and the abdominal wall.

> Inflammation of the peritoneum (peritonitis) is highly dangerous because it involves about as much surface area in a pathological process as all of the skin covering the body. It gives rise to a characteristic 'board-like rigidity' on palpation of the affected parts of the abdominal wall.

Anterior abdominal wall

The muscles that form the anterior part of the abdominal wall (**Fig. 4.2**) are the rectus abdominis, the external and internal oblique (abdominis) and the transversus abdominis, deep to which lie the transversalis fascia and parietal peritoneum.

Rectus abdominis – runs cranially (upwards) from the pubic crest (between symphysis and tubercle) to the fifth, sixth and seventh costal cartilages. It is enclosed by the rectus sheath (see below) and usually has three tendinous intersections that adhere to the anterior wall of the sheath. The two sheaths meet in the midline as the linea alba. Posteriorly in the sheath, midway between the umbilicus and the pubis, is the arcuate line, inferior to which the posterior rectus sheath is only represented by transversalis fascia. The muscle is innervated by the T7–T12 (intercostal) nerves.

> In thin muscular individuals the tendinous intersections may be seen as transverse depressions on the surface. This gives what is often referred to as a 'six pack' appearance.

External oblique, internal oblique and transversus abdominis – lie in that order from superficial (outside) to deep (inwards) between the iliac crest and the lower ribs. The aponeurotic medial part of the internal oblique splits to form the rectus sheath, with the aponeuroses of the external oblique and transversus joining the anterior and posterior layers of the sheath, respectively, except in the lowest part where all three aponeuroses lie anterior to rectus abdominis. The lowest part of the external oblique aponeurosis recurves and thickens to form the inguinal ligament, stretching between the anterior superior iliac spine and the pubic tubercle.

These muscles compress the abdominal contents to allow for raising intra-abdominal pressure and also support the

> The anterior superior iliac spine is at the anterior end of the iliac crest and easily palpable; the pubic tubercle is felt 2.5 cm lateral to the top of the midline pubic symphysis.

spine and hence body posture. Working on their own, rectus abdominis will flex the trunk while the obliques on each side will produce lateral flexion to the same side.

The external oblique is innervated (like rectus abdominis) by the T7–T12 intercostal nerves, and the other two muscles by T7–T12 but also by the L1 nerve carried in the iliohypogastric and ilioinguinal nerves.

Inguinal canal – an oblique gap, about 4 cm long, through the muscle aponeuroses above the medial end of the inguinal ligament (**Fig. 4.2**), which forms the floor of the canal. This short canal runs from the deep inguinal ring laterally to the superficial inguinal ring located medial to the pubic tubercle. External oblique aponeurosis forms the anterior wall throughout, reinforced laterally by the lowest fibres of internal oblique muscle (**Fig. 6.1**). Internal oblique fibres arch medially over the contents of the canal to form the roof of the canal and then form the posterior wall of the canal medially. The lowest fibres of transverse abdominis pass inferiorly to the pubis, blending with the internal oblique fibres posteriorly and forming the conjoint tendon, the posterior wall of the canal. The superficial ring is reinforced posteriorly by two muscle layers and the deep ring is reinforced anteriorly by two muscle layers. The intactness of the innervation of these muscle fibres, from the iliohypogastric and ilioinguinal nerves (L1), is important to maintain the canal's integrity, which otherwise depends largely on its obliquity. The canal is occupied by the contents of the spermatic cord (p. 201) in the male and the round ligament of the uterus in the female, with the ilioinguinal

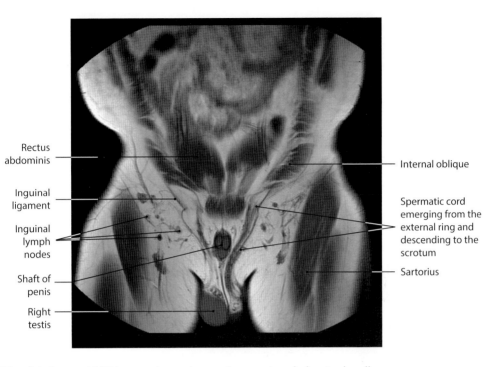

Rectus abdominis

Inguinal ligament

Inguinal lymph nodes

Shaft of penis

Right testis

Internal oblique

Spermatic cord emerging from the external ring and descending to the scrotum

Sartorius

Fig. 6.1 Coronal MR image through a male anterior abdominal wall.

nerve in both sexes. The canal is a potentially weak part of the abdominal wall, especially in males (because in foetal life the testis passed through it to reach the scrotum and there was a peritoneal pouch passing through the canal). It may, therefore, become the site of an inguinal hernia – a protrusion of abdominal contents (usually a loop of small intestine) that may extend into the scrotum.

Inguinal hernia are more common in males; femoral hernia (p. 213) are more common in females, in whom the inguinal canal is smaller. There are direct inguinal hernias, which pass through the conjoint tendon to reach the superficial ring, and indirect inguinal hernias, which pass through both the deep and superficial inguinal rings.

Damage to the ilioinguinal nerve in the canal (e.g. during the surgical repair of a hernia) does not affect the nerve supply to the muscle fibres guarding the canal, because the motor innervation arises from the nerve well before it reaches the canal; it is incisions in the lateral part of the abdominal wall (e.g. for appendectomy) that may damage it.

Surface features – a virtual grid of nine squares is used to divide the surface of the abdomen into regions (**Fig. 6.2**), so that the sites of pain, swellings, palpable masses etc. can be described by their location. The two vertical lines run down from the mid-point of the clavicle; the upper horizontal line, the transpyloric plane, joins the tips of the ninth costal cartilages and passes through the L1 vertebral body; the lower horizontal plane joins the tubercles on the

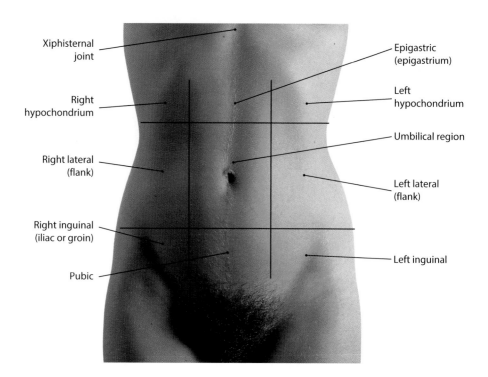

Xiphisternal joint

Right hypochondrium

Right lateral (flank)

Right inguinal (iliac or groin)

Pubic

Epigastric (epigastrium)

Left hypochondrium

Umbilical region

Left lateral (flank)

Left inguinal

Fig. 6.2 Regions of the abdomen. The upper transverse line is the transpyloric plane, level with the lower part of L1 vertebra and about a handsbreadth below the xiphisternal joint.

iliac crest (between the highest point of the ilium and the anterior superior iliac spine). The central regions are the epigastric superiorly, the umbilical and pubic inferiorly, and at the sides are the right and left hypochondrium superiorly and the lateral and inguinal regions inferiorly. The epigastric and lateral regions are sometimes called the epigastrium and lumbar (flank or loin) regions, respectively, the inguinal regions are also known as the iliac fossae, and the pubic region as the hypogastric regions; thus, a gastric ulcer may give rise to epigastric pain and an inflamed appendix to pain and tenderness in the right inguinal region or iliac fossa.

Occasionally, the subcostal plane is used instead of the transpyloric. It lies at the lower border of the rib cage to pass through L2, and is the lower point of the spinal cord in the adult. The supracristal plane joining

the highest points of the iliac crest passes through the L4 vertebra and can be used for the lower horizontal plane. A simpler and less precise way to divide the abdomen is to draw vertical and horizontal lines through the umbilicus, so dividing it into right and left upper and lower quadrants.

Lateral border of the rectus sheath – meets the costal margin at the ninth costal cartilage (**Fig. 6.3**). On the right, the fundus (lower end) of the gallbladder underlies this point, the region of maximal pain and tenderness in gallbladder disease (Murphy's sign).

Liver – may just be palpable at the right costal margin lateral to the rectus sheath when the patient takes a deep breath, although a liver enlarged and hardened by disease will be much more obvious on palpation.

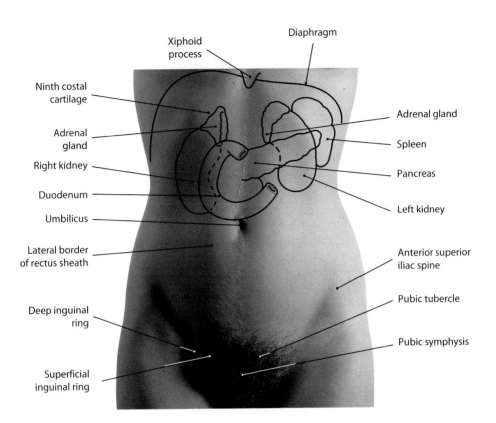

Fig. 6.3 Surface features of the abdomen.

> The size of the liver is usually estimated through percussion of the lower aspect of the right side of the rib cage.

Umbilicus – the midline, puckered scar that indicates the site of attachment of the foetal umbilical cord typically lies at the level of the disc between L3 and L4 vertebrae. The pulsation of the aorta may be felt (and in thin patients sometimes seen) just above or below the umbilicus by pressure on the overlying coils of the gut.

> It is in the umbilical region where one is able to palpate aneurysms of the abdominal aorta.

Duodenum – of the four parts that form the non-palpable C-shaped curve of the duodenum (**Figs. 6.3, 6.10, 6.11**), (often called by radiologists the duodenal loop), the first part lies at the level of the L1 vertebra, the second part at the right edge of the L2 vertebra, the third part crosses the L3 vertebra and the fourth part lies at the left margin of the L2 vertebra.

Head of the pancreas – lies within the C-shaped curve of the duodenum and the rest of the pancreas passes slightly upwards and to the left, with its tail reaching the hilum of the spleen in the left hypochondrium. The organ is not normally palpable.

Kidney – the lower pole may be felt in the lateral region by one hand on the anterior wall pressing backwards below the costal margin and the other pressing forwards from the back (referred to as 'balloting the kidney').

An enlarging kidney expands downwards towards the iliac crest; an enlarging spleen passes more obliquely towards the umbilicus and right iliac fossa.

Spleen – not normally palpable, since it is tucked up beneath the left dome of the diaphragm, in the long axis of the tenth rib. It must be 2 to 3 times its normal size to be palpable at the left costal margin.

Urinary bladder – being essentially a pelvic organ, it is only palpable, in the pubic region, when considerably distended.

In a female patient a distended bladder must not be mistaken for a pregnant uterus (or other pelvic mass such as an ovarian cyst).

Uterus – like the bladder it is a pelvic organ, but enlarges during pregnancy, reaching the top of the pubic symphysis at 3 months, the umbilicus at the fifth month and appearing to fill the whole abdomen at 9 months (full term).

Colon – in the left inguinal region, faecal material may be palpable in the descending or sigmoid colon ('loaded colon').

Posterior abdominal wall

This is the lumbar part of the vertebral column, which bulges forwards with the aorta and inferior vena cava anterior to it, forms the central part of the posterior abdominal wall

(Fig. 6.4) and has the right and left crus of the diaphragm (p. 132) arising from its upper part. On each side is psoas major, with psoas minor (if present) overlying it. More laterally, are quadratus lumborum, lying medial to the more laterally placed transversus abdominis, and iliacus, which lies lower on the inner aspect of the ilium.

Psoas major – runs caudally from the sides of the T12–L5 vertebrae and intervening discs to pass into the thigh deep to the inguinal ligament and attach to the lesser trochanter of the femur. The lumbar plexus of nerves is embedded within the muscle and the major branches emerge from it (see below), with twigs from L1–L3 nerves innervating the muscle. It is a powerful flexor of the hip (p. 217) (or, if the lower limb is fixed, it can flex the trunk). The small and unimportant psoas minor (absent in 40% of individuals) arises from the sides of the T12 and L1 vertebrae and the intervening disc and has a long tendon that passes down over psoas major, attaching to the iliopubic eminence of the hip bone, and is a weak flexor of the trunk.

Quadratus lumborum – lies lateral to psoas major and fills the gap between the medial part of the iliac crest and the medial half of rib 12, and will aid lateral flexion to the same side.

Transversus abdominis – attaches to the lower ribs, lateral edge of quadratus lumborum, the iliac crest and the outer third of the inguinal ligament before passing to the linea alba (p. 158).

Iliacus – covers the medial (inner) aspect of the iliac fossa and runs distally to enter the thigh on the lateral side of psoas major, attaching with it to the lesser trochanter. It is innervated by branches of the femoral nerve and is primarily a flexor of the

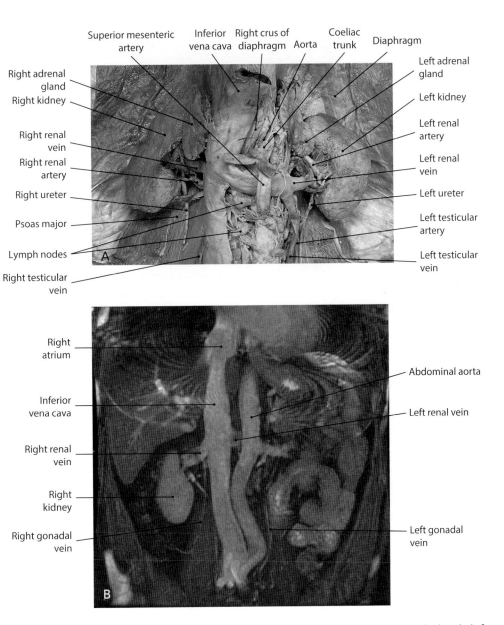

Fig. 6.4 (A) Posterior abdominal wall with major vessels, kidneys and adrenal glands left in place, (B) comparable coronal MR image.

hip joint. Occasionally considered together, the psoas and iliacus are referred to as ilio-psoas; although the two muscles have a common distal attachment and act to flex the hip, each does have a separate action.

Surface features – viewed from behind (**Fig. 6.5**), a line drawn between the highest points of the iliac crests passes through the spine of the L4 vertebra; other vertebrae can be counted upwards from here.

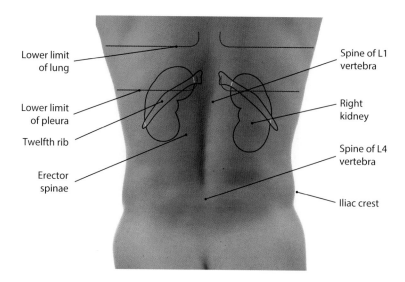

Fig. 6.5 Surface features of the lower back.

> Lumbar punctures (for obtaining specimens of cerebrospinal fluid) and epidural anaesthesia are commonly carried out between the spines of L3 and L4 vertebrae.

The position of each kidney can be visualised as a characteristic kidney shape about 12 cm high and 5 cm broad, with the hilum 5 cm from the midline and centred on the L1/2 vertebrae, the left kidney normally lying slightly higher than the right. The twelfth ribs are often too short to be palpable through the back muscles; because the costodiaphragmatic recess of the pleura crosses the twelfth rib at the level of the lateral border of the erector spinae, it is important not to misidentify the rib.

> The kidney is often approached surgically from behind, and it is important to remember the pleural cavity will separate the upper pole of the kidney from the twelfth rib and not to enter the pleural cavity.

Abdominal vessels and nerves

Abdominal aorta – enters the abdomen through the aortic opening (hiatus) of the diaphragm at the level of the T12 vertebra (p. 133). It runs down anterior to the lumbar vertebrae, terminating at the level of the L4 vertebra by dividing into the right and left common iliac arteries (**Figs. 1.4, 6.4, 6.6**).

The three large unpaired branches that arise from the anterior of the aorta supply the alimentary tract. Each artery supplies a length of gut that corresponds to three embryonic regions: foregut, from the lower oesophagus to just caudal to where the bile duct enters the second part of the duodenum (p. 172), by the coeliac trunk; midgut, from the caudal end of the second part of the duodenum to the transverse colon near the splenic flexure, by the superior mesenteric artery; and hindgut, from near the splenic flexure to the upper part of the anal canal, by the inferior mesenteric artery.

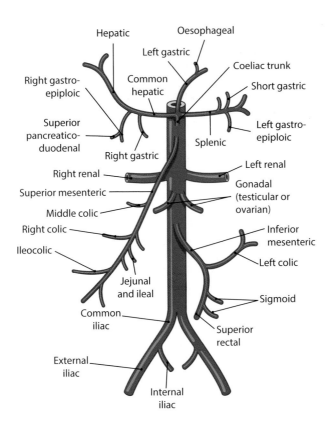

Fig. 6.6 The principal branches of the abdominal aorta.

The largest lateral paired branches of the aorta are the right and left renal arteries. Smaller paired branches include the gonadal vessels (testicular or ovarian), inferior phrenic and middle adrenal arteries, and four lumbar arteries.

Coeliac trunk – arises at the point where the aorta enters the abdomen to supply the foregut and associated organs and is usually a very short vessel that divides immediately into three branches: the left gastric, splenic and common hepatic arteries. The left gastric artery passes upwards on the diaphragm and to the left to reach the oesophagus and then descends on the lesser curvature of the stomach and gives off an oesophageal branch. The splenic artery runs on the posterior abdominal wall to the left along the upper border of the pancreas to the spleen, at which point it gives off the left gastroepiploic and short gastric arteries to the left side of the greater curvature and fundus of the stomach. The common hepatic artery passes on the posterior abdominal wall to the right and gives off the right gastric artery to the lesser curvature and the gastroduodenal artery (which in turn gives off the right gastroepiploic [on the greater curvature] and superior pancreaticoduodenal arteries). The common hepatic artery then turns cranially as the (proper) hepatic artery (also an origin for the right gastric artery) in the right free margin of the lesser omentum to reach the liver (p. 175); note the change of name from common hepatic to hepatic.

Superior mesenteric artery – arises from the aorta posterior to the body of the pancreas and passes caudally anterior to the uncinate process of the pancreas to supply the midgut. The principal branches are the numerous jejunal and ileal arteries (from its left side) and the inferior pancreaticoduodenal, ileocolic, right colic and middle colic arteries (from its right side).

Inferior mesenteric artery – arises from the aorta posterior to the third part of the duodenum to supply the hindgut. The principal branches are the left colic and sigmoid arteries; it ends by changing its name to the superior rectal artery, which passes down into the pelvis to reach the rectum and anal canal.

Portal vein – receives blood from all the structures supplied by the three large unpaired aortic branches just described. It is formed posterior to the pancreas by the union of the superior mesenteric vein with the splenic vein (**Fig. 6.7**); the inferior mesenteric vein usually drains into the splenic vein. The portal vein drains the gut from the lower end of the oesophagus to the upper part of the anal canal via the various tributaries of these vessels, thus conveying to the liver substances absorbed from the alimentary tract essential to ensure that anything absorbed by the intestinal tract can be processed by the liver before entering the systemic circulation. In addition, molecular components of red blood cells resulting from activities of the spleen pass

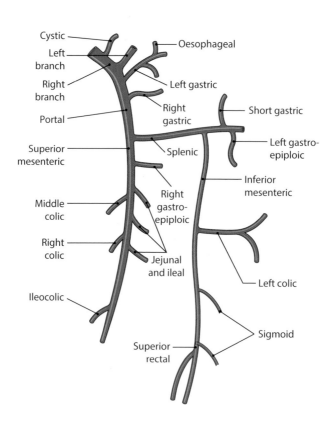

Fig. 6.7 The principal tributaries of the portal vein.

to the liver and help form bile fluid. The lower end of the oesophagus is the most important site of portosystemic anastomosis, between veins of the portal system and systemic veins. Diseases of the liver that lead to increased pressure in the portal vein (portal hypertension) result in dilatation of the veins (varacies) at the sites of portosystemic anastomoses.

Varices formed in the lower oesophagus are an important cause of severe bleeding from the upper gastrointestinal tract (haematemesis). Other sites of portosystemic anastomoses are around the umbilicus, anal canal and posterior to the ascending and descending colons.

Inferior vena cava – the principal vein of the body below the diaphragm, it lies on the right side of the aorta. It begins caudally at the level of the L5 vertebra by the union of the right and left common iliac veins (**Figs. 6.4, 6.8**) and runs cranially to pierce the central tendon of the diaphragm posterior to the liver at the level of the T8–T9 vertebrae. The largest tributaries are the right and left renal veins. The gonadal vein (testicular or ovarian) drains directly into the vena cava on the right, but on the left it enters the left renal vein. The highest

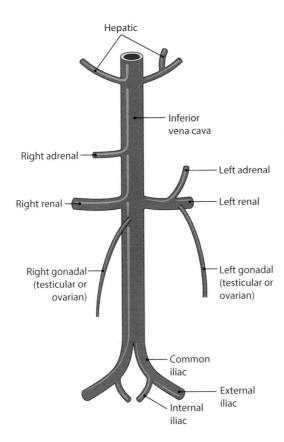

Hepatic

Inferior vena cava

Right adrenal

Left adrenal

Right renal

Left renal

Right gonadal (testicular or ovarian)

Left gonadal (testicular or ovarian)

Common iliac

External iliac

Internal iliac

Fig. 6.8 The principal tributaries of the inferior vena cava.

tributaries of the vena cava are the hepatic veins, which enter the vena cava where that vessel lies in the deep groove on the posterior of the liver (the hepatic veins therefore have no extrahepatic course). A number of small lumbar veins also enter the vena cava at various levels and connect with pelvic veins inferiorly, the azygos system superiorly and with the venous plexuses around the vertebral column.

Femoral nerve (L2, L3, L4) – the largest nerve on the posterior abdominal wall and the largest branch of the lumbar plexus (**Fig. 3.19**), which is within psoas major. It emerges from the *lateral* side of psoas low down and runs distally on the lateral side of the external iliac artery (which becomes the femoral artery in the thigh) to enter the anterior aspect of the thigh by passing deep to the inguinal ligament.

The nerve may be injured by stab wounds in the lower abdomen.

Lateral femoral cutaneous nerve (L2, L3) – smaller than the femoral nerve and emerging from psoas more cranially, it curls down superficial to iliacus, entering the thigh deep to the lateral part of the inguinal ligament.

Iliohypogastric and ilioinguinal nerves (L1) – smaller than the lateral femoral cutaneous nerve and emerging from psoas cranial to it, they run laterally to enter the lower anterior abdominal wall. The former supplies skin around the superficial inguinal ring and the latter passes through the inguinal canal. They are important because these first lumbar nerve fibres are the ones that supply the parts of the anterior abdominal wall muscles that guard the inguinal canal and skin around the pubis and external genitalia.

Genitofemoral nerve (L1/L2) – descends on the anterior surface of psoas to the abdominal wall. The genital branch passes through the inguinal canal to innervate the cremaster muscle (in the male), whereas the femoral branch passes deep to the inguinal ligament to innervate skin over the genitalia and femoral triangle.

Lumbosacral trunk – emerges from the deep *medial* border of psoas to join the anterior ramus of the S1 nerve anterior to piriformis on the posterior pelvic wall.

Obturator nerve – also emerges from the deep medial border of psoas to run along the side wall of the innominate bone (p. 191) passing through the obturator foramen to enter the medial compartment of the thigh.

Sympathetic trunks (p. 139) – continuing down from the thorax posterior to the diaphragm, these run anterior to the lumbar vertebral column, the left trunk *at the* left margin of the aorta and the right trunk *under cover of* (deep to) the right margin of the inferior vena cava. Branches from the ganglia join lumbar nerves and supply adjacent viscera and blood vessels.

Vagus nerves – entering the abdomen along the oesophagus as the anterior and posterior vagal trunks lying along the lesser curvature of the stomach in the lesser omentum, from which branches pass to the body of the stomach (to stimulate acid secretion) and to the gallbladder.

Abdominal viscera

Most of the abdominal cavity is occupied by viscera that belong to the digestive system (digestive tract, alimentary tract). The whole system comprises the mouth and pharynx (in the head and neck), the oesophagus (mainly in the thorax) and the stomach, small intestine and large intestine, which occupy the abdomen, and its lower part the rectum and anal canal in the pelvis. In the upper abdomen are the liver and pancreas, which are the largest of the digestive glands. The kidneys, which are the principal organs of the urinary system, and the adrenal glands, which are part of the endocrine system, are located posterior to the gastrointestinal system. Finally, the spleen (part of the lymphatic system) lies on the left under the costal margin.

The viscera and their blood supplies are considered individually. Although all receive autonomic nerve supplies, only a few details are clinically important:

- Sympathetic nerves (vasoconstrictor) carry pain fibres.
- Parasympathetic (vagal) fibres to the stomach stimulate motility and acid secretion in particular (also controlled by the hormone gastrin).
- Movement of the rest of the gut (peristalsis) depends on its own intrinsic nerve networks (the enteric plexus) and not on the external nerve supply.
- Lymph drainage, which follows the arteries supplying the structure, is to adjacent nodes, which eventually reach para-aortic nodes and in turn drain to the cisterna chyli (p. 134). Lymph drainage is most important for the stomach and colon (the more common sites for cancer) and for the transport of fat molecules from the small intestine. In the latter, fat is absorbed by the lacteals (lymphatic capillaries) of the gut mucosa and not into the blood capillaries, especially those in the ileum.

Stomach

The stomach, stimulated by the vagus nerves (p. 139), is where protein digestion begins. It is the most dilated part of the alimentary tract, situated between the oesophagus and the duodenum and lying in the epigastrium and left hypochondrium

> The word stomach (as in 'stomach ache') is often used by lay people to mean the abdomen rather than the specific organ.

(Figs. 6.9–6.11). It is roughly J-shaped, with the upper opening at the cardia or gastro-oesophageal junction to the left of the midline at the level of the T11 vertebra, and the lower opening at the pylorus or gastroduodenal junction to the right of the midline at the level of the L1 vertebra (transpyloric plane). The oesophagus joins the stomach at an acute angle (cardia), which has the effect of acting as a valve to prevent gastric contents refluxing into the lower oesophagus. The superior border is the lesser curvature, suspended from the liver by a fold of peritoneum, the lesser omentum (see below). Attached to the inferior border (the greater curvature) is another peritoneal fold, the greater omentum, hanging down like an apron anterior to the coils of intestine. The transverse mesocolon (the peritoneal support for the transverse colon – see below) and the transverse colon adhere to the posterior layer of the greater omentum. Deep to the stomach (and anterior to the pancreas and upper part of the left kidney) there is a peritoneal recess, the lesser sac (properly called the omental bursa); the only opening (like the vertical slot in a coin machine) into this closed space is the epiploic foramen (of Winslow). The relationships

> By placing a finger in the epiploic foramen during surgery it is possible to apply compression to the hepatic artery and portal vein, which run in the free margin of the lesser omentum, to control bleeding from an injured liver (Pringle's manoeuvre).

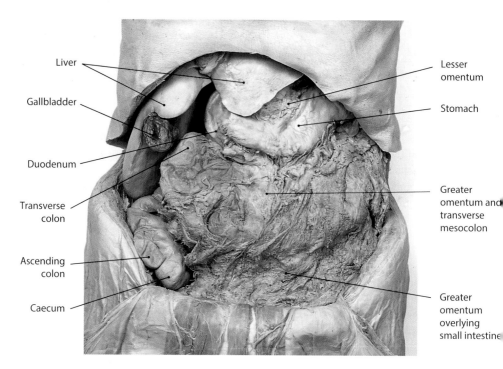

Fig. 6.9 Upper abdominal viscera, with the anterior abdominal wall turned downwards.

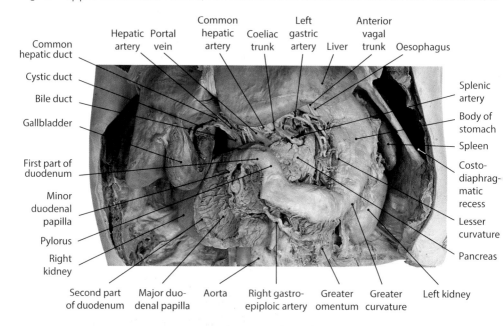

Fig. 6.10 Upper abdominal viscera. The lesser omentum (between the liver and stomach) and most of the greater omentum have been removed, together with part of the anterior wall of the duodenum.

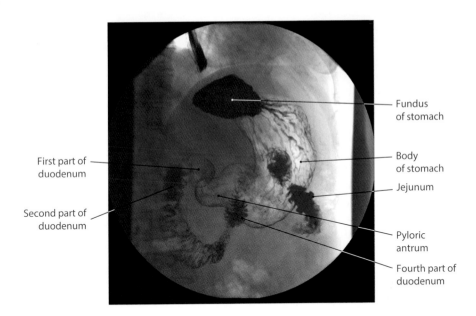

Fundus
of stomach

First part of
duodenum

Body
of stomach

Jejunum

Second part of
duodenum

Pyloric
antrum

Fourth part of
duodenum

Fig. 6.11 Radiographic barium study to demonstrate the stomach, duodenum and proximal jejunum.

of this opening, located on the right of midline, are the free margin of the lesser omentum anteriorly, the inferior vena cava posteriorly, the duodenum inferiorly and the liver superiorly. The lesser sac ensures free movement of the stomach against the structures posterior to it on the posterior abdominal wall.

The stomach has three parts: the fundus on the left (the part cranial to the cardia); the body (main part); and to the right the pyloric part (pyloric antrum, with the pyloric sphincter at the junction with the duodenum).

Blood supply – from the left and right gastric arteries along the lesser curvature, and from the short gastric and left and right gastroepiploic arteries along the greater curvature. Accompanying veins drain to the portal system (**Fig. 6.7**).

Small intestine

The small intestine consists of the duodenum, the jejunum and the ileum. It extends from the pylorus to the ileocaecal junction and is a hose-like tube about 4 m long (although longer after death due to relaxation of the muscular wall) and is concerned with the digestion and absorption of foodstuffs.

Gastric ulcers are treated with antibiotics in cases where they are caused by a bacterium (*H. pylori*) or with drugs to inhibit acid secretion (proton pump inhibitors) Surgical procedures are hardly ever done nowadays.

Cancer of the small intestine is rare; cancer of the stomach, colon and rectum is relatively common. The reason for the difference is not known.

Duodenum – 25 cm (or 12 finger breadths in length, as its name implies) long, is C-shaped, with four parts (usually called first to fourth) that run respectively posteriorly on the right of midline from the pylorus, down on the right of vertebrae L1 and L2, across the midline to the left at L3 and finally up on the left of vertebra L2 (posterior to the stomach), embracing the head of the pancreas and lying at the levels of L1–L3 vertebrae (**Figs. 6.3, 6.10, 6.11, 6.13**). The first part and the end of the fourth part, the duodenojejunal flexure, are intraperitoneal whereas the second, third and part of the fourth part are plastered onto the posterior abdominal wall by peritoneum (i.e. are retroperitoneal). It receives the bile and main pancreatic ducts that join at the hepatopancreatic ampulla (of Vater) embedded in the posteromedial wall of the second part and opening at the major duodenal papilla (**Fig. 6.17**). Occasionally, there may be an adjacent minor duodenal papilla receiving the opening of the accessory pancreatic duct (of Santorini).

> Duodenal ulcers occur in the first part, where acidic gastric contents first contact the bowel wall after passing through the pylorus.

Jejunum and ileum – suspended from the posterior abdominal wall by a fold of peritoneum, the mesentery (**Fig. 6.12**), which is only about 15 cm long at its attachment to the posterior abdominal wall, but becomes immensely frilled at the intestinal attachment. Referred to clinically as the small intestine, there is no clear junction between jejunum and ileum; the slightly thicker jejunum, the proximal two-fifths of the whole tube, is continuous with the fourth part of the duodenum at the duodenojejunal flexure, and the rest is the ileum, which joins the large intestine at the ileocaecal junction. The mesentery contains branches of the superior mesenteric vessels, lymphatics and lymph nodes, nerves and fat. The vessels passing to the mesenteric border of the jejunum have single arcades with long terminal branches, whereas those passing to the ileum have multiple arcades with short terminal branches.

> In 2% of the population there is a 4 cm long pouch (Meckel's diverticulum) located 60 cm proximal to the ileocaecal valve that represents an embryological remnant of the vitelointestinal duct. It may become blocked and inflamed, giving rise to symptoms suggesting appendicitis in the presence of a normal appendix.

Blood supply – of the duodenum down to the opening of the bile and pancreatic ducts, by the superior pancreaticoduodenal branch of the gastroduodenal branch of the common hepatic artery (**Fig. 6.6**). The rest of the duodenum is by the inferior pancreaticoduodenal branch from the superior mesenteric artery and the jejunum and ileum by branches from the left side of the superior mesenteric artery (**Fig. 6.13**). Veins drain to the portal system (**Fig. 6.7**).

Large intestine

The large intestine is involved in water absorption and the storage and evacuation of the waste products of digestion. It consists of the caecum (with the appendix), colon, rectum and anal canal, and is about 1.5 m long from the end of the ileum to the lower opening of the anal canal (anus) (**Figs. 6.12B, 6.14**). Of larger diameter than the small intestine, most of large intestine (caecum and colon) has three longitudinal bands of smooth muscle on the outer surface (taeniae coli) and small fatty tags (appendices epiploices), both of which features instantly distinguish it from the small intestine (**Figs. 6.12–6.14**).

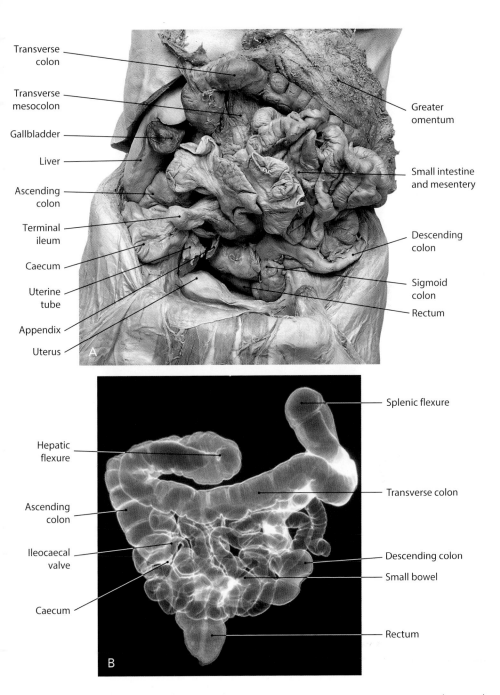

Fig. 6.12 Small and large intestines: (A) the greater omentum, transverse colon and transverse mesocolon have been lifted upwards (over the stomach), so the posterior surfaces of these structures are seen here. Some coils of small intestine have also been displaced upwards to show female pelvic structures, (B) CT colonography illustrating the central small bowel surrounded by the large bowel (green/blue tinged).

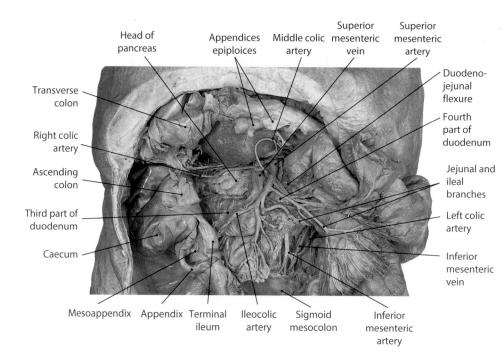

Fig. 6.13 Mesenteric vessels and adjacent viscera. The transverse colon has been lifted upwards and coils of small intestine have been displaced to the left, with the mesentery of the small intestine dissected away to demonstrate the inferior mesenteric vessels.

Caecum – the blind rounded start of the large intestine (**Figs. 6.12, 6.15**), it continues cranially as the ascending colon. The ileum joins on its left (medial) side at the ileocaecal junction. This acts as a one-way valve, allowing passage of contents into the caecum but preventing caecal contents (e.g. faeces or gas) passing into the ileum. The caecum normally lies in the right iliac fossa.

Appendix – (properly called vermiform appendix – worm-like) is a narrow blind-ended tube (the narrowest part of the whole alimentary tract), with its base opening into the caecum 2 cm caudal to the ileocaecal junction (**Figs. 6.12, 6.15**). Its length varies, but is often about 8 cm, with the tip in any position from posterior to the caecum to hanging caudally into the pelvis. It has its own small mesentery, the mesoappendix, containing the appendicular artery (**Fig. 6.15**). The

three taeniae coli (longitudinal muscle) of the caecum all converge onto the base of the appendix – a useful guide to finding it if hidden behind coils of gut.

> Acute appendicitis is the commonest abdominal emergency requiring an operation. It is usually due to the narrow lumen of the appendix becoming blocked, leading to infection and inflammation distal to the blockage.

Colon – consists of ascending, transverse, descending and sigmoid parts (**Figs. 6.9, 6.12, 6.13**). The ascending colon, which is retroperitoneal, continues upwards from the caecum to the liver, where it turns medially at the right colic flexure (hepatic flexure) to become the transverse colon

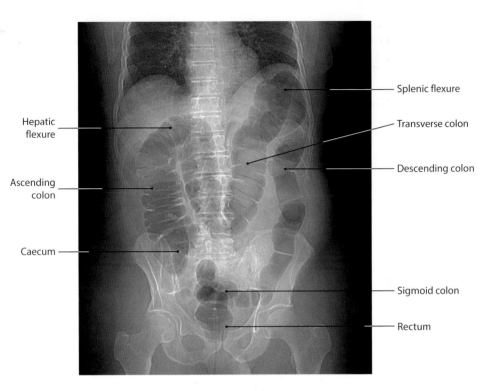

Splenic flexure

Hepatic flexure

Transverse colon

Descending colon

Ascending colon

Caecum

Sigmoid colon

Rectum

Fig. 6.14 MR image (scout colonography) of the colon visualised as air was injected into the colon via the rectum.

(intraperitoneal). This is suspended by peritoneum (transverse mesocolon) from the lower border of the pancreas, which is attached to the deep layer of the greater omentum. At the spleen it turns caudally at the left colic flexure (splenic flexure) as the descending colon (retroperitoneal) to the left iliac fossa, where it regains a mesentery (sigmoid mesocolon) to become the sigmoid colon.

> The sigmoid part is the commonest site for colonic cancer.

Rectum and anal canal – see p. 196.

Blood supply – from caecum to near the splenic flexure by colic branches of the superior mesenteric artery, then the remainder by the inferior mesenteric artery (**Figs. 6.6, 6.13**). These branches all anastomose one with the other to form what is referred to as the marginal artery (of Drummond). The posterior caecal branch of the superior mesenteric gives off the appendicular artery. Veins drain to the portal system (**Fig. 6.7**).

Liver

The liver is the largest gland in the body, with many metabolic and storage functions, including the secretion of bile, which assists in fat digestion. It is wedge-shaped, tapering and extending to the left, largely under the right dome of the diaphragm (**Figs. 6.16, 6.18, 6.19**); it thus lies mostly in the right hypochondrial and epigastric regions. It has peritoneal attachments to the diaphragm (the coronary ligament with triangular

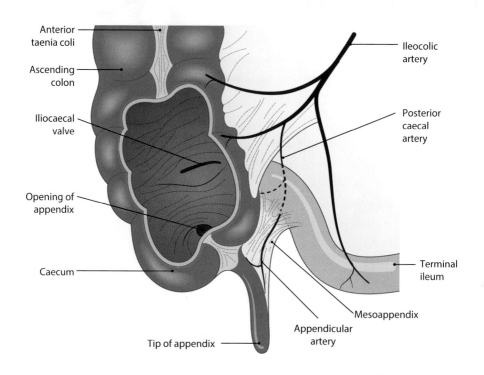

Fig. 6.15 The caecum and appendix, with a window cut in the anterior wall of the caecum.

ligaments at its left and right edges) and anterior abdominal wall (falciform ligament), but is also kept in place by the hepatic veins that run directly into the inferior vena cava from the bare area (posterior part of liver with no peritoneal covering) lying in a deep groove on the posterior aspect of the liver. It has a large right and a small left lobe, but the caudate and quadrate lobes, which topographically are part of right lobe, are *functionally* part of the left lobe because, like the left lobe, they receive their blood supply from *left* branches of the hepatic artery and portal vein; the main part of the right lobe receives blood from the right branches of these vessels. The caudal (inferior) surface, also known as the visceral surface, has near its centre the porta hepatis, where vessels and ducts enter and leave. The lesser omentum, the peritoneal fold that runs between the stomach and liver, is attached to the

margins of the porta hepatis. Running in the right margin of the lesser omentum is the hepatoduodenal ligament in which lies the portal vein (posteriorly), hepatic artery (anteriorly) and bile duct (below and **Fig. 6.10**).

Note: The liver can be divided into 10 'lobes', knowledge of which is used when doing a partial liver transplant, especially from a living donor.

Blood supply – by the hepatic artery for arterial blood (~20%) and by the portal vein for portal blood (~80%) from the alimentary tract and spleen (**Figs. 6.6, 6.7**). The right and left branches of these vessels enter at the porta hepatis. Three or more hepatic veins drain posteriorly directly into

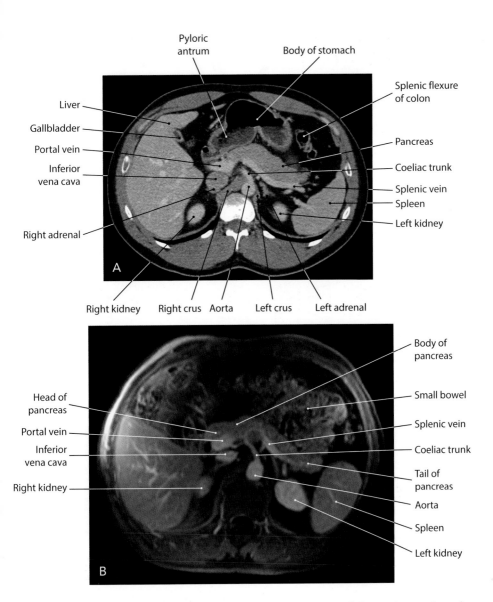

Figs. 6.16 Axial images of the upper abdomen at the level of the T12 vertebra, from below: (A) CT image, (B) MR image for comparison.

the inferior vena cava (not via the porta hepatis) and are hidden from an anterior view unless the liver is removed.

Gallbladder and biliary tract

Bile from liver cells reaches the right and left hepatic ducts, which leave the liver at the porta hepatis and unite to form the common hepatic duct, which is joined by the cystic duct from the gallbladder to form the common bile duct (**Figs. 6.10, 6.17**) lying in the free edge of the lesser omentum along with the hepatic artery and the portal vein.

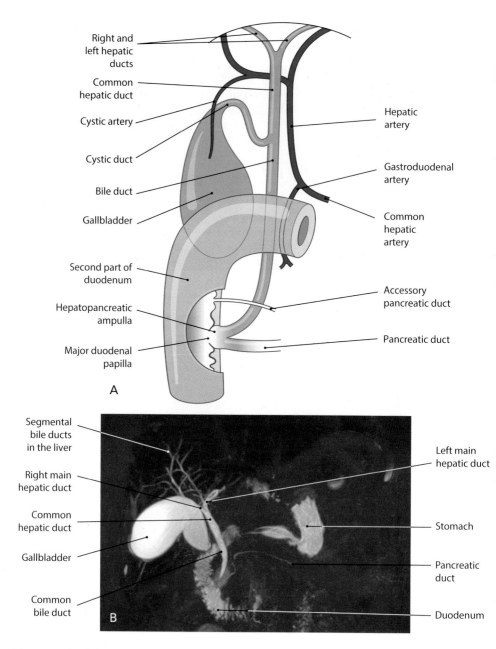

Right and left hepatic ducts

Common hepatic duct

Cystic artery

Cystic duct

Bile duct

Gallbladder

Second part of duodenum

Hepatopancreatic ampulla

Major duodenal papilla

Hepatic artery

Gastroduodenal artery

Common hepatic artery

Accessory pancreatic duct

Pancreatic duct

A

Segmental bile ducts in the liver

Right main hepatic duct

Common hepatic duct

Gallbladder

Common bile duct

Left main hepatic duct

Stomach

Pancreatic duct

Duodenum

B

Fig. 6.17 The biliary tract: (A) diagram with a window cut in the second part of the duodenum, (B) MR retrograde cholecystopancreatogram (note: the cystic duct is not visible).

Gallbladder – where bile is concentrated, stored and released under the influence of an intestinal hormone. The gallbladder is pear-shaped and about 10 cm long, attached to the visceral surface of the right lobe of the liver, with the lowest part, the fundus, lying against the anterior abdominal wall where the right margin of the rectus sheath meets the costal

> The right ninth costal margin is the region of abdominal pain and tenderness in gallbladder disease.

margin (ninth costal cartilage). Posteriorly, the fundus overlaps the junction of the first and second parts of the duodenum (hence the green postmortem staining of this part of the gut by bile that seeps through the gallbladder wall), and a high transverse colon may lie just below the fundus.

> Stones (calculi) in the gallbladder (gallstones) may escape into the cystic and bile ducts and cause spasms of pain (biliary colic). They are not usually visible unless a contrast medium is used in a radiological examination.

Bile duct – about 8 cm long and 8 mm in diameter, it lies in the right margin of the lesser omentum, where it lies anterior to the portal vein, with the hepatic artery on the duct's left side. Correct identification of the bile duct and adjacent structures is vital to the understanding of diseases of, and operations on, the stomach, duodenum, pancreas, liver and biliary tract. The bile duct then passes posterior to the first part of the duodenum to reach the second part, where it enters the posteromedial part of the wall to join the pancreatic duct at the hepatopancreatic ampulla (of Vater), which opens at the major duodenal papilla (about 10 cm distal to the pylorus).

> One of the most important areas in the whole abdomen. Obstruction of the bile duct (e.g. by a gallstone or cancer of the head of the pancreas) is one cause of jaundice (yellow pigmentation of the skin and cornea).

Blood supply – the gallbladder receives the cystic artery, which is normally a branch of the right hepatic artery and must be correctly identified prior to removal of the gallbladder (cholecystectomy). It supplements small vessels passing from the gallbladder bed of the liver to the gallbladder. The cystic artery is highly variable and has been described passing from most of the surrounding vessels. Because of this special care must be taken to identify it during cholecystectomy in order to avoid ligating the hepatic artery (in error). Usually venous blood from the gallbladder drains through a series of small veins directly into the liver (gallbladder bed); a cystic vein draining to the right branch of the portal vein is uncommon (**Figs. 6.6, 6.7**). The bile duct is supplied by branches from the gastroduodenal and hepatic vessels.

Pancreas

The pancreas secretes (under the control of intestinal hormones) digestive enzymes and also has endocrine cells (in the pancreatic islets of Langerhans) whose products, mainly insulin and glucagon, are essential for carbohydrate metabolism. It is a hook-shaped gland, about 15 cm long, that lies transversely across the upper abdomen, with the head in the C-shaped curve of the duodenum, extending to the left deep (posterior) to the stomach as the body before ending as the pancreatic tail near the hilum of the spleen (**Figs. 6.10, 6.13, 6.16, 6.18**). Inferiorly the head has a small process projecting to the left and lying deep to the superior mesenteric artery (uncinate process). It is retroperitoneal, with the transverse mesocolon attached in a line from the lower border.

The main pancreatic duct (of Wirsung) runs from the tail to the lower part of the head and normally joins the bile duct at the hepatopancreatic ampulla

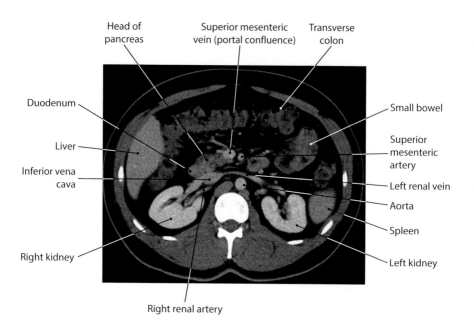

Fig. 6.18 Axial CT scan of the upper abdomen through the L1 vertebra, from below.

> Carcinoma of the head of pancreas may compress the bile duct, causing obstructive jaundice. Conversely, a gallstone may block the ampulla and give rise to pancreatitis.

(of Vater). Interestingly, in a small number of individuals an accessory pancreatic duct (of Santorini) runs from the lower part of the head and uncinate process into the duodenum, about 2 cm proximal to the main duct (**Fig. 6.17**). These may be so close they appear as one, or may be separate. This is useful to remember when reviewing radiological investigations of the pancreatic duct system. The ducts convey the pancreatic enzymes concerned with digestion; the endocrine secretions from the islets are secreted directly into the venous blood.

Blood supply – mainly from the splenic artery, which runs just posterior to

the upper border of the pancreas, with some branches from the superior mesenteric artery to its head (**Fig. 6.6**). Veins drain to the portal system (**Figs. 6.7, 6.16**).

> It is worth remembering that the superior mesenteric artery commences posterior to the pancreas but then lies anterior to the uncinated process as it passes distally, especially when reviewing CT scans of the upper abdomen.

Nerve supply – there are relatively few autonomic nerves to the pancreas. This is of clinical importance because cancer of the pancreas usually does not present symptoms such as pain until the pathology is advanced. This may be the reason that pancreatic cancer typically has a poor prognosis.

Kidneys and ureters

The urinary system in both sexes consists of the kidneys, ureters, urinary bladder and urethra, all concerned with the production, storage and elimination of urine.

The main function of the kidneys is to produce urine, so maintaining the body's fluids and electrolytes in their proper concentrations and helping to keep blood pressure within normal limits, a state of homeostasis. Each kidney is about 12 cm long, 6 cm wide and 4 cm thick. They lie posteriorly in the peritoneum in the 'paravertebral gutters' at the sides of the vertebral column (**Figs. 6.4, 6.18, 6.19**) and are surrounded by a special layer of perinephric fat and fascia. The upper pole of the left kidney rises as high as the eleventh rib, with the diaphragm and the lowest part of the pleural cavity intervening; the right kidney only rises as high as the twelfth rib (due to the bulk of the liver on the right). The hilum of the kidney (a notch on the medial aspect, where vessels and ureter enter or leave) varies but is usually on a level with the intervertebral disc between the first and second lumbar vertebra (but can be as high as just above the transpyloric plane on the left and just below the transpyloric plane on the right); on each side it lies 5 cm from the midline. The second part of the duodenum overlies the hilum on the right side; the body of the pancreas crosses the left hilum or upper pole.

> Occasionally, in a healthy individual, the kidney can be found in the iliac fossa because it did not ascend as usual during development; in this location it is referred to as a pelvic kidney.

The ureter, which conducts urine from the kidney to the bladder, runs down posterior to the peritoneum lying on psoas major, to enter the pelvis by crossing anterior to the origin of the external iliac vessels level with the sacroiliac joint. The expanded upper end of the ureter (the part that leaves the hilum of the kidney) is the renal pelvis and is normally level with the first lumbar intervertebral disc, but could be higher or lower.

> Using contrast radiography of the renal tract the ureters run distally level with the tips of the vertebral transverse processes. Any displacement from this position suggests some retroperitoneal pathology.

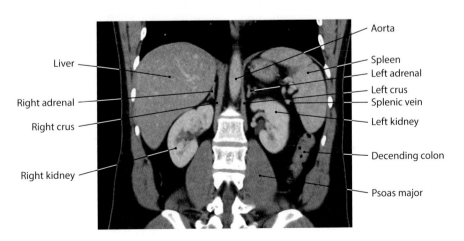

Fig. 6.19 Coronal CT scan of the posterior abdominal wall demonstrating the organs.

Blood supply – from the paired large renal arteries that leave the aorta at right angles. Usually a single vessel on each side running into the hilum, where each divides into several branches (**Fig. 6.6**). The origin of the renal arteries, usually level with the upper border of the second lumbar artery, but can arise anywhere between here and level with the origin of the superior mesenteric artery at the upper border of the first lumbar vertebra. Occasionally, one or more accessory renal arteries are seen leaving the aorta caudal to the main renal artery and run to supply the lower pole. Veins unite in the hilum to form the single renal vein that drains to the inferior vena cava (**Figs. 6.4, 6.8**); the left renal vein crosses anterior to the aorta to reach the inferior vena cava (**Fig. 6.18**). Branches from the renal, gonadal, iliac and vesical vessels supply the adjacent parts of the ureter, depending on the level.

Adrenal glands

The adrenal (suprarenal) glands (**Figs. 6.4, 6.16, 6.19**) are endocrine organs with two distinct parts: an outer cortex that produces hormones, such as cortisol, concerned with blood and fluid volumes and their electrolyte contents; and an inner medulla, which secretes the hormones noradrenaline and adrenaline (catecholamines), which are part of the activity of the sympathetic nervous system and act systemically via a hormonal process rather than via nerves directed to a target organ. The right suprarenal gland is shaped like a three-sided pyramid, about 3 cm high and 3 cm thick, that lies partly behind the peritoneum against the upper pole of the right kidney, but with its uppermost part in contact with the posterior aspect of the liver. The left gland, often more crescentic in shape, is posterior to the peritoneum of the lesser sac (see above), on the medial side of the left kidney above the hilum. The adrenal chromaffin cells of the medulla are modified post-ganglionic sympathetic neurons

that receive preganglionic sympathetic fibres directly from lateral horn cells (p. 9).

Blood supply – several small arteries from the inferior phrenic, aorta and renal (from superior to inferior) arteries. There is usually only one vein on each side; on the right it is very short and runs directly into the inferior vena cava, which is just beside the gland, but on the left it is longer and drains into the left renal vein, although veins from each gland can follow the arteries that supply it (**Fig. 6.8**).

> Surgery to remove a tumour of the adrenal medulla (phaeochromocytoma) normally isolates the blood supply before the gland is touched. This is especially important as they are hormone producing and handling the gland before the blood supply is controlled results in a surge of adrenaline or noradrenaline, which may lead to a dangerous rise in blood pressure.

Spleen

The spleen, the largest of the lymphoid organs, lies tucked up against the left half of the diaphragm (which separates it from the pleura and ribs 9–11), along the upper pole of the left kidney and posterior to the stomach (**Figs. 6.16, 6.18, 6.19**). It is surrounded by peritoneum whose folds (splenorenal ligament and gastrosplenic ligament) anchor it to the kidney and stomach, respectively.

Blood supply – by the splenic artery, often a tortuous vessel running posterior to the upper border of the pancreas (**Fig. 6.10**). The straighter splenic vein runs posterior to the pancreas to the right to join the superior mesenteric vein and form the portal vein (**Figs. 6.7, 6.16**). Thus, although the spleen is not part of the alimentary tract, its blood unexpectedly drains to the portal system, perhaps explained as it develops in association with structures of the foregut, hence sharing a common blood supply. Functionally, the spleen breaks down red blood cells and the liver processes those breakdown products.

Summary

- The *umbilicus* normally lies at the level of the disc between vertebrae L3 and L4, and most of the important abdominal structures lie superior to this level. The other important area is the *right iliac fossa*, where the pain of appendicitis becomes localised.
- The *hilum of each kidney* is about 5 cm from the midline, just cranial to and just caudal to the transpyloric plane on the left and right, respectively. The usual order of structures at the hilum is vein, artery, ureter from anterior to posterior. The *adrenal glands* are found against the upper and medial part of each kidney.
- The C-shaped curve of the *duodenum* lies between the levels of vertebrae L1 and L3, and embraces the head of the pancreas, whose body and tail pass to the left across the left kidney to the hilum of the spleen.
- The *lesser omentum* of peritoneum runs from the liver to the lesser curvature of the stomach, and contains in its right free margin the portal vein with the bile duct anterior to the right edge of the vein and the hepatic artery to the left of the duct.
- The *bile duct* is formed cranial to the first part of the duodenum by the union of the cystic duct from the gallbladder with the common hepatic duct, which resulted from the union of the right and left hepatic ducts that emerge from the visceral surface of the liver.
- The *caudate* and *quadrate lobes of the liver* belong functionally to the left lobe; they receive blood from the left branches of the hepatic artery and portal vein, and drain bile to the left hepatic duct. The right branches supply the right lobe, and bile drains to the right hepatic duct.
- The three large unpaired branches from the anterior of the abdominal aorta are those that supply gut: *coeliac trunk* at T12 (from lower oesophagus to where the bile duct enters the duodenum), *superior mesenteric artery* at L1 (from duodenum to near the splenic flexure of the colon) and *inferior mesenteric artery* at L3 (from splenic flexure to the upper part of the anal canal). The above areas of supply, supplemented by the splenic vein, comprise the drainage area of the portal vein.
- Of the main tributaries of the inferior vena cava, those most frequently overlooked are the *hepatic veins*; they have no extrahepatic course and cannot be seen unless the liver is removed.
- The most important site of *portal–systemic anastomosis* is the lower end of the oesophagus, where enlarged veins may burst (oesophageal varicies).
- The left and right *gastric arteries* anastomose along the lesser curvature of the stomach, and the left and right *gastroepiploic arteries* anastomose along the greater curvature; the short *gastric arteries* supply the fundus.
- The main blood supply to the pancreas is the *splenic artery*, with the smaller pancreaticoduodenal vessels supplying the head.

Continued

Continued

- The root of the *mesentery of the small intestine* (15 cm in length) runs from the duodenojejunal flexure downwards and to the right towards the right iliac fossa.
- The transverse colon and sigmoid colon have their own mesenteries (*transverse mesocolon* and *sigmoid mesocolon*), but the ascending and descending colon are retroperitoneal.
- *McBurney's point*, a third of the way along a line from the anterior superior iliac spine to the umbilicus, is the point of maximum tenderness in a patient with appendicitis. It indicates the position of the base of the appendix, where it opens into the caecum; the tip of the appendix is very variable in position.

Questions

Answers can be found in Appendix A, p. 247.

Question 1

When operating on the inguinal canal to repair a hernia it is important for the surgeon to understand the relevant anatomy. Identify which wall is being described if it is composed of medially the conjoint tendon and transversalis fascia throughout.

(a) Anterior wall.

(b) Roof.

(c) Posterior wall.

(d) Floor.

(e) Lateral wall.

Question 2

An indirect inguinal hernia emerges through the deep inguinal ring. Identify in the statement below the correct description of the point of emergence of an indirect inguinal hernia.

(a) Above and medial to the pubic tubercle.

(b) Above and lateral to the pubic tubercle.

(c) Below and lateral to the pubic tubercle.

(d) Below and medial to the pubic tubercle.

(e) Midpoint of the inguinal ligament.

Question 3

When examining the abdomen it is useful to be able to relate internal structures to the abdominal wall. Which statement below gives the most accurate normal relationship?

(a) In the pubic region, the abdominal aorta divides to form common iliac arteries at the fifth lumbar vertebral body.

(b) The origin of the femoral artery occurs at the level of the superficial inguinal ring.

(c) The hilum of both kidneys, the pancreas and the first part of the duodenum all lie along the transpyloric plane.

(d) On the posterior abdominal wall, the ureter, as it passes distally, runs along the tips of the transverse processes and crosses the sacroiliac joint deep to the bifurcation of the common iliac arteries.

(e) The spleen is palpable under the right costal margin level with the 9th costal cartilage.

Question 4

All the structures located in the abdomen have relationships to the surrounding structures. In the statements below, identify the one that gives the most accurate description of normally expected relationships.

(a) Lying along the lesser curvature of the stomach are the gastric branches of the vagus nerve accompanied by the left gastroepiploic artery.

(b) The body of the gallbladder is normally related posteriorly to the third part of the duodenum and the fundus lies in contact with the ascending colon.

(c) The right renal vein lies in the transverse plane anterior to the aorta before entering the inferior vena cava.

(d) The left adrenal gland lies lateral to psoas at the upper border of L1 and anterior to the upper pole of the left kidney.

(e) The epiploic foramen lies anterior to the inferior vena cava with the liver above and the ascending colon below. In its free edge lies the common bile duct and right colic artery anterior to the hepatic vein.

Question 5

With regard to the intestinal tract, which of the statements below best describes the feature seen in the majority of individuals?

(a) The appendices epiploicae are all small pouches of colonic mucosa located along the ante-mesenteric border of the colon and are a distinguishing feature.

(b) The taenia coli are found as three discrete bundles of smooth muscle along the length of the colon and are not found on the caecum, where they form a complete sheet of muscle.

(c) The greater omentum attaches cranially to the greater curvature of the stomach lying anterior to all of the small intestine. It is mobile and is often referred to as the 'policeman of the abdomen', as it tends to wrap around areas of inflammation within the peritoneal cavity.

(d) Meckel's diverticulum is normally present and is located 60 cm proximal to the ileocaecal valve in the left iliac fossa.

(e) The porta hepatis is located to the left of mid-line and marks the position where the greater omentum joins the lesser curvature of the stomach to the visceral surface of the liver.

Question 6

The abdominal aorta is located on the posterior abdominal wall and gives rise to a number of important branches. Which statement below best describes the normal anatomy related to this vessel?

(a) It commences in the abdomen at the lower border of the diaphragm at the level of the lower edge of the first lumbar vertebral body.

(b) The inferior mesenteric artery is an unpaired artery that passes to the right to supply the descending colon lying in the related iliac fossa.

(c) The gonadal arteries are paired branches arising from the aorta at the level of the third lumbar vertebra and lie anterior to the branches of the two mesenteric arteries as they pass laterally to supply the colon.

(d) The left renal vein passes anterior to the aorta as it passes to the inferior vena cava from the hilum of the left kidney.

(e) The coeliac artery, one of the four unpaired branches, running anteriorly to supply the foregut through its main branches, the left gastric, splenic and common hepatic artery.

Question 7

An 85-year-old woman is admitted with a 24-hour history of abdominal pain. At laparotomy she is found to have an infarction of the proximal jejunum due to thrombosis in branches of a major artery. Which artery is most likely to be involved?

(a) Coeliac axis.

(b) Superior mesenteric.

(c) Inferior mesenteric.

(d) Inferior pancreaticoduodenal.

(e) Gastroduodenal.

Question 8

In tall thin patients, the superior mesenteric artery may compress a vein that crosses the midline behind this artery. Which of the following veins is most likely to be compressed between the superior mesenteric artery and the aorta?

(a) Left hepatic vein.

(b) Right adrenal vein.

(c) Left renal vein.

(d) Right gonadal vein.

(e) Left common iliac vein.

Question 9

A slightly overweight 58-year old patient is diagnosed with gallbladder disease. Her presenting pain is most likely to be in the:

(a) Right hypochondrium.

(b) Right lumbar region.

(c) Right iliac region.

(d) Epigastrium.

(e) Left hypochondrium.

Question 10

An infant male is diagnosed with a congenital (indirect) inguinal hernia? The hernia sac is most likely to begin at the:

(a) Anterior superior iliac spine.

(b) Deep inguinal ring.

(c) Inguinal canal.

(d) Superficial inguinal ring.

(e) Femoral ring.

Question 11

A 55-year-old homeless male presents in the Emergency Department vomiting dark red blood. On physical examination he is found to have an enlarged, hard liver. From which of the following vessels is he most likely bleeding?

(a) Cystic vein.

(b) Common hepatic artery.

(c) Portal vein.

(d) Superior mesenteric vein.

(e) Oesophageal vein.

Question 12

A 50-year-old woman presents with painless jaundice. Which of the following diagnoses is most likely?

(a) Renal calculus (kidney stone).

(b) Appendicitis.

(c) Tumour in the head of the pancreas.

(d) Inguinal hernia.

(e) Gastric ulcer.

Question 13

An 18-year-old female comes to the Emergency Department complaining of epigastric pain. She has a fever and laboratory tests show an elevated white blood cell count. After 12 hours of observation, the pain suddenly shifts to the right lower quadrant. Which of the following diagnoses is most likely to be confirmed?

a) Biliary stone.

b) Gastric ulcer.

c) Appendicitis.

d) Renal colic.

e) Infarcted small bowel.

Question 14

A 20-year-old woman deliberately goes on an extreme diet and loses a great deal of weight. She now comes to the clinic complaining of nausea, vomiting, severe pain after eating and diarrhoea. A diagnosis of superior mesenteric artery (SMA) syndrome is made. Which of the following structures is most likely compressed between the SMA and the aorta?

(a) Pylorus.

(b) Gallbladder.

(c) Right renal vein.

(d) Third part of the duodenum.

(e) Left common iliac vein.

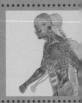
Introduction

The word pelvis, as in bony pelvis, means a basin, but it can also be used as a term to mean the lower part of the abdominal cavity. When in the anatomical position, the bony pelvis is structured so that body weight is transmitted from the vertebral column to the lower limbs through the bony pelvis. In addition, in the female the lower aperture of the bony pelvis must provide sufficient accommodation for the passage of a foetus on its birth journey to become a newborn child in a vaginal delivery.

The bony pelvis – consists of the sacrum and coccyx posteriorly, which unite at each side with the hip bone (old name: innominate) at the sacroiliac joint (**Figs. 7.1, 7.2**).

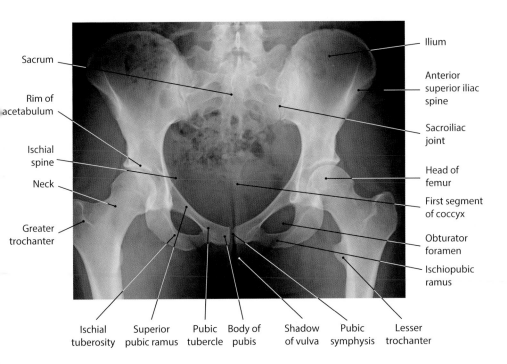

Sacrum

Rim of acetabulum

Ischial spine

Neck

Greater trochanter

Ilium

Anterior superior iliac spine

Sacroiliac joint

Head of femur

First segment of coccyx

Obturator foramen

Ischiopubic ramus

Ischial tuberosity · Superior pubic ramus · Pubic tubercle · Body of pubis · Shadow of vulva · Pubic symphysis · Lesser trochanter

Fig. 7.1 Anteroposterior radiograph of the female pelvis.

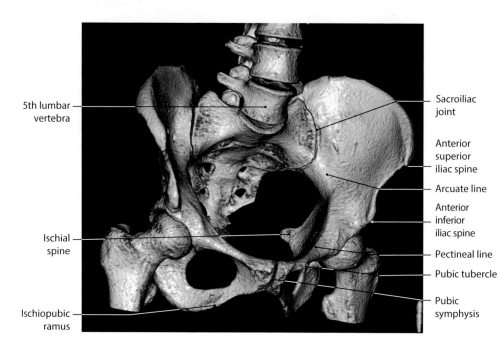

5th lumbar vertebra

Ischial spine

Ischiopubic ramus

Sacroiliac joint

Anterior superior iliac spine

Arcuate line

Anterior inferior iliac spine

Pectineal line

Pubic tubercle

Pubic symphysis

Fig. 7.2 Oblique reformat, from CT of the abdomen, demonstrating features on the medial side of the innominate bone.

The hip bone is formed from three fused bones: the ilium, the ischium and the pubis. Anteriorly the two hip bones join at the pubic symphysis. The pelvic brim (or pelvic inlet) is formed by the superior edge of the sacrum (with the sacral promontory in the midline), the arcuate line of the ilium, the superior ramus and body of the pubis and the pubic symphysis; this is the boundary between the true pelvis or pelvic cavity, inferior to the brim, and the false pelvis, bounded laterally by the wings of the ilium, which is the part above the brim and more properly belongs to the abdominal cavity. **Note:** When the bony pelvis is correctly orientated, it is tilted forwards so that the anterior superior iliac spines and the superior aspect of the pubic symphysis are in the same vertical plane (as when holding the bony pelvis against a wall with these bony points touching the wall). The pelvic cavity runs posteriorly almost at a right angle to the abdominal cavity.

Pelvic muscles – several are located within the pelvic cavity. On the anterior aspect of the sacrum, on each side, is piriformis and lying laterally on the inner aspect of the hip bone is obturator internus; both muscles belong to the gluteal region of the lower limb as lateral rotators of the hip joint. In contrast, levator ani and coccygeus form the highly important pelvic floor or pelvic diaphragm designed to retain abdominal and pelvic structures within the peritoneal cavity.

The muscular pelvic diaphragm must not be confused with the fibrous urogenital diaphragm (p. 194), which contains the external urethral sphincter.

Pelvic nerves – the sacral plexus (**Fig. 3.20**) lies anterior to piriformis; most of its branches are examined in dissections of the gluteal region or radiologically (**Figs. 7.3, 8.5**). The sacral parts of the sympathetic

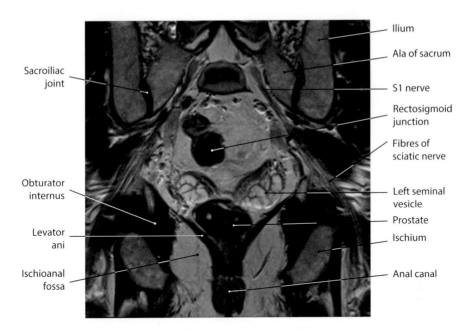

Fig. 7.3 Coronal MR image of the male pelvis demonstrating the levator ani.

trunks lie medial to the anterior sacral foramina and S2–S4 nerves give off parasympathetic branches. The internal iliac vessels and their branches lie anterior to the nerves and supply the pelvic viscera (**Figs. 7.4A, 7.5A**), although the ovarian artery arises superiorly from the abdominal aorta and reaches the ovary through its own fold of peritoneum, the suspensory ligament of the ovary. The corresponding testicular artery is part of the spermatic cord in the inguinal canal.

Perineum – found below the pelvic diaphragm, it is the very lowest part of the trunk in both sexes. It contains the external genital organs, some small perineal muscles and the voluntarily controlled external anal and urethral sphincters.

Viewed from below the perineum is diamond-shaped, bounded by the pubic symphysis anteriorly, the ischial tuberosities laterally and the coccyx posteriorly (**Figs. 7.6, 7.7**). It is divided into two triangles by a line joining the ischial tuberosities. Posteriorly, containing the opening of the anal canal (anus), is the anal region/triangle, and anteriorly, containing the external genital organs, is the urogenital region/triangle.

The male external genital organs are the scrotum (containing the testis, epididymis and start of the ductus deferens) and penis. The female external genital organs consist of the mons pubis, the paired labia majora and labia minora, the bulb of the vestibule, the vestibule of the vagina and the clitoris; collectively, they form the vulva.

The hip (innominate) bone – superiorly lies the crest of the ilium, which terminates anteriorly as the anterior superior iliac spine and just inferior to which is the anterior inferior iliac spine (**Figs. 7.1, 7.2**). On the inner aspect of the ilium, level with the acetabulum, lies an edge, the arcuate line. The pubic bone anteriorly has on its superior edge a swelling, the pubic

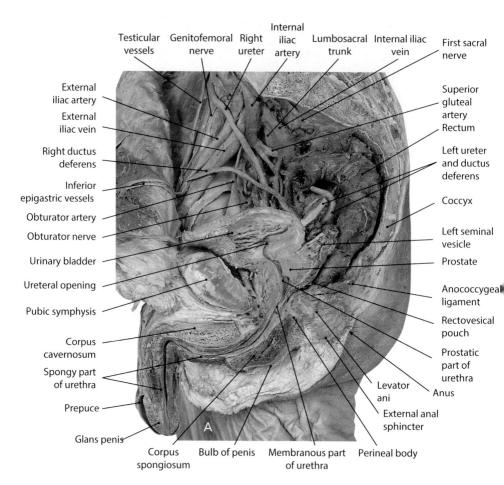

Internal
Testicular Genitofemoral Right iliac Lumbosacral Internal iliac First sacral
vessels nerve ureter artery trunk vein nerve

External
iliac artery

External
iliac vein

Right ductus
deferens

Inferior
epigastric vessels

Obturator artery

Obturator nerve

Urinary bladder

Ureteral opening

Pubic symphysis

Corpus
cavernosum

Spongy part
of urethra

Prepuce

Glans penis

Superior
gluteal
artery

Rectum

Left ureter
and ductus
deferens

Coccyx

Left seminal
vesicle

Prostate

Anococcygeal
ligament

Rectovesical
pouch

Prostatic
part of
urethra

Levator
ani Anus

External anal
sphincter

A

Corpus Bulb of penis Membranous part Perineal body
spongiosum of urethra

Fig. 7.4 (A) Right half of a sagittal section of the male pelvis. The cut has passed through the whole length of the urethra, but the rectum and anal canal have not been sectioned and the external anal sphincter covers the left side of the anal canal. The lower ends of the left ureter and ductus deferens are seen, together with part of the left seminal vesicle.

(Continued)

tubercle, and two extensions projecting laterally – the superior and inferior rami. Posteriorly and inferior to the ilium lies the ischium, formed by a tubercle, on which we sit, a spine projecting medially and an inferior ramus. The large opening within is the obturator foramen, mostly closed by the obturator membrane, which has a small gap, the obturator canal, superiorly. Posteriorly between the ischium, ilium and sacrum lies the greater and lesser sciatic notches, turned into foramina by the sacro-spinous and sacrotuberous ligaments.

Piriformis – arises from the middle three segments of the anterior of the sacrum and runs laterally to leave the pelvis through the greater sciatic foramen and become attached to the medial aspect of the greater trochanter of the femur (**Fig. 8.5**). It is a lateral rotator of the femur and is important as a landmark in the gluteal region (p. 215).

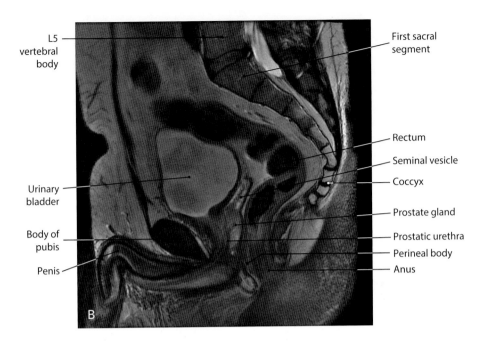

L5 vertebral body

First sacral segment

Rectum

Seminal vesicle

Coccyx

Urinary bladder

Prostate gland

Body of pubis

Prostatic urethra

Perineal body

Penis

Anus

B

Fig. 7.4 *(Continued)* (B) Sagittal MR image of a male pelvis.

Obturator internus – arises from the lateral wall of the inside of the pelvis and the obturator membrane (**Figs. 7.3, 7.8**), and turns at 90° through the lesser sciatic notch, between the ischial tuberosity and spine, to reach the medial aspect of the greater trochanter of the femur. The obturator nerve runs below the pelvic brim to pass into the thigh through the obturator canal on the upper edge of this muscle.

Coccygeus – is really the anterior muscular part of the sacrospinous ligament, passing from the coccyx and ligament to the ischial spine and forming the posterior part of its own half of the pelvic floor.

Levator ani – this pair of muscles form most of the pelvic floor (**Figs. 7.3, 7.4A, 7.5A, 7.6A, 7.7A**). The levator ani has two bony attachments: anteriorly to the body of the pubis, and posterolaterally to the ischial spine. In between the bony attachments, it arises from a thickening

> Stretching of the pelvic floor during childbirth (parturition) may lead to urinary incontinence (e.g. when coughing, which suddenly increases abdominal pressure).

in the fascia that overlies the obturator internus muscle – the tendinous arch of the levator ani. The front half of the levator ani is often called the pubococcygeus and the rest of it the iliococcygeus. The muscle fibres run downwards, inwards (medially) and posteriorly to form a gutter, which converges on the midline raphe containing the perineal body (see below), the anococcygeal body, and the coccyx, but there is a gap anteriorly between the medial borders of each muscle, through which passes the urethra, while the anal canal passes through the muscle in both sexes. In the female, the vagina lies just posterior to the urethra and anterior to the perineal body. The most anterior of the medial fibres of pubococcygeus attach the pubis to the perineal body to form the levator prostatae muscle, below the male prostate; similar fibres in the female constitute the pubovaginalis muscle, which acts as a vaginal sphincter and assists in maintaining urinary continence. The next thickened group of these medial fibres unite with their fellows of the opposite side, attaching at the perineal body, anococcygeal body and the anal sphincters in between, so forming the important puboanalis (puborectalis) muscle, a sling around the anorectal junction that maintains an angle of about 120° between, the rectum and anal canal (see below) to maintain faecal continence. The innervation of the levator ani is by S3 and S4 nerves.

> Patients who suffer from faecal incontinence may be taught 'pelvic exercises' to strengthen the perineal muscles in order improve their symptoms.

Pelvic splanchnic nerves – parasympathetic branches from S2–S4 nerves that innervate the pelvic viscera. In particular, they are the motor nerves to the smooth muscle of the bladder (detrusor), cause relaxation of the internal urethral (involuntary) sphincter and are also responsible for the vasodilatation that causes vascular congestion of the erectile tissue located in the perineum for the male penis and female clitoris (hence their old Latin name: *nervi erigentes*).

Perineal body – a mass of midline tissue (old name: central perineal tendon) anterior to the anus (**Fig. 7.4**) and so in the female between the anus and the vagina (**Fig. 7.5**).

> Obstetricians and gynaecologists use the term 'perineum' in a restricted sense to mean the perineal body and not the whole of the genital and anal regions, as defined anatomically.

Anococcygeal body (ligament) – similar midline tissue between the anus and coccyx.

Ischioanal fossa – the fat-filled space (formerly called the ischiorectal fossa) below the pelvic diaphragm on either side of the anal canal (**Figs. 7.3, 7.6–7.8**), together forming the anal triangle of the perineum. In the lateral wall of the fossa, against the ischial tuberosity and obturator internus, is the pudendal (Alcock's) canal, a fascial channel through which runs vessels and nerves that supply the perineum. Crossing the fossa from lateral to medial are the inferior rectal nerve and accompanying vessels passing to innervate the external anal sphincters. The fossa allows distension of the anal canal during defaecation. In the female the fossa also facilitates the great expansion of the vagina during childbirth.

> The ischioanal fossa is a common site for abscesses to occur. Care must be taken when draining an abscess as damage to the innervation of the anal sphincters will result in faecal incontinence.

Urogenital triangle – the anterior part of the perineum and forming its floor is the urogenital diaphragm, a sheet of fascia joining the ischiopubic rami together. Between this fascia and the more superficial skin is the superficial perineal pouch. However, the

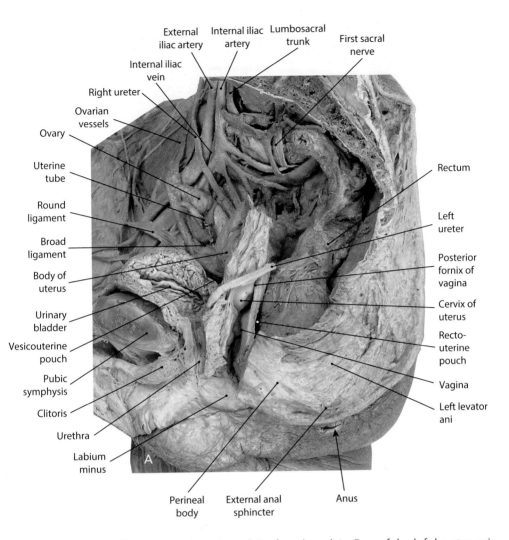

Figs. 7.5 (A) Right half of a sagittal section of the female pelvis. Part of the left levator ani muscle overlies the lower end of the rectum and blends with the left side of the external anal sphincter. The vagina has been opened to show the cervix of the uterus, and the lower part of the left ureter has been dissected out as it passes through the bladder wall.

(Continued)

urogenital diaphragm can be thought of as containing a space, known as the deep perineal pouch, where the important voluntarily controlled sphincter urethrae (external urethral sphincter), through which the urethra passes, is located. Posteriorly the urogenital diaphragm has a free edge to which attaches the posterior edge of the membranous fascia (which lies just deep to the skin over the urogenital skin, closing off the superficial perineal pouch [space]), which contains the erectile tissues that attach to the inferior layer of the diaphragm (see below) and, in the male, to the testis.

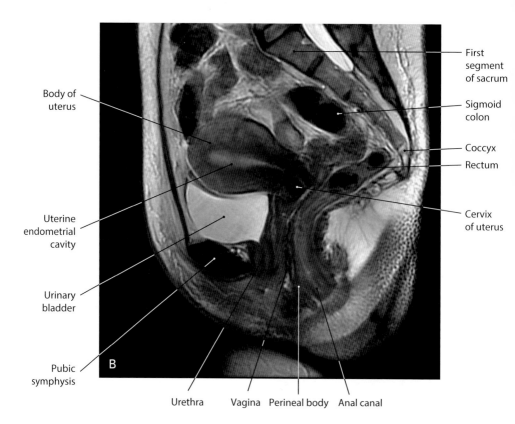

Body of
uterus

First
segment
of sacrum

Sigmoid
colon

Coccyx

Rectum

Uterine
endometrial
cavity

Cervix
of uterus

Urinary
bladder

Pubic
symphysis

B

Urethra   Vagina Perineal body Anal canal

Figs. 7.5 *(Continued)* (B) Sagittal MR image of a female pelvis.

Pelvic organs

Rectum and anal canal

The rectum is the continuation of the sigmoid colon, beginning at the level of the
third segment of the sacrum and lying in
the concavity of the lower sacrum and coccyx (**Figs. 7.4, 7.5**). It is about 12 cm long
and is retroperitoneal and distinguished
from the rest of the colon by having a complete longitudinal muscle coat rather than
three taenia coli. The upper third has peritoneum anteriorly and laterally, the middle
third anteriorly only and the lower third is
deep to the peritoneum.

The anal canal continues from the
lower end of the rectum as the last 4 cm
of the alimentary tract, ending at the anus
just posterior to the perineal body. The
canal has an internal sphincter of smooth
muscle and is surrounded by an external
sphincter of skeletal muscle, composed
of deep, superficial and subcutaneous
portions (**Fig. 7.6, 7.7**) (innervated by
branches of the pudendal nerve). The
junction between rectum and anal canal is
marked by the anorectal ring, a palpable
landmark on rectal examination (U-shaped
rather than a complete ring), due to the
sling of the puborectalis part of levator ani
muscle (p. 193), which maintains an angle
of 120°, important for faecal continence;
during defaecation this muscle relaxes and
the angle becomes less acute.

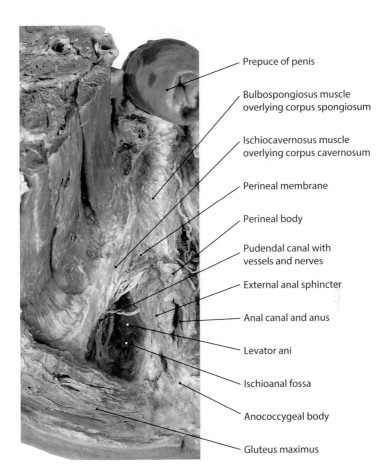

- Prepuce of penis
- Bulbospongiosus muscle overlying corpus spongiosum
- Ischiocavernosus muscle overlying corpus cavernosum
- Perineal membrane
- Perineal body
- Pudendal canal with vessels and nerves
- External anal sphincter
- Anal canal and anus
- Levator ani
- Ischioanal fossa
- Anococcygeal body
- Gluteus maximus

Fig. 7.6 Dissection of the central and right parts of the male perineum.

Using an old fashioned rigid sigmoidoscope, the clinician is only able to view the rectum and anal canal. In order to view the sigmoid colon a flexible fibre optic instrument is required.

Blood supply – the terminal branch of the inferior mesenteric artery (superior rectal) supplies the rectum and upper part of the anal canal, but the lower part is supplied by branches of the pudendal artery, the inferior rectal). There are corresponding veins, so that the upper part of the canal drains to the portal system and the lower part to systemic veins. The anal canal is thus a site for portosystemic anastomosis (p. 167), and is also an important watershed for lymph drainage – the upper part to pelvic nodes, but the lower part to inguinal nodes. In addition, there are also middle rectal vessels that supply the muscle layer of the middle part of the rectum, but do not pass deep to interfere with the portosystemic anastomosis.

Carcinoma of the anal canal may present with palpable lymph nodes in the inguinal region.

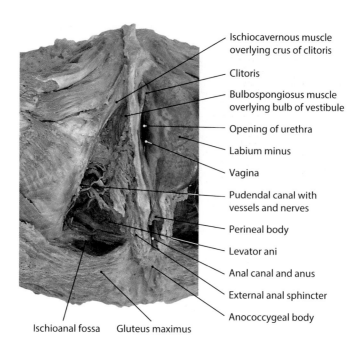

Ischiocavernous muscle overlying crus of clitoris

Clitoris

Bulbospongiosus muscle overlying bulb of vestibule

Opening of urethra

Labium minus

Vagina

Pudendal canal with vessels and nerves

Perineal body

Levator ani

Anal canal and anus

External anal sphincter

Anococcygeal body

Ischioanal fossa   Gluteus maximus

Fig. 7.7 Dissection of the central and right parts of the female perineum.

Rectal examination – means digital examination by a (gloved and lubricated) index finger inserted through the anus and upwards as far as possible. Palpable structures are the anorectal ring posteriorly, prostate (normal or enlarged) in the male or the cervix in the female anteriorly and cancerous growths in the lower rectum or cancerous tumours in the rectovesical pouch of peritoneum in the male or within the recto-uterine pouch in the female (p. 204).

> Haemorrhoids are swellings of the cushions of vascular submucosal soft tissue in the lower part of the anal canal that help to maintain faecal continence. They may become enlarged (haemorrhoidal disease or piles) and may prolapse or bleed.

Male pelvic organs

Ureter – enters the pelvis by *crossing* the external iliac vessels and then running inferiorly down the posterior aspect of the lateral wall *anterior to* the internal iliac vessels (**Fig. 7.4A**) before turning *forwards (anteriorly) at the ischial spine on the superior aspect of the pelvic floor*. Here the *ureter is crossed* by the ductus deferens, passing from lateral to medial, before reaching the posterior corner of the base of the bladder. There is no sphincter as such as it passes through the bladder wall. However, the obliquity of its passage through the bladder wall ensures that as the bladder fills the urethra is effectively closed.

> The pain of renal colic is usually due to a small stone (calculus) getting stuck in the ureter on its way between kidney and bladder.

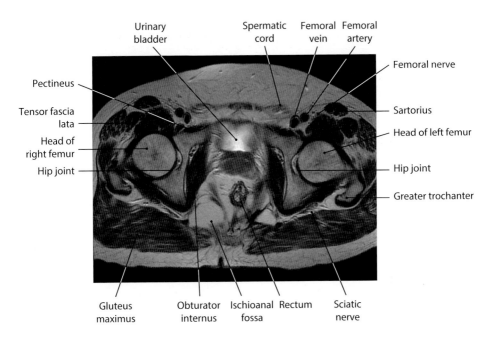

Fig. 7.8 Axial MR image of the male pelvis at the level of the greater trochanters of the femurs, from below.

Urinary bladder – when empty lies posterior to (behind) the pubic symphysis and anterior to the lower part of the rectum (**Figs. 7.4, 7.8**). The lowest part of the peritoneal cavity is formed by a fold of peritoneum reflecting from the anterior of the rectum to the upper part of the base of the bladder and its superior surface, the rectovesical pouch. This pouch is highly important, since it falls within reach of the examining finger in rectal examination (see above). The lower posterior part of the bladder base is the trigone, the most fixed part and shaped like an inverted triangle with the ureters entering at each upper posterior angle and the urethra leaving at the lower anterior angle (internal urethral meatus, also the location of smooth muscle that acts as an internal sphincter). The innervation is parasympathetic, from the pelvic splanchnic nerves.

As the bladder fills with urine, it rises above the level of the pubic symphysis behind the lower part of the anterior abdominal wall, pushing the peritoneum away from the anterior abdominal wall as it rises. It then becomes possible to insert a needle or drainage tube into the bladder just superior to the pubic symphysis without entering the peritoneal cavity, should it be impossible to drain the bladder via the urethra.

Prostate – consists of glands embedded in a mass of connective tissue and smooth muscle arranged as a peripheral zone with a central zone around and posterior to the urethra. The prostate secretes about 30% of the seminal fluid (p. 201), is about the size and shape of a chestnut (normally there is a midline groove, lies inferior to the bladder (**Figs. 7.3, 7.4**) and is supported inferiorly by the urogenital diaphragm. The urethra runs through the gland (see below) and about 12 minute prostatic ducts discharge the secretion into it, in addition to the two larger ejaculatory ducts (see below).

> Enlargement of the prostate (benign prostatic hypertrophy: BPH) is common after the age of about 50 and may lead to obstruction of urinary outflow and distension of the bladder.

Examining the prostate is an important part of digital rectal examination in men. The normal prostate is smooth with a palpable distinct groove or sulcus between the lateral lobes – loss of the groove is indicative of cancer.

> Cancer of the prostate is less common but it often begins in the posterior portion of the organ where it can be palpated during rectal examination.

Urethra – the common channel for urine and seminal fluid (semen), it leaves the lowest part of the bladder (**Fig. 7.4**) and runs through the prostate (prostatic urethra U-shaped in cross-section) and then through the urogenital diaphragm (membranous urethra, where it is surrounded by skeletal muscle that forms the voluntary external urethral sphincter, responsible for urinary continence), and finally enters the root of the penis to become the penile urethra (a total length of about 18 cm). There is a 90° change of direction between the proximal end of the penile part of the urethra and the membranous part. Some smooth muscle at the junction of the bladder and prostatic urethra forms the internal urethral sphincter and also probably prevents retrograde ejaculation of seminal fluid into the bladder.

> When complete obstruction of outflow occurs (acute retention) it may be necessary to insert a urinary catheter through the urethra into the bladder. A cystoscope can be passed through the urethra to examine the bladder.

> If the penile urethra is damaged, urine can leak into the superficial perineal pouch, where its spread is limited by the membranous fascia lining the scrotal pouch.

> The combined testis and epididymis are sometimes called the testicle.

Testis and epididymis – the testis, roughly egg-shaped and about 3 cm long, contains a mass of seminiferous tubules that produce the male germ cells, spermatozoa, which pass into the epididymis, a very long coiled tubular structure that adheres to the *posterolateral side* of the testis and where spermatozoa are stored as they mature. The front and sides of the testis are covered by a closed serosal sac derived from peritoneum, the tunica vaginalis.

> An accumulation of fluid in the tunica vaginalis (hydrocele) produces a swelling surrounding the front and sides of the testis; an enlarged epididymis lies towards the top and back of the testis, an important distinction. A hydrocele transilluminates (i.e. it transmits light if a light source is placed behind it).

The testes also contain groups of endocrine cells that produce the male sex hormone, testosterone. The testis and epididymis of both sides lie within the superficial perineal pouch (space), which contributes to the scrotum. The testicular arteries arise from the abdominal aorta; the corresponding veins drain on the right to the inferior vena cava and on the left usually to the left renal vein. Lymphatic channels accompany the testicular vessels, so that testicular lymph drains directly to para-aortic nodes and not to the overlying scrotal skin or inguinal nodes.

> This drainage pattern is clinically significant when diagnosing tumour spread, as the tumour spreads to nodes that are not palpable and is why in the past testicular cancer often had a poor prognosis.

Ductus (vas) deferens – the direct continuation of the epididymis, leaves the *lower*

> Vasectomy (removing a short length of ductus deferens [old name was vas deferens] to produce male sterilisation is carried out at the top of the scrotum on each side by dissecting out the ductus from the rest of the spermatic cord structures.

end of the epididymis to ascend in the spermatic cord (**Fig. 6.1**) and through the inguinal canal. Emerging from the lateral end of the inguinal canal (p. 158) through the deep inguinal ring, the ductus deferens runs down the anterior part of the lateral wall of the pelvis and crosses *superficial to the ureter* to reach the posterior of the prostate (**Fig. 7.4**). Here it dilates, forming the ampulla, before joining the duct of the seminal vesicle to form the ejaculatory duct that enters the prostatic part of the urethra.

Seminal vesicle – produces much of the seminal fluid (rich in fructose) and lies lateral to the ampulla of the ductus deferens in contact with the posterior wall of the bladder base (**Figs. 7.3, 7.4**), with its upper end just below the point of entrance of the ureter into the bladder. The very short duct

leaves the lower end to join the ductus deferens at the edge of the prostate and form the ejaculatory duct.

> Normal seminal vesicles are not usually palpable on rectal examination.

Seminal fluid – the fluid vehicle for transport of spermatozoa. It is produced by the seminal vesicles (60%) and prostate (30%), with only a small amount coming from the testes. However, this latter contribution contains the spermatozoa.

Spermatic cord – the collective name for the deferens, the testicular and other vessels and nerves, and various connective tissue and muscular (cremaster) coverings derived from the abdominal musculature that form the inguinal canal (**Fig. 6.1**). It therefore only lies between the superficial inguinal ring and the testis.

Scrotum – the wrinkled sac of skin and some smooth muscle (dartos) that enclose the testis, epididymis and the start of the ductus deferens bilaterally.

Penis – the male organ of micturition (urination) and copulation (sexual intercourse), whose root lies anterior to the anus (**Figs. 7.4, 7.6**). It consists of three columnar masses of vascular tissue: a single corpus spongiosum with an expanded part proximally (bulb attached to the urogenital diaphragm) and at the distal end (glans penis); and the paired corpora cavernosum on each side attached to the urogenital diaphragm and ischiopubic ramus. Each corpus is surrounded by muscle, the spongiosum by the muscle bulbospongiosus, the cavernosus by the muscle ischiocavernosus, all bound together in a tubular sheath of skin and connective tissue (deep fascia of the penis; Buck's fascia). The fold of skin covering the glans is the prepuce (foreskin, **Fig. 7.4A**). The urethra (see above) runs through the corpus spongiosum and glans to open at the tip of the glans; it serves at different times for the passage of urine or seminal fluid. Erection is due to (parasympathetic) vasodilatation of the arteries of the corpora and is a necessary prelude to ejaculation, the discharge of seminal fluid (semen) containing sperm (spermatozoa). Ejaculation depends on the (sympathetic) contraction of the smooth muscle of the prostate and each seminal vesicle and ductus deferens, supplemented by contraction of the bulbospongiosus (skeletal) muscle that overlies the bulb of the penis.

> Circumcision is the operation to remove the foreskin.

Female pelvic organs

Ureter – enters the pelvis by *crossing* the external iliac vessels and then runs inferiorly down the posterior part of the lateral pelvic wall, anterior to the internal iliac vessels, to the ischial spine. It then turns forwards, passing under the broad ligament of the uterus, where it is crossed by the uterine artery, to enter the posterior aspect of the bladder base, crossing the lateral vaginal fornix as it does so 1 cm lateral to the cervix (**Fig. 7.5A**).

> Chronic obstruction may lead to dilatation of the ureters and renal pelvises (hydronephrosis) as a result of back pressure. Kidney function may be adversely affected.

Urinary bladder – lies posterior to the pubic symphysis (**Fig. 7.5**), as in the male, and anterior to the middle third of the vagina, with the body of the uterus usually lying on its superior surface.

Urethra – is straight, only 4 cm long, and surrounded by the voluntarily controlled external urethral sphincter lying within the deep perineal pouch. Most of the urethra is embedded within the connective tissue of the anterior wall of the distal third of the vagina and it opens into the vaginal vestibule (**Fig. 7.5**) (see below), 2.5 cm posterior to the clitoris.

> The shortness of the female urethra predisposes to ascending infection into the bladder, leading to cystitis.

Ovary – produces the female germ cells (ova) and also the hormones oestrogen and progesterone, which control the female reproductive system. An almond-shaped structure (**Fig. 7.5A**), it is suspended by a fold of peritoneum, the mesovarium, from the posterior aspect of the broad ligament. The open (fimbriated) end of the uterine (Fallopian) tube lies nearby, so that discharged ova may enter it. Within the mesovarium and posterior aspect of the broad ligament lies the ligament of the ovary, which

> Uterine tubes can become blocked either by clipping or dividing them bilaterally, as in female sterilisation, or through chronic inflammation, which may lead to obstruction and a fertilised egg becoming implanted in the tube (tubal or ectopic pregnancy).

is an embryological remnant associated with the descent of the gonad. The ovarian artery arises (like the testicular artery) from the abdominal aorta and reaches the ovary by passing over the pelvic brim in its own fold of peritoneum, accompanied by (a) the ovarian vein, which (like the testicular vein) drains on the right into the inferior vena cava and on the left into the left renal vein, and (b) lymphatic vessels draining lymph to para-aortic lymph nodes. As with the testes, ovarian cancer often has a poor prognosis.

Cancer of the ovary and uterus are among the commonest female cancers.

Cervical screening (smear test) may detect precancerous changes in the cervical mucosa, which if treated will prevent cervical cancer.

Uterus – the womb, whose lining during reproductive life undergoes the monthly changes of the menstrual cycle, and where the fertilised ovum if present will normally become implanted and develop into a new individual. The uterus (**Figs. 6.12A, 7.5**) is a pear-shaped, thick-walled organ of smooth muscle, about 8 cm long, usually tilted forwards (anteverted) and folded anteriorly (anteflexed) to overlie

Bimanual examination of the uterus involves placing the flat of one hand above the pubic symphysis and pressing downwards while the index and middle fingers of the other hand (as in vaginal examination, below) press the cervix upwards.

the bladder. The main part is the body, whose upper end is the fundus; the lower end is the cervix (about 3 cm long), which projects into the vagina and opens into it through the external os at the lower end of the cervical canal. From the junction of the body and fundus a uterine (Fallopian) tube projects at each side towards the lateral pelvic wall; it is the draping of peritoneum over these tubes that forms the broad ligament. The cavity of the uterus is lined by a specialised mucous membrane, the endometrium, which responds to cyclical hormonal changes (although the lining of the cervix does not take part in these changes). Below the uterine tube, the round ligament (a continuation of the ligament of the ovary) runs laterally to enter the inguinal canal through the deep inguinal ring as it passes to attach to labia majora).

The uterine artery runs medially from the internal iliac and crosses the ureter superficially, accompanied by corresponding veins. This artery will anastomose with branches of the ovarian artery along the uterine tube. Lymph from the cervix and body of the uterus normally drains to pelvic nodes, but some from the fundus may travel via lymphatics that accompany the round ligament and so reach inguinal nodes.

A loose fold of peritoneum, the broad ligament, attaches the uterus to the side wall of the pelvis. However, the main factors that hold the uterus in its normal position are condensations of connective tissue deep to the peritoneum in the region of the cervix and upper vagina. These pass laterally to the lateral pelvic wall as the transverse cervical ligaments (cardinal ligament or Mackenrodt's ligament), backwards on either side of the rectum to the sacrum as uterosacral ligaments, and anteriorly either side of the urethra as pubocervical ligaments. These ligaments are difficult to appreciate in dissections, but are highly important in the living woman to prevent uterine prolapse.

The uterosacral ligaments may be detected on rectal (not vaginal) examination, since they pass backwards on either side of the rectum.

The hymen is a mucosal fold at the vaginal margin that is usually ruptured during the first sexual intercourse.

If particularly dense or interfering with the discharge of menstrual products, the hymen may have to be surgically incised.

Vagina – the female copulatory organ, and also the birth canal and passage for the discharge of menstrual products (**Figs. 7.5**). About 12 cm long when undistended, it lies posterior to the bladder and urethra, although the urethra is more accurately described as being embedded within the connective tissue of the anterior third of the vaginal wall. The cervix of the uterus projects into the upper end (deepest third) of the vagina; the furrow surrounding the cervix here is the vaginal fornix, named anterior, lateral and posterior. Posterior to the vagina is the lower part of the rectum, and stretching between the posterior vaginal fornix with the uterus anteriorly and rectum posteriorly is the recto-uterine pouch of peritoneum (pouch of Douglas). This corresponds to the rectovesical pouch in the male and is, likewise, the lowest part of the peritoneal cavity in the female when upright. The lower end of the vagina is the introitus or vestibule, and has the urethra opening into it anteriorly, 2.5 cm behind the clitoris. The bladder is related to the middle third of the anterior wall of the vagina. There are no glands in the vagina; the moisture that occurs during sexual excitement is largely due to a transudation of fluid through the vaginal walls.

> On vaginal examination, using the index and middle fingers (gloved and lubricated), the uterine cervix can be palpated in the deepest third of the vagina, with the recto-uterine pouch of peritoneum as a possible site for cancerous deposits posteriorly. The ovary and part of the uterine tube may be palpated at each side of the vagina, especially if enlarged. Also, an ultrasonic transducer can be inserted into the vagina to image the pelvic organs.

Mons pubis – the fatty tissue anterior to the pubic symphysis, covered by hairy skin, continues posteriorly on each side of the vaginal opening as the labia majora (singular, labium majus).

Labia minora – smaller, fat-free skin folds (singular, labium minus), internal to the labia majora (**Fig. 7.7**) and covered by hairless skin, that form the immediate boundaries surrounding the vaginal opening (vestibule). On either side of the opening is the bulb of the vestibule, an elongated mass of erectile tissue (male equivalent bulb of penis).

Clitoris – the corresponding structure to the penis of the male, but although the male urethra runs through the penis, the female urethra does not run through the much smaller clitoris (**Fig. 7.7**), which is an organ concerned only with sexual arousal. It has a crus on each side (male equivalent corpus cavernosum and ischiocavernosus). The urethra opens into the vestibule of the vagina 2.5 cm behind the clitoris.

Greater vestibular (Bartholin's) glands – small mucous glands under cover of the posterior part of the bulb of the vestibule, which lubricate the vestibule. They open on the inside of the labia minora by a single duct on each side, in the 4- and 8-o'clock positions when looking from below with the patient lying on her back.

> Infection of the greater vestibular glands may lead to painful abscesses in these positions.

> When using the clock to describe this part of the perineum, the pubis is at 12 o'clock and the perineal body (or anococcygeal body if describing anal pathology) lies at six o'clock.

Summary

- The cavity of the *true pelvis*, below the pelvic brim, runs posteriorly at almost 90° from the abdominal cavity.
- The two levator ani and the two coccygeus muscles form the *pelvic diaphragm* or *pelvic floor* (skeletal muscle, supplied by S3 and S4 nerves), separating the pelvic cavity from the perineum, and must not be confused with the *urogenital diaphragm*, which is a much smaller fibromuscular mass (below and separate from the pelvic diaphragm) containing the *sphincter urethrae* (external urethral sphincter, skeletal muscle, innervated by the pudendal nerve).
- The *ureter* enters the pelvis by crossing the external iliac vessels at the pelvic brim and then runs inferiorly on the lateral pelvic wall anterior to the internal iliac artery before turning forwards anteriorly (crossed superficially by the ductus deferens or uterine artery) to enter the bladder and open at the posterior angle of the trigone. The *ductus deferens* runs down the lateral pelvic wall anteriorly.
- The empty *bladder* is a pelvic organ, lying posterior to the pubic symphysis, but when distended it may rise above the level of the symphysis. The smooth muscle of the bladder is supplied by the pelvic splanchnic (parasympathetic) nerves, which empty it, and sympathetic nerves, which allow it to fill.
- The *male urethra* is about 18 cm long and has prostatic, membranous and spongy (penile) parts; the external urethral sphincter surrounds the membranous part. The *female urethra* is straight and only 4 cm long, surrounded by the external urethral sphincter.
- Each *seminal vesicle* lies postero-inferior to the bladder and its duct joins the ductus deferens to form the ejaculatory duct, which runs through the prostate to open into the prostatic urethra.
- The junction of the rectum and anal canal is marked by the *palpable anorectal ring* produced by the sling of the puborectalis muscle. The lowest part of the peritoneal cavity (rectovesical or recto-uterine pouch) is in reach of the fingertip during rectal examination.
- The upper part of the *anal canal* is a site of portosystemic anastomosis and a watershed for the drainage of lymph. From the lower part it drains to inguinal nodes, like other parts of the perineum, including the lower vagina and vulva and the scrotum (but not the ovary or testis, whose lymphatics accompany its blood vessels and therefore drain to aortic nodes within the abdomen).
- The *body of the uterus* usually overlies the bladder and the *cervix* projects into the upper end of the vagina. The *ovary* is suspended from the back of the broad ligament of the uterus, and the *round ligament* of the uterus enters the inguinal canal. The main uterine supports are the lateral cervical, anterior pubocervical and posterior uterosacral ligaments. Most uterine lymph drains to pelvic nodes, but some from the fundus may reach inguinal nodes via the round ligament.

Questions

Answers can be found in Appendix A, p. 249.

Question 1

The pelvic diaphragm is an important divide between the pelvic cavity above and the perineum below. Which statement below most accurately describes its structure?

(a) Attaching to the body of the pubis and the fascia covering obturator internus and the ischial tuberosity, its fibres pass posteriorly, inferiorly and medially to form a midline raphe.

(b) Attaching to the fascia covering obturator internus and the ischial spine, the muscle fibres pass posteriorly, inferiorly and medially to form a midline raphe.

(c) Attaching to the fascia covering obturator internus and the ischial spine, the muscle fibres pass posteriorly, inferiorly and laterally to form a midline raphe

(d) Attaching to the back of the pubic bone, the fascia covering obturator internus and the ischial spine, the muscle fibres pass posteriorly, inferiorly and laterally to form a midline raphe.

(e) Attaching to the back of the pubic bone, the fascia covering obturator internus and the ischial spine, the muscle fibres pass posteriorly, inferiorly and medially to form a midline raphe.

Question 2

Unlike organs elsewhere in the body, which all lie within the central trunk, the testis is located external to the trunk. Which statement most accurately describes the testicular anatomy?

(a) The two testes lie within the superficial perineal pouch with a single serosal covering, both known as the tunica vaginalis.

(b) The epididymis lies on the posterior aspect of the testis and both are surrounded by the tunica vaginalis.

(c) In the adult, there is normally a serosal link between the tunica vaginalis and the peritoneal cavity through the spermatic cord, which links the testis to the inside of the pelvis.

(d) The membranous fascia lines the scrotal skin, deep to which the serosal tunica vaginalis surrounds the anterior and sides of each testis.

(e) The arterial supply to the testis and its venous drainage both connect the testis to the vessels of the posterior abdominal wall, while the lymphatic drainage links it to the inguinal group of lymph nodes.

Question 3

The ovary is located within the pelvic cavity. Which statement below most accurately describes the anatomy of the ovary?

(a) The ovary is located lateral to the body of the uterus, hanging on the anterior aspect of the broad ligament and connected to the uterus by the round ligament.

(b) The ovary lies on the posterior aspect of the broad ligament, suspended by the mesovarium but not covered by peritoneum, and is connected to the uterus by the ovarian ligament.

(c) The ovary receives its blood supply normally through the mesovarium as a branch of the uterine artery.

(d) The ovary is covered in peritoneum suspended on the posterior aspect of the broad ligament by the mesovarium through which the ovarian artery passes.

(e) The ovary is located on the anterior aspect of the broad ligament and is suspended via the mesovarium through which the ovarian artery passes. It is connected to the uterus by the ovarian ligament.

Question 4

The male perineum is a triangular space bounded by the ischiopubic rami. Which statement most accurately describes the structures involved?

(a) The deep perineal pouch lies deep to the urogenital diaphragm.

(b) The floor of the superficial perineal pouch comprises the anterior fibres of levator ani to which the membranous fascia attaches.

(c) The bulb of the penis lying in the superficial pouch is covered by the smooth muscle ischiocavernosus.

(d) The deep perineal pouch lies within the urogenital diaphragm and contains erectile tissue.

(e) The crus of the penis is composed of erectile tissue covered by a layer of skeletal muscle innervated through the pudendal nerve.

Question 5

Which statement below most accurately describes the anatomy of the prostate?

(a) The prostate is located posterior to the symphysis pubis and inferior to the bladder, and the ureter passes through it.

(b) The seminal vesicles and the ductus deferens are located laterally to the prostate and the ejaculatory ducts they form enter the urethra from a lateral position.

(c) The prostate has a groove on its posterior surface, inferior to the seminal vesicles, which is palpable on rectal examination.

(d) The membranous urethra passes through the prostate gland and has openings for the ejaculatory ducts and the 12 ducts from the gland itself.

(e) Sitting on the pelvic diaphragm, the prostate is located inferior to the body of the pubis.

Question 6

The relationships of the external part of the female genital tract are important when performing a clinical examination. Which statement describes accurately the anatomy?

(a) The anterior fibres of levator ani sweep around the vagina to attach to the anal sphincters and anococcygeal body only.

(b) The cervix is related to the middle third of the anterior vaginal wall.

(c) The clitoris lies 1 cm posterior to the opening of the urethra.

(d) In the deepest reaches of the vagina one can palpate masses lying in the rectovesical pouch.

(e) The anterior wall of the vagina is related superficially to the urethra and then the bladder is related to the middle third.

Question 7

A 55-year-old man presents with palpable lymph nodes in both groins. Cytology of the glands confirms a diagnosis of secondary carcinoma. Which is the most likely site for the primary tumour?

(a) Lower anal canal.

(b) Prostate.

(c) Testis.

(d) Upper third of the rectum.

(e) Urinary bladder.

Question 8

A varicoele is an abnormal dilatation of the pampiniform venous plexus within the spermatic cord. It is much more commonly found on the left side. What is the most likely reason for this?

(a) The left testicular vein lies behind the external iliac artery and is likely to be compressed by it.

(b) The left testicular vein drains into the left renal vein, where it is most likely compressed.

(c) The left testicular vein drains directly into the inferior vena cava, where it is most likely compressed by the aorta.

(d) The left testicular artery lies anterior to the left testicular vein and compresses it.

(e) The left testicular vein lacks valves to prevent back flow, unlike the right testicular vein.

Question 9

Severe intraperitoneal sepsis may result in a pelvic abscess, which in the female will collect in the recto-uterine pouch. Where can this be palpated?

(a) Anterior to the vagina during digital per vaginal examination.

(b) Posterior to the vagina during digital per vaginal examination.

(c) Posterior to the rectum during digital rectal examination.

(d) Superior to the uterus during bimanual examination.

(e) In the lateral vaginal fornices during bimanual examination.

Question 10

A 22-year-old pregnant woman who is due to give birth reports to her obstetrician that she feels "wobbly in the hips" when she walks. The doctor tells her that this is common in women near the time for delivery. Which of the following is the most likely explanation?

(a) Dislocation of one or both hips.

(b) Torn or strained ligaments of the hip capsule.

(c) Loosening of the pubic symphysis.

(d) Her centre of gravity has shifted too far forward.

(e) This is a psychosomatic sensation ('It's all in her head').

Question 11

A 78-year-old man with advanced bladder cancer complains of difficulty walking. Physical examination reveals weakness of the adductors of his left thigh. Which of the following nerves is most likely being compressed by the tumour and causing this symptom?

(a) Femoral.

(b) Sciatic.

(c) Obturator.

(d) Tibial.

(e) Common fibular.

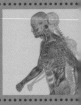

Introduction

The lower limb accounts for 10% of the body weight. The delicate pirouette of the ballet dancer and the relentless plod of the marathon runner are different examples of lower limb movement (locomotion) and control of the centre of body mass (posture). When standing upright, gravity pulls on the centre of body mass to create the line of gravity passing just posterior to the axis of movement of the hip joint but anterior to the knee and ankle joints, working with these well designed joints to keep the weight-bearing foot in place. Various trunk and limb muscles routinely make unconscious adjustments to maintain this upright position. Like so much of normal health, locomotion is taken for granted and only fully appreciated when injury or disease impose a limit on accustomed movement.

The two hip bones are firmly united anteriorly, in the midline by the pubic symphysis, and posteriorly each articulates with the sacrum at the sacroiliac joints (**Fig. 2.7**), so forming the bony pelvis (**Figs. 7.1, 7.2**). Although synovial, the sacroiliac joints are atypical in that they allow negligible movement between the bones (although there is a slight increase in the later stages of pregnancy to assist in childbirth by allowing the pelvis to get larger). Compared with the shoulder, the ball-and-socket hip joint is very stable, since the bones of the hip girdle are firmly united and the head of the femur is lodged deeply in the cup-shaped acetabulum of the hip bone which, with the labrum, extends over the equator of the femoral head to provide the near perfect base for locomotion.

Hip and thigh

Muscles passing anterior to the hip are the flexors of the hip joint and are closely associated with the femoral vessels and nerve. As they pass more distally they are associated with the main anterior muscle of the thigh, quadriceps femoris, made up of rectus femoris and the three vastus muscles – medialis, lateralis and intermedius – innervated by the femoral nerve. The medial part of the thigh is the adductor compartment, whose nerve is the obturator nerve. Posterior to the hip, is the gluteal region (buttocks) containing the extensors and lateral rotators of the hip joint and, more distally, the compartment contains the flexor muscles of the knee joint, commonly called the hamstrings and innervated by the largest nerve in the body, the sciatic nerve.

Bony prominences – at the junction between the thigh and abdomen (**Figs. 8.1, 2.7A**), the two important bony landmarks are the anterior superior iliac spine, at the anterior end of the iliac crest, and the pubic tubercle, which is 2.5 cm lateral to the top

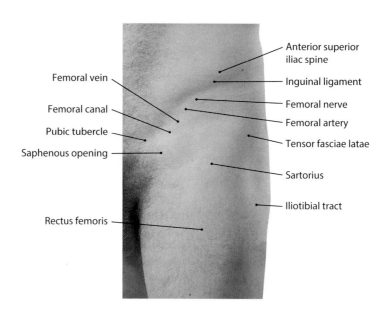

Fig. 8.1 Surface features of the front and left side of the left thigh.

The anterior superior iliac spine can be seen and felt easily; the pubic tubercle cannot be seen but can be felt in a thin person.

The femoral nerve lies lateral to the palpable artery; the femoral vein lies medial to the artery.

of the pubic symphysis. The inguinal ligament extends between these two points. Lateral to the upper thigh, a hands length below the iliac crest, the greater trochanter of the femur can be felt, forming the most lateral part of the hip. Posteriorly, the ischial tuberosity is deep to the lower edge of gluteus maximus (**Fig. 8.2**); it can be felt when sitting by leaning to one side and slipping a hand under the raised side.

Femoral triangle – a descriptive region (**Fig. 8.3**) bounded superiorly by the inguinal ligament, laterally by the medial border of sartorius and medially by the medial border of adductor longus. It contains the femoral nerve, artery, vein and canal, in that order from lateral to medial distal to the inguinal ligament. The upper parts of the artery and vein and the canal are surrounded by the connective tissue

known as the femoral sheath, but the nerve lies outside the sheath. All are deep to the deep fascia of the thigh, known as the fascia lata, the most lateral part of which forms a particularly thick and strong band, the iliotibial tract (p. 213).

Femoral nerve – lies *lateral* to the artery (**Fig. 8.3**) and divides into a sheaf of muscular and cutaneous branches, which supply the muscles and skin of the anterior thigh. It has contributions from lumbar nerves 2–4. The saphenous nerve is a long cutaneous branch that runs as far distally as the base of the great toe – the only femoral nerve branch that extends below the knee.

Femoral artery and vein – a continuation under the inguinal ligament, of the corresponding external iliac vessels, the vein lies medial to the artery (**Fig. 8.3**) within

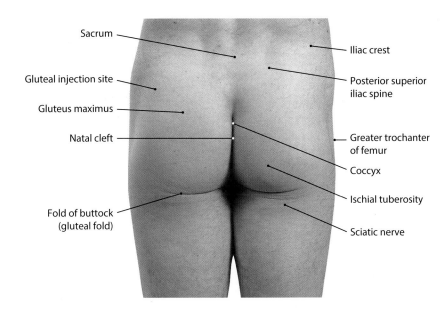

Fig. 8.2 Surface features of the lower back and gluteal region.

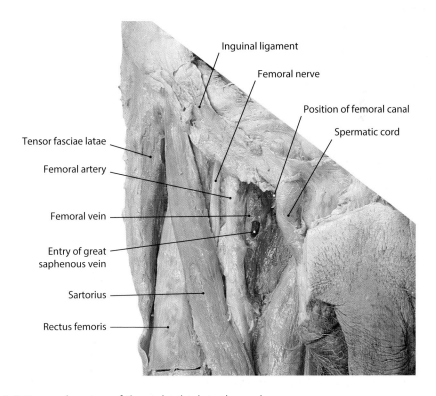

Fig. 8.3 Femoral region of the right thigh in the male.

a sheath of fascia (femoral sheath), which is an extension of transversalis fascia in the abdomen. The largest branch of the artery, the deep femoral (profunda femoris) artery, passes posteriorly between the adductor muscles to branch and (including the circumflex femoral arteries) supply muscles of the thigh. In the lower thigh, the femoral artery pierces adductor magnus to become the popliteal artery.

> The femoral pulse can be felt at a point midway between the anterior superior iliac spine and the pubic tubercle.

It is in the femoral triangle that variations are commonly seen. It is not uncommon for one or both of the circumflex femoral branches to arise from the proximal part of the femoral artery instead of branching from the more commonly recognised site of the deep femoral artery.

> Clinically, the term 'common femoral' describes the femoral artery from the inguinal ligament to its deep (profunda) branch. The remaining part of the femoral artery continuing distally is referred to as the superficial femoral artery.

Great saphenous vein – the largest tributary of the femoral vein (also known as the long saphenous), which it enters by passing through the saphenous opening (**Fig. 8.4**), a gap in the fascia lata 4 cm below and lateral to the (palpable) pubic tubercle. It receives several tributaries (superficial branches from the external genitalia, anterior thigh,

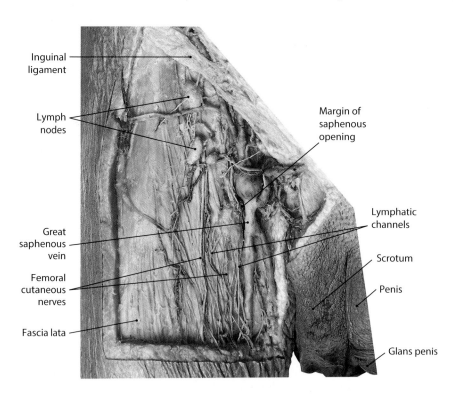

Inguinal ligament

Lymph nodes

Margin of saphenous opening

Lymphatic channels

Great saphenous vein

Femoral cutaneous nerves

Scrotum

Penis

Fascia lata

Glans penis

Fig. 8.4 Superficial dissection of the upper right thigh in the male. There is a large varicosity at the upper end of the great saphenous vein.

teral thigh and lower abdominal wall) efore passing through the opening (see lso p. 227).

emoral canal – the most medial com- artment of the femoral sheath (8.3), about cm long, with an opening (femoral ring) ito the abdominal cavity deep to the ingui- al ligament. The canal exists to allow lym- hatics to pass from the lower limb into the elvis, and also to allow the femoral vein o expand for increased venous return from ie lower limb.

> A loop of intestine may pro- trude through the ring with a peritoneal covering into the canal, so forming a femoral hernia.

nguinal lymph nodes – about 15 or so, ing superficially along the great saphe- ous vein and inferior to the nearby part f the inguinal ligament (Fig. 8.4), with vo or three deep to the deep fascia beside ie femoral vein. Efferent channels pass rom these deep nodes through the femo- al canal to the external iliac nodes. Apart rom draining the whole of the lower limb ncluding the gluteal region), the nodes eceive lymph from the trunk wall (front nd back) below the umbilical level and rom the perineum, thus including the ower vagina and anal canal.

> Inguinal nodes may become involved as a result of disease in the perineum and gluteal region as well as from the lower limb and lower abdominal wall.

Quadriceps femoris – collective name for ectus femoris and the three vasti muscles. Rectus femoris (Fig. 8.3) arises proximally rom the hip bone above the acetabulum nd the anterior inferior iliac spine and is he most anterior muscle. Vastus medialis

and vastus lateralis arise from the medial and lateral surfaces of the femur, respec- tively, and vastus intermedius (the deepest muscle) arises from the anterior aspect of the femur. All converge distally to form the quadriceps tendon, attaching to the top of the patella, which in turn is anchored to the tuberosity of the tibia by the patellar ligament (often called patellar tendon clin- ically) (Figs. 8.7–8.10). Since only the rec- tus crosses the hip it can flex the hip joint, but both the rectus and the vasti extend the knee (pp. 222, 223). All four muscles are innervated by the femoral nerve.

> The lower oblique fibres of vas- tus medialis pull on the patella medially, as the rest of quad- riceps try to pull it laterally. This ensures the patella tracks normally on the anterior femur preventing it impinging on the lateral aspect of the femoral condyle, giving rise to anterior knee pain.

Tensor fasciae latae – short muscle on the lateral side of the anterior thigh (Fig. 8.3) arising from the anterior 5 cm of the outer edge of the iliac crest and running distally to blend into the iliotibial tract. It helps to brace the iliotibial tract and keep the knee extended by working with gluteus maximus (p. 214). It is innervated by the superior gluteal nerve.

Sartorius – the muscle with the lon- gest parallel fibres in the body, it passes obliquely across the thigh (Fig. 8.3) from the anterior superior iliac spine laterally to the medial surface of the tibia (ante- rior to the distal attachments of gracilis and semitendinosus). It assists in flexion of the hip and knee joints and laterally rotates the hip, and is innervated by the femoral nerve.

Pectineus – in the medial part of the floor of the femoral triangle, it runs from the pectineal line of the pubis to the femur along a line between the lesser trochanter and the linea aspera. It separates the femoral vein and canal from the hip joint, and is usually innervated by the femoral nerve (sometimes by the obturator nerve).

Adductor muscles – the most superficial and medial of the group and thigh is gracilis, with adductor longus adjacent and adductor brevis placed deep to longus (**Fig. 8.6**). All attach proximally to the pubis and its inferior ramus; gracilis reaches the medial surface of the tibia (between sartorius and semitendinosus), whereas the other two are attached distally into the linea aspera of the femur. Adductor magnus is the largest and deepest of the group, running from the ischial tuberosity and adjacent ramus to the whole length of the linea aspera, the medial supracondylar line and to the adductor

tubercle of the femur. The distal part contains the opening (adductor hiatus) through which the femoral artery passes posteriorly to enter the popliteal fossa, where it changes its name to popliteal artery. This group is innervated by the obturator nerve with part of adductor magnus attaching to the adductor tubercle receiving innervation from the sciatic nerve.

Gluteal fold – fold of the buttock (**Fig. 8.2**) a transverse, but downwardly curved, skin crease due to hip joint movement; it does *not* correspond to the lower border of gluteus maximus.

Gluteus maximus – the muscle that forms the bulk of the buttock (**Figs. 7.8, 8.2, 8.5**) and whose fibres run down at 45° from the posterior of the ilium, sacrum, coccyx and sacrotuberous ligament to

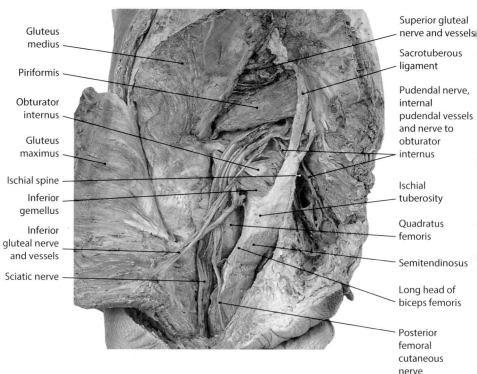

Gluteus medius —
Piriformis —
Obturator internus —
Gluteus maximus —
Ischial spine —
Inferior gemellus —
Inferior gluteal nerve and vessels —
Sciatic nerve —

Superior gluteal nerve and vessels
Sacrotuberous ligament
Pudendal nerve, internal pudendal vessels and nerve to obturator internus
Ischial tuberosity
Quadratus femoris
Semitendinosus
Long head of biceps femoris
Posterior femoral cutaneous nerve

Fig. 8.5 Dissection of the left gluteal region, with gluteus maximus turned laterally.

ross the gluteal fold obliquely. The fibres from the ilium are mostly inserted into the iliotibial tract of the fascia lata; all other fibres insert on the gluteal tuberosity on the posterior of the proximal femur. The muscle is a powerful extensor of the flexed hip, as in climbing stairs and running, and is the only muscle innervated by the inferior gluteal nerve.

Gluteus medius and gluteus minimus – arise proximally from the lateral side of the ilium and converge on to the greater trochanter of the femur (**Fig. 8.6**). They are described as abductors of the hip, but are much more important as preventers of adduction (see Hip joint, below). They are innervated by the superior gluteal nerve.

Piriformis – functionally relatively unimportant (p. 192), but the guide to the gluteal region; nerves and vessels coming from the pelvis do so either superior to or inferior to this muscle (**Fig. 8.5**). Those lying superior are the superior gluteal nerve and vessels; all the rest lie inferior to it. The muscle arises proximally from the middle portion of the sacrum and passes laterally through the greater sciatic foramen (p. 26) to the tip of the greater trochanter of the femur. The surface marking of the lower border is along a line from midway between the posterior superior iliac spine and the coccyx to the tip of the trochanter.

Sciatic nerve – the most important structure in the gluteal region, it usually emerges from the pelvis inferior to piriformis (**Figs. 7.3, 8.5**) and runs down the posterior thigh deep to the hamstring muscles (biceps laterally and semitendinosus and semimembranosus medially), innervating them and part of adductor magnus. At the upper angle of the popliteal fossa it divides into the tibial and common fibular (peroneal) nerves (pp. 223 and 225). Occasionally, the branches forming the sciatic nerve (p. 61) can split the

> The surface marking of the sciatic nerve at the top of the thigh is midway between the ischial tuberosity and the tip of the greater trochanter of the femur.

piriformis into two slips before forming the single sciatic nerve distal to piriformis. It has contributions from L4 to S3.

Posterior femoral cutaneous nerve – runs distally superficial to the hamstrings (**Fig. 8.5**) to supply a strip of skin in the middle of the posterior thigh and calf, a long narrow area of supply.

Superior gluteal nerve – innervates gluteus medius and minimus and tensor fasciae latae (**Fig. 8.5**).

Inferior gluteal nerve – innervates only gluteus maximus (**Fig. 8.5**).

Pudendal nerve, internal pudendal vessels and nerve to obturator internus – these structures (**Fig. 8.5**) have a very short course in the gluteal region, leaving the pelvis through the greater sciatic foramen inferior to piriformis, then crossing behind the ischial spine and sacrospinous ligament to enter the perineum through the lesser sciatic foramen.

Gluteal intramuscular injection – the correct site is the *upper outer quadrant* of the gluteal region (**Fig. 8.2**). The quadrants are defined by measuring from the highest point of the iliac crest to the gluteal fold, and from the midline to the outer edge of the greater trochanter. Correctly defined, the upper outer quadrant is well away from the sciatic nerve.

> The most common cause of sciatic nerve injury is misplaced gluteal injections.

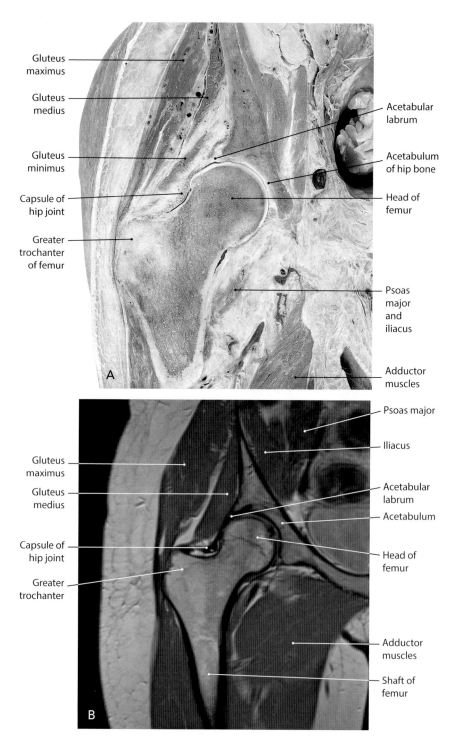

Fig. 8.6 (A) Coronal section of the right hip joint, (B) comparable MR image.

Hamstrings – muscles that span the hip joint and knee joint – the semitendinosus, semimembranosus and long head of biceps femoris (**Fig. 8.11**). All attach proximally to the ischial tuberosity (except the *short* head of biceps, which arises from the posterior femur and hence is not a true hamstring, since it does not span the hip joint). Biceps runs distally to the lateral side to the head of the fibula, with the common fibular (peroneal) nerve posterior to its lower part.

> With the knee flexed to a right angle, the biceps tendon is easily felt on the lateral side behind the knee, with the tendon of semitendinosus overlying the broader semimembranosus on the medial side.

The 'semi' muscles run distally on the medial side, semimembranosus attaching to the medial condyle of the tibia and semitendinosus to the medial surface inferior to the condyle, deep to the gracilis attachment. The hamstrings act as extensors of the hip and flexors of the knee and are innervated by the sciatic nerve.

> As the hamstrings cross two joints, they can be damaged by trying to flex the hip joint with the knee in full extension, resulting in a torn hamstring.

Hip joint – the best example of a ball-and-socket joint. The head of the femur fits snugly into the acetabulum of the hip bone (**Figs. 7.1, 7.8, 8.6**), which is deepened around the periphery by the cartilaginous acetabular labrum and across the acetabular notch by the fibrous transverse acetabular ligament. The ligament of the head of the femur runs from the non-articular fossa close to the transverse ligament to the fovea of the head, carrying important blood vessels to the femoral head in the young child; however, these usually degenerate before adulthood. The capsule is attached to the hip bone around the margins of the acetabulum; on the femur, it attaches *anteriorly* to the intertrochanteric line, but *posteriorly* it attaches halfway along the neck. The capsule reflects back on itself towards the femoral head carrying the retinacular blood vessels that supply the femoral head in adults. Thus, much of the neck is intracapsular and covered by synovial membrane.

> Fractures of this part of the neck may tear the retinacular vessels, causing avascular necrosis of the head and delaying or preventing healing.

Iliofemoral ligament – most important of the ligaments that reinforce the capsule and one of the strongest in the body (because the body's centre of gravity passes posterior to the joint, so the ligament resists the tendency to tilt backwards – hip extension), it is shaped like an inverted Y and attaches from the anterior inferior iliac spine to the lateral and medial ends of the intertrochanteric line. (**Note:** Its eponym is the 'inverted' Y ligament of Bigelow.)

Pubofemoral and ischiofemoral ligaments – reinforce the capsule anteriorly and posteriorly, respectively.

The principal muscles that produce movements at the hip joint are:

- **Flexion** – psoas major, iliacus, rectus femoris, sartorius and, to a minor extent, tensor fasciae latae.
- **Extension** – hamstrings, gluteus maximus and ischial part of adductor magnus.
- **Abduction** – gluteus medius and minimus.
- **Adduction** – adductor longus, brevis and magnus, and gracilis.

- **Lateral rotation** – gluteus maximus, piriformis, obturator externus, obturator internus and gemelli, and quadratus femoris.
- **Medial rotation** – gluteus medius and minimus and, to a minor extent, tensor fasciae latae. This is a more powerful movement than lateral rotation.

The types of movement possible at the hip joint are similar to those at the shoulder, but are more limited because of the shapes of the bones constraining the range of motion. Note that, in walking, the rather small amount of hip extension is produced by the hamstrings; only with greater ranges of movement, as when climbing stairs or running, does gluteus maximus play an important part.

The abducting action of gluteus medius and minimus is less important than the way these muscles *prevent adduction*. During walking those on the side of the limb that is on the ground prevent the pelvis from tilting (due to gravity acting on the centre of body mass) to the opposite side. They also produce medial rotation of the femur; the

long-standing belief that psoas major is medial rotator is not supported by electro myographic studies.

Knee, leg and foot

Bony prominences – the patella is th obvious feature anterior to the knee, wit the tuberosity of the tibia inferior to i (**Figs. 2.7A, 8.7**). With the knee flexe to a right angle, the patella is easy to fee anterior to the medial and lateral condyle of the femur and tibia and the joint gap i between. On the lateral side, the head o the fibula has the tendon of biceps fem oris attaching to it. In the leg the media surface of the tibia, commonly called th shin, is subcutaneous and can be traced dis tally (down) to the medial malleolus at th ankle (**Figs. 8.13, 8.14**). On the lateral side most of the fibula is encased in muscles, bu becomes subcutaneous distally, ending a the lateral malleolus.

Knee joint – the joint between the condyle of the femur and tibia, with the patella als taking part anteriorly by articulating wit

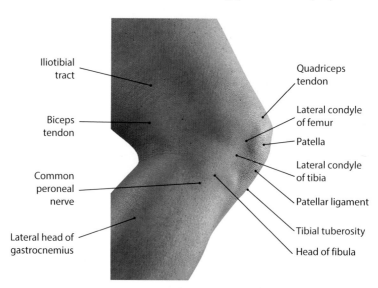

Fig. 8.7 Surface features of the lateral side of the right knee, partly flexed.

ne condyles of the femur (but not with the bia) (**Figs. 8.8–8.10**). The femur and tibia re held together mainly by the lateral and medial collateral ligaments and the anterior nd posterior cruciate ligaments.

The joint capsule is replaced anteriorly y the patella and patellar ligament; the ligament keeps the patella at a constant distance from the upper end of the tibia, although the position of the patella in relation to the femur changes as the knee joint flexes and extends. The popliteus tendon penetrates the lateral side of the capsule posteriorly to reach its attachment to the

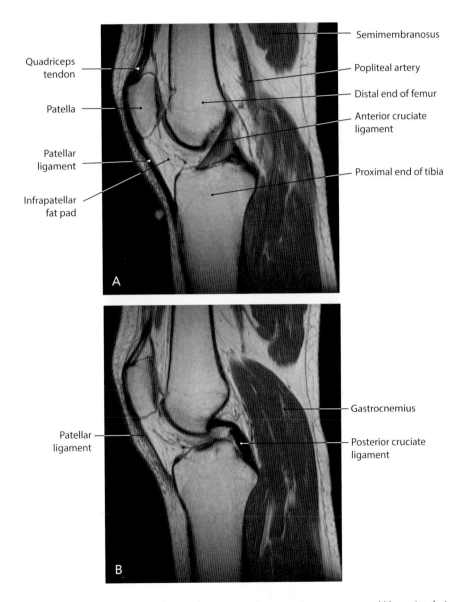

Fig. 8.8 MR images of the right knee demonstrating cruciate anatomy: (A) sagittal view of anterior cruciate ligament, (B) sagittal view of posterior cruciate ligament. *(Continued)*

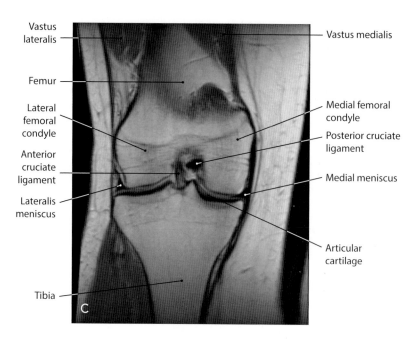

Fig. 8.8 (Continued) MR images of the right knee demonstrating cruciate anatomy (C) coronal view showing both cruciate ligaments.

side of the lateral epicondyle. Although intracapsular, it remains extrasynovial, with a sleeve-like extension of synovial membrane around it.

Lateral ligament – properly called the fibular collateral ligament, is a rounded cord-like structure, about 5 cm long, and is easily felt when 'put on the stretch' (e.g. when sitting down, bring the left ankle up to rest on the right knee, and feel the left lateral ligament running from the head of the fibula to the lateral epicondyle of the femur).

Medial ligament – properly called the tibial collateral ligament, it is a broad band-like structure, about 12 cm long, passing from the medial epicondyle of the femur to a broad area of the tibia distal to the medial condyle. It has superficial and deep layers and is not easily felt.

Cruciate ligaments – named for the fact that they cross each other and from their attachments to the tibia: the *anterior* cruciate (**Figs. 8.8, 8.10**) passes from the *anterior* of the upper surface of the tibia to the inside of the lateral condyle of the femur and the *posterior* cruciate passes from the *posterior* of the upper surface of the tibia to the inside of the medial condyle of the femur. The anterior cruciate ligament is the most frequently injured of the knee ligaments.

> The integrity of the anterior cruciate ligament is tested clinically by the anterior draw sign, in which the patient lies on a couch while their knee is bent to a right angle, then the examiner attempts to pull the tibia anteriorly.

Medial and lateral menisci – the 'cartilages of the knee' are C-shaped structures (although the lateral meniscus is almost circular) attached to the upper surface of

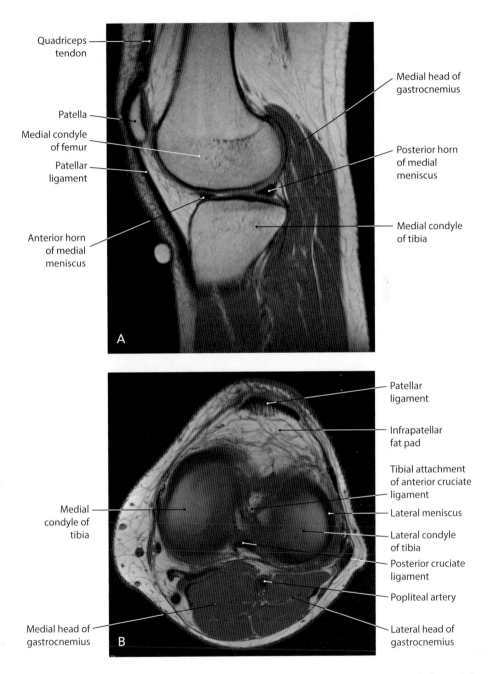

Fig. 8.9 Menisci as visualised using MRI: (A) sagittal section through the medial condyles of the femur and tibia, (B) axial view of both menisci.

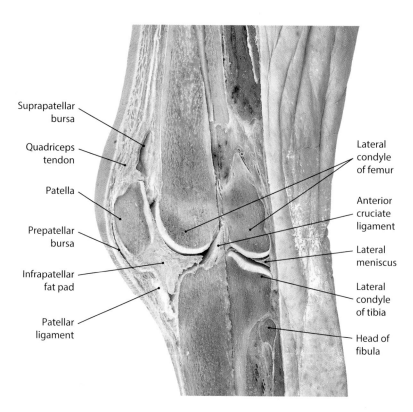

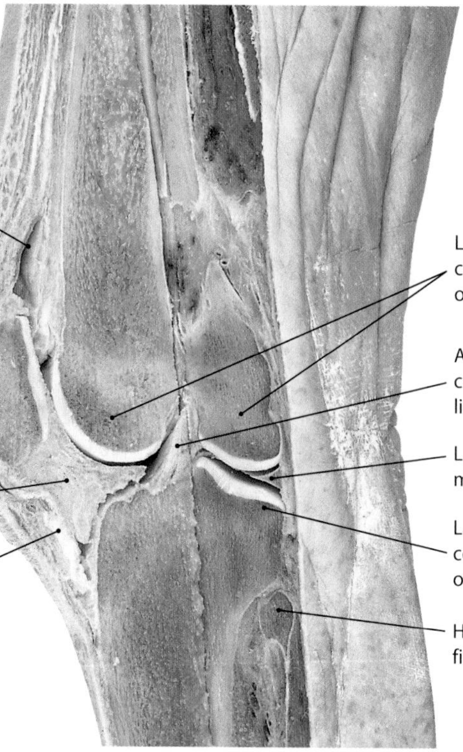
Suprapatellar bursa
Quadriceps tendon
Patella
Prepatellar bursa
Infrapatellar fat pad
Patellar ligament
Lateral condyle of femur
Anterior cruciate ligament
Lateral meniscus
Lateral condyle of tibia
Head of fibula

Fig. 8.10 Section of the left knee. Combined coronal and sagittal section (anterior lateral quadrant removed), showing the lateral condyles of the femur and tibia.

the tibia. The *medial meniscus is also firmly attached to the tibial collateral ligament*, but the lateral one is *not* attached to the lateral ligament. The medial meniscus is thus the more firmly anchored and so more liable to be trapped and torn during twisting movements of the knee than the lateral meniscus (**Figs. 8.8, 8.9**).

> In 'twisting' injuries of the knee the medial meniscus is 20 times more liable to damage than the lateral.

Bursae – numerous in the knee region, but the largest is the suprapatellar bursa (**Fig. 8.10**), which is not a true bursa as it is continuous with the upper end of the synovial cavity and extends deep to the quadriceps tendon for three finger breadths superior to the upper border of the patella.

> Effusions into the knee joint ('water on the knee') inevitably distend this bursa as well.

Others include the semimembranosus bursa behind the tendon, which may communicate with the joint, and the subcutaneous prepatellar bursa anterior to the lower part of the patella and upper part of the patellar ligament (the bursa of 'housemaid's knee' when it is inflamed – bursitis).

The principal muscles that produce movements of the knee joint are:

- **Flexion** – hamstrings, gastrocnemius and weakly popliteus.

- **Extension** – quadriceps femoris.
- **Medial rotation (of tibia, when partially flexed)** – semimembranosus and semitendinosus.
- **Lateral rotation (of tibia, when partially flexed)** – biceps.

Flexion and extension of the knee are hinge-like movements between the femur and tibia, although the movements are not identical with those of a simple hinge, but are complicated by a slight rotation between the two bones. To begin flexion from the fully extended position (and assuming the tibia to be fixed), popliteus (p. 230), passing from the upper part of the posterior tibia to the side of the lateral epicondyle, first 'unlocks' the joint by laterally rotating the femur on the tibia, and then the other flexors carry on the movement. From the flexed position, there is medial rotation of the femur on the tibia towards the end of extension (due to the shape of the joint surfaces and tension in the ligaments) – referred to as 'locking', hence the need for the 'unlocking' movement by popliteus to initiate flexion. In the partially flexed position, the hamstrings can produce some rotation of the leg on the thigh (e.g. with the femur fixed, biceps can cause some lateral rotation of the tibia on the femur, and the semimembranosus and semitendinosus some medial rotation). As part of quadriceps femoris, the lowest fibres of vastus medialis are of great importance for the last few degrees of extension to ensure normal tracking of the patella by pulling medially to prevent it displacing laterally.

> Even a few days of bed rest causes a measurable loss of size and power in the quadriceps muscles, hence the feeling of unsteadiness on getting up and walking again.

Popliteal fossa – a diamond-shaped area posterior to the knee (**Fig. 8.11**), its upper boundaries are the biceps, with the common fibular (peroneal) nerve deep to it on the lateral side, and the semimembranosus, with the tendon of semitendinosus deep to it on the medial side. Its lower boundaries are the lateral head of gastrocnemius and plantaris laterally and the medial head of gastrocnemius medially. The three large structures in the fossa passing vertically in the mid-line of the fossa are the tibial nerve, popliteal vein and popliteal artery, *in that order from superficial to deep.*

> Tearing of the muscular or tendinous fibres of biceps femoris behind the knee is a common sports injury.

Tibial nerve – a direct continuation of the sciatic nerve that runs straight down the middle of the fossa (**Fig. 8.11**) and disappears into the calf between the heads of gastrocnemius to run deep to the soleus. It supplies all the calf muscles and divides inferior to the medial malleolus into the medial and lateral plantar nerves for the cutaneous and muscular innervation of the sole of the foot (**Fig. 8.12**).

Popliteal vein – often double, it runs between the tibial nerve and popliteal artery and receives the small (short) saphenous vein, which pierces the fascial roof of the fossa (**Fig. 8.11**). It accompanies and runs posterior to the popliteal artery.

Popliteal artery – a continuation of the femoral artery that enters the fossa through the opening in adductor magnus (adductor hiatus) and enters the calf deep to gastrocnemius. The depth of the artery (**Fig. 8.11**) makes the popliteal pulse difficult to feel. It is fixed in place by the medial and lateral pairs of genicular branches. This artery is

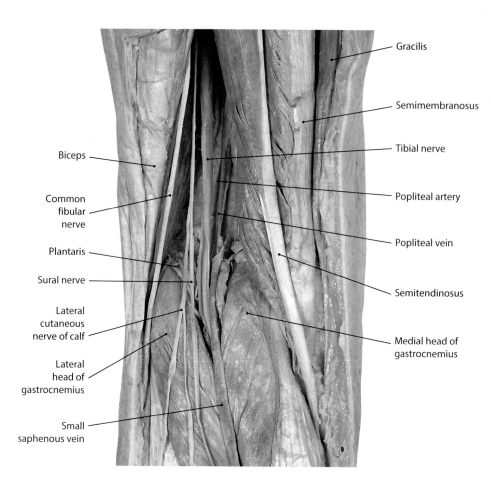

Fig. 8.11 Dissection of the left popliteal fossa.

at risk of laceration in distal fractures of the femur. The artery divides in the upper calf into the anterior and posterior tibial arteries, which supply the leg and foot.

> The popliteal pulse is best felt from the front with the knee flexed, with the examiner's thumbs on the front of the knee and the fingers of both hands pressing forwards into the middle of the fossa.

Anterior tibial artery – runs superior to the interosseous membrane to lie between the extensor muscles of the anterior leg. At the ankle it lies between the tendons of extensor hallucis longus medially and

extensor digitorum longus laterally. As the anterior tibial artery passes across the ankle joint it changes its name to the dorsalis pedis artery (**Fig. 8.13A**). Its metatarsal branches provide dorsal digital vessels for the sides of the toes.

> The dorsalis pedis pulse can be palpated along the upper part of a line from the midpoint between the malleoli towards the first toe cleft (but note that the artery is absent in about 12% of feet).

Posterior tibial artery – runs deeply between the calf muscles on the tibial side to reach the posterior aspect of the medial

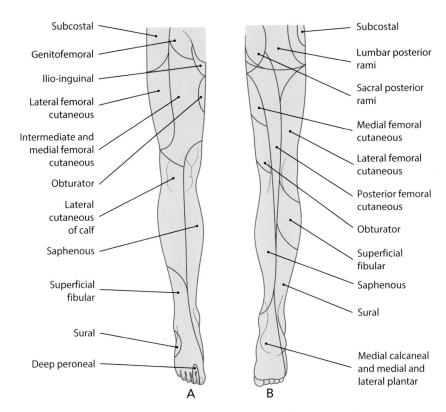

Fig. 8.12 Cutaneous nerves of the right lower limb: (A) front, (B) back.

malleolus (**Fig. 8.14A**). It gives off the fibular (peroneal) artery that runs laterally, posterior to the fibula. The posterior tibial artery ends by dividing inferior to the sustentaculum tali of the calcaneus into the medial and lateral plantar arteries, which enter the sole. Distally, the lateral plantar artery turns medially as the plantar arch (level with the bases of the middle metatarsal bones) to anastomose with the dorsalis pedis artery through the first intermetatarsal space. The metatarsal branches provide plantar digital vessels for the sides of the toes.

> The posterior tibial pulse is palpated behind the medial malleolus 2.5 cm anterior to the medial border of the calcaneal (Achilles') tendon.

> The common fibular nerve wraps around the neck of the fibula and is liable to injury (e.g. by a tight plaster cast or fracture of the fibular neck), giving rise to foot drop and loss of sensation over the lateral dorsum of the foot.

Common fibular (peroneal) nerve – arising from the sciatic nerve at the apex of the popliteal fossa, it runs down deep to the biceps tendon and curls anteriorly around the neck of the fibula (**Fig. 8.7**), where it lies superficial, easily palpable and in contact with the bone where it is vulnerable to injury. Here it divides into the superficial fibular (peroneal) nerve, which innervates skin on the anterior of the distal leg and dorsum of the foot and the lateral group

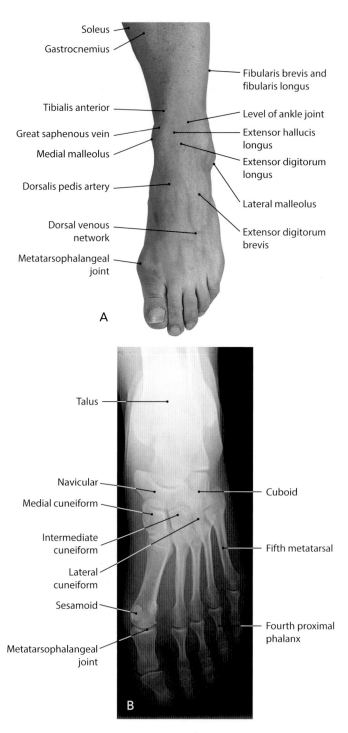

Fig. 8.13 The left leg, ankle and dorsum of the foot: (A) surface features, (B) anteroposterior radiograph.

of muscles fibularis (peroneus) longus and brevis. The deep fibular (peroneal) nerve continues anteriorly into the anterior compartment of the leg to run with the anterior tibial artery and innervates the ankle extensor muscles and a small area of skin of the dorsal first toe web space.

Tibialis anterior – forms the bulge on the anterolateral side of the upper part of the shin (leg). Its tendon passes distally anterior to the ankle joint (**Fig. 8.13A**) to attach to the medial side of the medial cuneiform and base of the first metatarsal. It is innervated by the deep fibular (peroneal) nerve.

Extensor hallucis longus and extensor digitorum longus – relatively smaller muscles with the latter lying superficially from the anterior fibula and the former deeper from the fibula and adjacent interosseous membrane. Anterior to the ankle these tendons lie lateral to that of tibialis anterior (**Fig. 8.13A**) and pass to the great toe and other toes, respectively, to form dorsal digital expansions similar to those of the fingers (p. 119). The lateral part of the digitorum muscle distally is fibularis (peroneus) tertius, which reaches the base and/or shaft of the fifth metatarsal. In some people it appears to be absent, as it blends with the extensor expansion of the fifth digit. All are innervated by the deep fibular (peroneal) nerve.

Superior and inferior extensor retinacula – thickenings of deep fascia at the ankle and on the dorsum of the foot, respectively, they prevent underlying ankle extensor tendons from bowing forwards. The order of the tendons at the ankle from medial to lateral is tibialis anterior, extensor hallucis longus, extensor digitorum longus and fibularis (peroneus) tertius (**Fig. 8.13A**). The palpable anterior tibial

vessels and deep fibular (peroneal) nerve lie between the hallucis and digitorum tendons.

Extensor digitorum brevis – the only muscle of the dorsum of the foot, from the dorsal surface of the calcaneus it gives off tendons that join the hallucis and digitorum tendons to the four medial toes. The part going to the great toe is sometimes called the extensor hallucis brevis. It is innervated by the deep fibular (peroneal) nerve.

Great saphenous vein – passing proximally from the medial side of the foot, it lies at the ankle *anterior to the medial malleolus* (**Fig. 8.14A**). This was formerly the common site for intravenous infusions, which may still be given here, but upper limb veins are now preferred since there is a greater risk of thrombosis in the leg veins, although in an emergency for a short time it can provide easy access, especially in the younger patient. The vein runs proximally subcutaneously and at the knee lies a hand's breadth posterior to the medial border of the patella. Continuing proximally, it drains into the femoral vein after passing through the saphenous opening of the superficial fascia covering the femoral triangle (p. 210).

> The great saphenous vein runs anterior to the medial malleolus; the small saphenous vein runs posterior to the lateral malleolus.

Small saphenous vein and sural nerve – passing proximally from the lateral side of the foot, the vein lies at the ankle posterior to the lateral malleolus and runs subcutaneously to reach the popliteal fossa where it drains into the popliteal vein (**Fig. 8.11**). It is accompanied by the sural nerve,

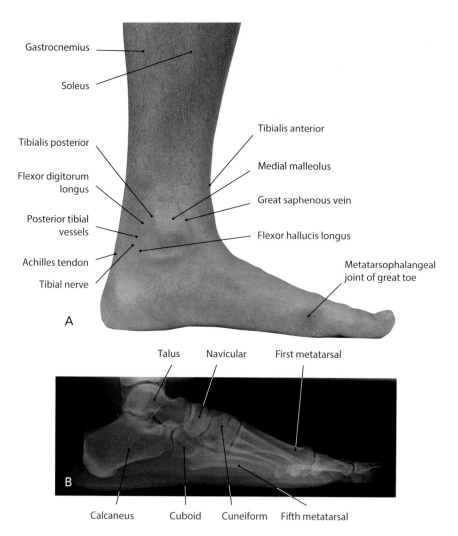

Fig. 8.14 Medial side of the left foot: (A) surface features, (B) radiograph of a weight-bearing foot.

a cutaneous branch of the tibial nerve. Since it only supplies the skin on a small part of the heel, the sural nerve is considered expendable and is harvested for biopsy or for a nerve graft.

Perforating veins – mostly posterior to the lower part of the tibia and medial malleolus, uniting deep and superficial veins. Some perforators are joined together by the posterior arch vein, which runs into the great saphenous at a higher level. These veins and their tributaries are the ones that may become dilated and tortuous – varicose veins. The perforating veins have valves that direct blood from superficial to deep, so that the 'muscular pump' of the muscles of sole and calf can help the return of blood to the top of the limb.

posterior of the femur superior to the medial condyle and a lateral head from superior to the lateral condyle (**Fig. 8.11**). It forms, with the tendon of soleus, the tendo calcaneus or Achilles tendon, attached to the posterior of the calcaneus (**Figs. 8.14, 8.15**). Gastrocnemius is innervated by the tibial nerve.

> Incompetence of the valves in perforating veins allows the hydrostatic pressure in the deep venous system to be transmitted to the superficial veins, resulting in varicose veins (dilated, tortuous veins). Varicose veins are more common in females, perhaps due to pressure on abdominal veins during pregnancy, and may lead to ulceration of the skin above the medial malleolus (venous ulcers).

> A ruptured Achilles tendon, a painful injury, gives a palpable gap above the calcaneus. It results in the loss of ability to plantar flex the foot so that it is impossible to stand on tiptoe on the affected side.

Gastrocnemius – the most superficial calf muscle, with a medial head from the

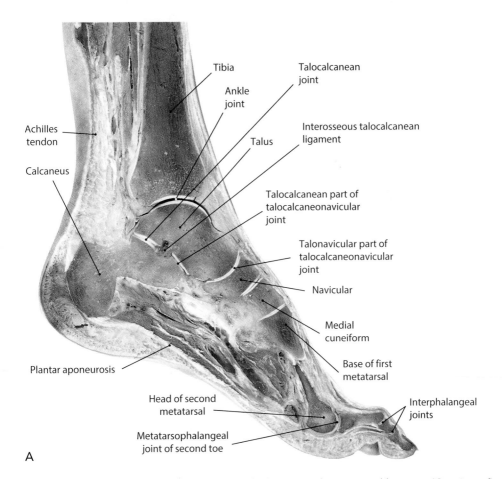

A

Fig. 8.15 Left foot: (A) sagittal section through the second metatarsal bone.   *(Continued)*

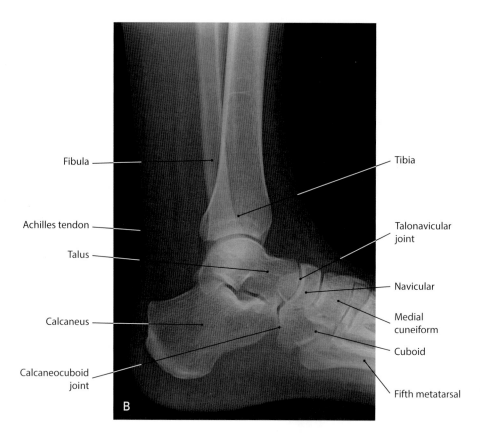

Fibula — Tibia

Achilles tendon — Talonavicular joint

Talus —

Navicular

Calcaneus — Medial cuneiform

Cuboid

Calcaneocuboid joint —

Fifth metatarsal

B

Fig. 8.15 (Continued) Left foot: (B) radiograph of the ankle and hindfoot.

Soleus – immediately deep to the gastrocnemius, with an arched attachment from the posterior of the proximal tibia (creating the soleal line) and fibula, distally it becomes tendinous to blend with gastrocnemius. Viewed from behind it bulges slightly beyond the gastrocnemius at each side (**Fig. 8.14A**). The many veins located especially in this muscle form part of the muscle pump designed to aid venous return to the top of the limb. It is innervated by the tibial nerve.

> In and around the soleus muscle is a plexus of veins within which, in patients who are confined to bed, blood may stagnate and lead to deep vein thrombosis, with the possibility of pulmonary emboli (p. 151).

Plantaris – a very small muscle belly from the posterior of the femur superior to the lateral condyle, with a very long thin tendon running down between gastrocnemius and soleus to join the medial side of the Achilles tendon. Rupture causes pain, but no palpable gap. It is innervated by the tibial nerve.

> Clinically, plantaris is harvested to act as a tendon graft for tendon or ligament reconstruction where needed.

Popliteus – triangular-shaped muscle that arises from the upper posterior part of the tibia above the soleal line, and passes upwards and laterally to the lateral part of the lateral condyle of the femur, with an attachment also to the lateral meniscus. It plays the vitally important role of 'unlocking' the knee joint to initiate knee flexion (p. 223). It is innervated by the tibial nerve.

Tibialis posterior – deepest muscle of the calf, from the posterior of the *tibia* and *fibula* and interosseous membrane, which stretches between the two bones, with a tendon that passes medially to lie posterior to the medial malleolus (**Fig. 8.14A**) and runs to the tuberosity of the navicular bone. It is innervated by the tibial nerve.

Flexor digitorum longus – from the posterior of the *tibia*, with a tendon that runs superficial to tibialis posterior at the ankle (**Figs. 8.14A**) and forms the tendons for the lateral four toes (corresponding to flexor digitorum profundus in the hand), where they are attached to the bases of the distal phalanges. It is innervated by the tibial nerve.

Flexor hallucis longus – from the posterior of the *fibula*, with a tendon that grooves the posterior of the talus and then crosses medially in the sole (deep to flexor digitorum longus) to reach the base of the distal phalanx of the great toe (**Fig. 8.18**). It is innervated by the tibial nerve.

Flexor retinaculum – from the medial malleolus to the side of the calcaneus, it keeps the flexor tendons in place. The order of tendons *behind the medial malleolus*, from medial to lateral, is tibialis posterior, flexor digitorum longus, flexor hallucis longus (**Fig. 8.14A**). The posterior tibial vessels and tibial nerve lie between the digitorum and hallucis tendons and divide just distal to the malleolus into the medial and lateral plantar vessels and nerves, which supply the muscles and skin of the sole.

Fibularis (peroneus) longus and fibularis (peroneus) brevis – arising from the fibula, they form the muscles of the small lateral compartment of the leg. At the ankle the brevis tendon is in contact with the posterior surface of the lateral malleolus, and runs distally to attach to the base of the fifth metatarsal. The longus tendon is superficial to that of brevis, and enters the sole where it lies in the groove on the cuboid bone (**Fig. 8.16A**) before attaching to the medial cuneiform and the base of the first metatarsal (on the sides of these bones opposite the attachment of tibialis anterior). Both muscles flex the ankle and evert the foot and are innervated by the superficial fibular (peroneal) nerve.

Superior fibular (peroneal) retinaculum – from the lateral malleolus to the side of the calcaneus, it keeps the tendons of fibularis (peroneus) longus and brevis in place, with brevis deep to longus *posterior to the lateral malleolus*, where the small saphenous vein and sural nerve also lie.

Inferior fibular (peroneal) retinaculum – holds the fibular (peroneal) tendons against the side of the calcaneus, above and below the fibular (peroneal) tubercle, respectively.

Ankle joint – between the lower ends of the tibia and fibula and the talus (**Figs. 8.15, 8.16**). The joint capsule is reinforced by the medial (deltoid) ligament, which runs from the medial malleolus to the side of the talus and the sustentaculum tali of the calcaneus (deep fibres) and navicular (superficial layer of fibres). It is very strong. On the lateral side there is not one ligament, but three small ones: anterior and posterior talofibular, and calcaneofibular. The anterior talofibular is the most commonly injured ankle ligament.

Severe injuries at the ankle usually cause an avulsion fracture of the attached bone rather than tearing the ligament put under strain. However, lesser injuries are more common and result in partial tearing of the ligament (sprain).

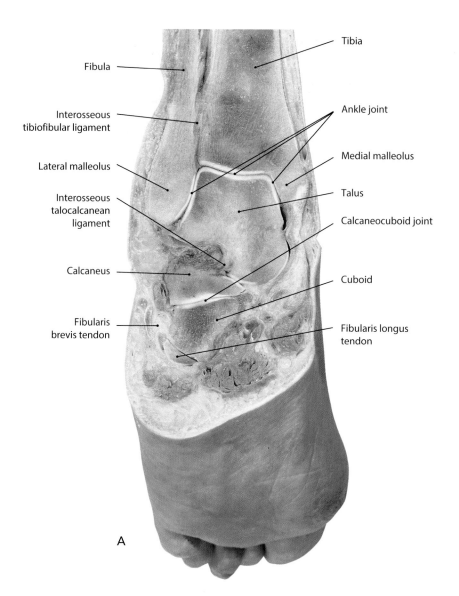

Fibula

Interosseous
tibiofibular ligament

Lateral malleolus

Interosseous
talocalcanean
ligament

Calcaneus

Fibularis
brevis tendon

Tibia

Ankle joint

Medial malleolus

Talus

Calcaneocuboid joint

Cuboid

Fibularis longus
tendon

A

Fig. 8.16 Left ankle joint: (A) coronal section.   *(Continued)*

The principal muscles that produce movements at the ankle joint are:

- **Extension (dorsiflexion)** – tibialis anterior, extensor hallucis longus, extensor digitorum longus and fibularis (peroneus) tertius.

- **Flexion (plantarflexion)** – gastrocnemius, soleus, tibialis posterior, flexor hallucis longus, flexor digitorum longus, fibularis (peroneus) longus and brevis.

The way the talus is gripped between the tibia and fibula means that the only

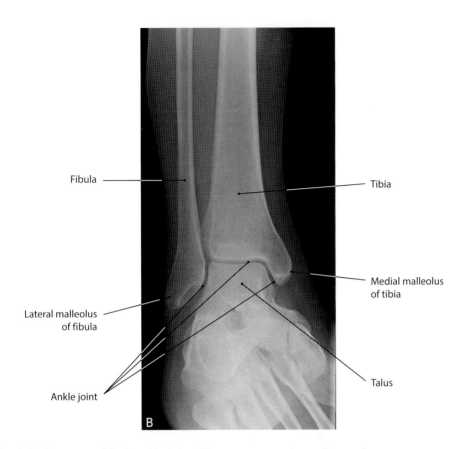

Fibula

Tibia

Medial malleolus
of tibia

Lateral malleolus
of fibula

Talus

Ankle joint

B

Fig. 8.16 *(Continued)* Left ankle joint: (B) anteroposterior radiograph.

movements possible are extension and flexion (see below for other foot movements).

Subtalar joint – collective name for joints beneath the talus, which are the talocalcaneal joint posteriorly (sometimes itself called the subtalar joint) and the talocalcaneonavicular joint (with two parts – talocalcaneal and talonavicular) anteriorly (**Figs. 8.15, 8.16**). It is at these joints that most of the movements of inversion and eversion of the foot occur. The interosseous talocalcaneal ligament (**Figs. 8.15A, 8.16A**), which passes between the adjacent grooves on the lower surface of the talus and upper surface of the calcaneus, is a strong band that

holds the talus and calcaneus together. Imagine the talus gripped between the malleoli and the whole of the rest of the foot swivelling inwards (inversion) or outwards (eversion) underneath the talus.

Mid-tarsal joint – collective name for the calcaneocuboid joint and the talonavicular joint (front part of the talocalcaneonavicular joint) (**Fig. 8.20**), where a small amount of inversion and eversion occurs.

The principal muscles that produce movements at the subtalar and mid-tarsal joints are:

- **Inversion** – tibialis anterior and tibialis posterior.

- **Eversion** – fibularis (peroneus) longus, brevis and tertius.

Plantar aponeurosis – from the medial and lateral tubercles of the calcaneus, it divides distally into five slips, one for each toe, and fuses with the fibrous flexor sheaths and the metatarsophalangeal joint capsules (**Fig. 8.17**). It acts as a strong tie-beam that helps to preserve the longitudinal arches of the foot; it has numerous septa, which run into the skin and subcutaneous tissue of the sole to give a firm union between these structures. Plantar fasciitis is a common painful inflammation of this fascia.

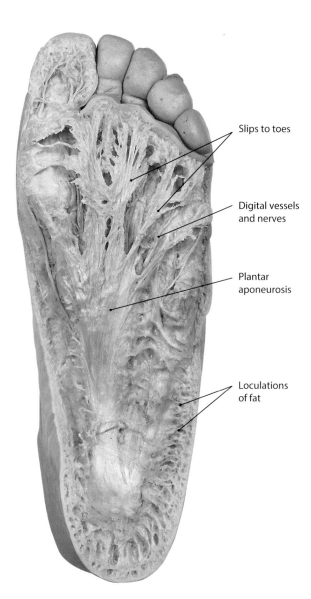

Slips to toes

Digital vessels and nerves

Plantar aponeurosis

Loculations of fat

Fig. 8.17 Dissection of the plantar aponeurosis of the left foot.

Muscles of the sole – like the palm of the hand, the sole has separate muscles for the great and little toes, as well as others with multiple tendons. Of the larger and more important muscles, flexor digitorum brevis is the central superficial muscle of the sole, immediately deep to the plantar aponeurosis (it corresponds to flexor digitorum superficialis in the hand), with tendons to the middle phalanges of the four lateral toes splitting to allow the tendons of flexor digitorum longus to pass through to the distal phalanges (**Fig. 8.18**). Quadratus plantae, sometimes called flexor accessorius, is deep to brevis, attaching to flexor digitorum longus (just before that muscle

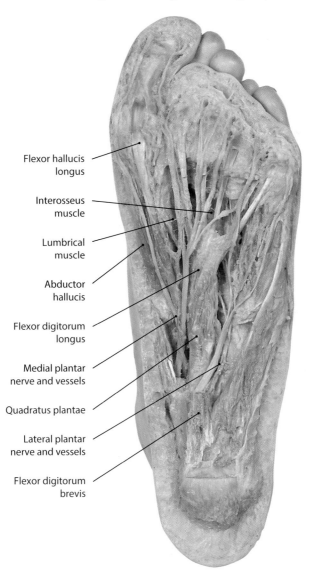

Fig. 8.18 Dissection of the sole of the left foot after removal of the plantar aponeurosis and most of the flexor digitorum brevis.

splits into its four tendons) and supposedly counteracts the slightly oblique pull of longus. The lumbrical and interosseous muscles have similar attachments to those of the hand, and are important in keeping the toes straight (i.e. flexing the metatarsophalangeal joints and extending the interphalangeal joints).

Medial and lateral plantar nerves – the nerves of the skin and muscles of the sole (**Fig. 8.18**). The medial plantar innervates abductor hallucis, flexor digitorum brevis, flexor hallucis brevis and the first lumbrical; *all the others* are innervated by the lateral plantar nerve, mostly by its deep branch, which curls around the lateral border of quadratus plantae. Cutaneous branches from the lateral plantar nerve innervate the lateral side of the sole and lateral one-and-a-half toes, with medial plantar branches going to the medial three-and-a-half toes and the medial part of the sole.

Ligaments of the foot – many ligaments unite the various foot bones; because of the arched shape of the foot, those of the sole are particularly strong. The interosseous talocalcaneal ligament is mentioned above. Others of particular importance are the long and short plantar ligaments and the spring ligament.

Long plantar ligament – a strong band that runs from the calcaneus to the cuboid and the bases of the middle three metatarsals. It converts the groove on the cuboid into a tunnel for the fibularis (peroneus) longus tendon.

Short plantar ligament – (properly called the plantar calcaneocuboid ligament) is deep to the long plantar ligament.

Spring ligament – (properly called the plantar calcaneonavicular ligament) runs from the sustentaculum tali of the calcaneus to the navicular, blending at the side with the deltoid ligament of the ankle and forming an important support for the head of the talus on its upper surface.

> Despite its common name, the spring ligament does not contain an unusual amount of elastic tissue.

Joints of the toes – structurally similar to those of the fingers, the most important is the metatarsophalangeal joint of the great toe (**Figs. 8.19, 8.20**), which is particularly involved in the 'push-off' phase of walking and running. Ill-fitting shoes can produce a lateral deformity of the toe, hallux valgus, which once begun is enhanced by the pull of the long flexor and extensor tendons to cause undue prominence of the head of the first metatarsal – a bunion.

Maintenance of arches – in the static foot the maintenance of the arches (p. 31) depends largely on ligaments (which cannot change their tension, although they may become stretched), mainly on the long and short plantar and spring ligaments, and on the plantar aponeurosis. During gait (walking and running), muscles assume an important role since they can contract and vary the tension exerted by their tendons as required. The important muscles are the small muscles of the foot, together with tibialis anterior and tibialis posterior on the medial side and fibularis (peroneus) longus and brevis on the lateral side. Muscles tend to contract to raise the arches before they are loaded with body weight and then gradually relax as the ligaments start to take the load.

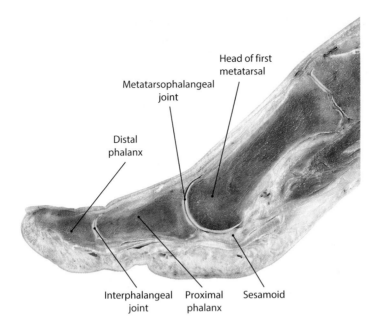

Head of first metatarsal

Metatarsophalangeal joint

Distal phalanx

Interphalangeal joint   Proximal phalanx   Sesamoid

Fig. 8.19 Sagittal section of the left great toe.

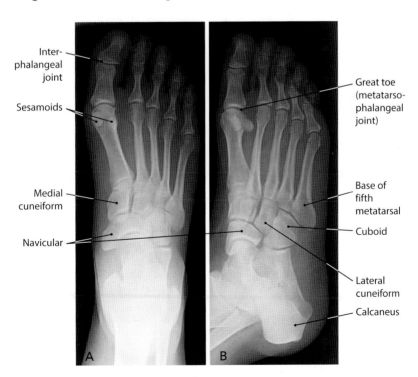

Inter-phalangeal joint

Sesamoids

Medial cuneiform

Navicular

Great toe (metatarso-phalangeal joint)

Base of fifth metatarsal

Cuboid

Lateral cuneiform

Calcaneus

A   B

Fig. 8.20 Radiographs of a left foot: (A) anteroposterior view, (B) oblique view demonstrating the tarsal bones more clearly.

Summary

- Deep to gluteus maximus, the *piriformis muscle* is the key to locating structures in the gluteal region. Of the vessels and nerves that emerge from the pelvis to enter the region, all do so by passing inferior to piriformis except for the superior gluteal nerve and vessels, which emerge superiorly. The most important structure in the region is the *sciatic nerve*, the largest in the body. At the top of the back of the thigh it lies midway between the ischial spine and the greater trochanter of the femur, and then runs distally deep to the hamstrings, which it innervates, to end at the top of the popliteal fossa by dividing into the tibial and common fibular (peroneal) nerves.
- The anterior of the capsule of the *hip joint* is attached to the intertrochanteric line, but posteriorly the capsule does not reach as far as the intertrochanteric crest, being attached halfway along the back of the femoral neck. Fracture of the neck disrupts blood vessels that supply the head of the femur.
- The *iliofemoral ligament*, reinforcing the hip joint capsule anteriorly, is one of the strongest in the body. The flexors of the hip (psoas major, rectus femoris) are mainly innervated by the *femoral nerve*, the adductors by the *obturator nerve* and the hamstrings by the *sciatic nerve*, with *gluteus maximus* extending the flexed hip (as in standing from a seated position and climbing stairs) being innervated by the inferior gluteal nerve. *Gluteus medius* and *minimus*, which prevent tilting of the pelvis when the opposite foot is off the ground during walking, are innervated by the superior gluteal nerve.
- At the front of the upper thigh, the *femoral nerve* lies lateral to the palpable *femoral artery*, with the *femoral vein* on the medial side of the artery and the femoral canal (the site of a possible femoral hernia) medial to the vein. Other palpable arteries in the lower limb are the popliteal, dorsalis pedis and posterior tibial.
- The *quadriceps tendon* is attached to the upper end of the patella; the patellar ligament attaches the lower end to the tuberosity of the tibia.
- The *tibial nerve* passes down among the muscles of the posterior or flexor compartment of the leg, which it supplies, to divide, inferior to the medial malleolus, into the medial and lateral plantar nerves, which supply the foot.
- The *common fibular (peroneal) nerve* divides at the neck of the fibula into the superficial fibular (peroneal) nerve, supplying skin of the leg and dorsum of the foot and the lateral fibular (peroneal) compartment of muscles, and the deep fibular (peroneal) nerve, which is the motor nerve of the muscles of the anterior extensor compartment of the leg.
- *Hinge movements* during flexion and extension of the knee are complicated by rotation between the femur and tibia; with the knee in extension, the popliteus muscle (tibial nerve) is required to 'unlock' the joint to initiate flexion. The medial meniscus of the knee joint is firmly fixed to the medial ligament, and is more frequently damaged than the lateral meniscus, which has an attachment to the popliteus tendon.
- Lying anterior to the *ankle* the order of structures from medial to lateral is: tibialis anterior, extensor hallucis longus, anterior tibial vessels, deep fibular (peroneal) nerve and extensor digitorum longus.
- Lying posterior to the *medial malleolus* the order of structures from medial to lateral is: tibialis posterior, flexor digitorum longus, posterior tibial vessels, tibial nerve and flexor hallucis longus.

- Lying posterior to the *lateral malleolus*, fibularis (peroneus) brevis lies deep to fibularis (peroneus) longus.
- The *great saphenous vein* lies anterior to the medial malleolus and ends by joining the femoral vein, passing through the saphenous opening, which lies 3.5 cm below and lateral to the pubic tubercle.
- The *small saphenous vein* lies posterior to the lateral malleolus and runs up the posterior of the leg to drain into the popliteal vein in the popliteal fossa, where the order of structures from superficial to deep is: tibial nerve, popliteal vein and popliteal artery.
- At the ankle joint only flexion and extension occur; inversion and eversion of the foot take place at the joints beneath the talus, with the two tibialis muscles (anterior and posterior) producing inversion and the two fibularis (peroneal) muscles (longus and brevis) producing eversion.
- The segments of the *spinal cord* mainly concerned in supplying major limb muscles are: L2 – psoas major; L3 – quadriceps femoris; L4 – tibialis anterior and posterior; L5 – fibularis (peroneus) longus and brevis; S1 – gastrocnemius; S2 – small muscles of the foot.

Questions

Answers can be found in Appendix A, p. 250.

Question 1

The femoral triangle is an important region in the upper thigh and is frequently explored surgically. Which of the statements below is anatomically accurate?

(a) The femoral artery lies lateral to the femoral nerve beside the femoral canal.

(b) The femoral canal is bounded anteriorly by the inguinal ligament and posteriorly by the superior pubic ramus and contains lymphatic channels and nodes.

(c) The femoral artery has only one branch in the distal part of the femoral triangle and this is the circumflex femoral artery.

(d) The femoral vein lies lateral to the femoral artery and receives the great saphenous vein as its tributary.

(e) The femoral nerve lies within the femoral sheath lateral to the femoral vein before it starts to branch distal to the sheath.

Question 2

The hip joint is a very stable joint. Which of the statements below most accurately describes the related anatomy?

(a) When the right limb is supporting body weight, it is gluteus medius and minimus on the unsupported left limb that prevent falling to the unsupported left limb.

(b) When walking upstairs, it is the action of the extensor muscles of the hip and knee to counter the effects of gravity in the limb taking the load that will raise the body up.

(c) When sitting down, the hip flexor muscles, psoas and rectus femoris actively control the rate of descending from the standing position.

(d) When standing upright, the hip joint is in the extended position and the degree of extension is actively controlled by psoas and rectus femoris.

(e) Adduction of the hip joint by the adductor group of muscles is limited by the iliofemoral and ischiofemoral ligaments.

Question 3

The innervation of the muscles of the lower limb follows a clear pattern. In the statements below, identify the one that most accurately describes the anatomy of lower limb innervation?

(a) Sectioning the sciatic nerve at the apex of the popliteal fossa will denervate all muscles of the leg and posterior thigh.

(b) Sectioning the obturator nerve at the obturator foramen as it enters the thigh will prevent hip abduction.

(c) If the common fibular nerve is sectioned at the neck of fibula, there will be a weakness in ankle inversion and loss of ankle extension.

(d) If the posterior tibial nerve is sectioned, there will be a loss of active ankle flexion.

(e) Sectioning of the common fibular nerve in the popliteal fossa will cause problems, with popliteus being unable to unlock the extended knee.

Question 4

The knee joint is basically a hinge joint maintained by ligaments rather than bony shape. Which statement most accurately describes knee ligaments?

(a) The fibular collateral ligament is a broad flat band that is not palpable.

(b) The anterior cruciate ligament passes from the anterior of the intercondylar notch of the femur to the posterior of the tibial intercondylar ridge.

(c) The posterior cruciate passes from the posterior of the upper surface of the tibia to the posterior aspect of the intercondylar notch of the femur.

(d) The tibial collateral ligament is a broad flat band to which the medial meniscus gains attachment.

(e) The patellar ligament passes from the tibial tuberosity to the patella and is important in preventing the femur slipping forwards on the tibia.

Question 5

The popliteal fossa is a diamond-shaped space posterior to the knee joint. Identify the statement below that most accurately describes popliteal anatomy.

(a) Biceps femoris forms the medial border superiorly and the common fibular nerve lies deep to its medial edge.

(b) The tibial nerve lies in the midline just deep to the popliteal vein.

(c) The inferior boundary is formed by the two heads of gastrocnemius and plantaris arising from the medial femoral condyle.

(d) The popliteal artery is the deepest structure in the fossa and is held in place by pairs of genicular arteries passing medially and laterally.

(e) The popliteal vein lies deep to the popliteal artery and the tibial nerve is the most superficial structure within the fossa.

Question 6

Muscles of the leg have actions mostly seen at the ankle and foot joints. Which statement is anatomically accurate?

(a) Flexor hallucis longus passes most laterally behind the medial malleolus to run and attach to the proximal phalanx of the big toe and only flexes the metatarsophalangeal joint.

(b) Flexor digitorum longus passes posterior to the medial malleolus to run obliquely across the foot, splitting to attach to the middle phalanx of each, and flexes only the joints it crosses.

(c) Tibialis posterior runs posterior to the medial malleolus to attach to the tuberosity of the navicular and flexes and inverts the ankle.

(d) Fibularis longus attaches to the base of the fifth metacarpal and will flex and invert the foot.

(e) Tibialis anterior attaches to the tuberosity of the navicular and allows flexion and inversion of the ankle joint.

Question 7

The main ligaments of the foot have clear attachments, functions and descriptive names. Of the statements below, which most accurately describes the anatomy of the named ligament?

(a) The head of the talus is supported by the plantar calcaneonavicular (spring) ligament.

(b) The long plantar ligament attaches to the cuboid proximal to the peroneus longus tendon.

(c) The interosseous ligament of the talus joins it to the navicular bone.

(d) The plantar aponeurosis joins the calcaneus to the metatarsals.

(e) The spring ligament is designed to maintain the lateral longitudinal arch.

Question 8

A 32-year-old woman injured her right superior gluteal nerve in a road traffic accident. On physical examination it was noted that she had a waddling gait and a positive Trendelenburg sign. Which of the following is the most likely physical finding in this patient?

(a) The right side of the pelvis sags or droops when she attempts to stand on her left foot.

(b) The left side of the pelvis sags or droops when she attempts to stand on her right foot.

(c) She cannot stand from a seated position.

(d) She has difficulty flexing her right thigh at the hip.

(e) She has difficulty extending her left thigh at the hip.

Question 9

A 19-year-old man was struck by an automobile while crossing a road. In the Emergency Department a radiograph showed a fracture of his proximal fibula. Physical examination revealed that he was unable to dorsiflex his foot on the injured side, a condition known as 'foot drop'. Which of the following nerves is most likely injured?

(a) Saphenous.

(b) Superficial fibular.

(c) Deep fibular.

(d) Tibial.

(e) Sciatic.

Question 10

A 72-year-old woman is undergoing a total hip replacement (hip arthroplasty). After incising the gluteal musculature the orthopaedic surgeon identifies the underlying structures. Which of the following structures is used as a key landmark in this region?

(a) Sciatic nerve.

(b) Piriformis muscle.

(c) Gemellus muscles.

(d) Ischial tuberosity.

(e) Obturator externus.

Question 11

After suffering an injury to her right knee during a soccer match, a 22-year-old woman is seen at the local orthopaedic clinic. She is seated during the physical examination and the examining physician holds her right leg with both hands. The right leg can be pulled anteriorly but not posteriorly. The left leg does not move when the same test is performed on that side. Which of the following structures is most likely injured in this patient?

(a) Medial meniscus.

(b) Lateral meniscus.

(c) Anterior cruciate ligament.

(d) Posterior cruciate ligament.

(e) Medial collateral ligament.

Question 12

A 20-year-old man suffers a laceration to the posterior portion of his foot when walking barefooted. The examining physician performs a physical examination. Movements of the foot at the toes are normal except the patient is unable to abduct his toes. Which of the following nerves has most likely been transected (cut)?

(a) Superficial fibular.

(b) Deep fibular.

(c) Medial plantar.

(d) Lateral plantar.

(e) Saphenous.

Question 13

A 23-year-old woman injures her ankle after tripping on an uneven surface. Radiographs reveal no broken bones in her foot. Physical examination reveals a severe inversion sprain of her ankle. Which of the following structures has most likely been injured in this patient?

(a) Anterior talofibular ligament.

(b) Posterior talofibular ligament.

(c) Medial plantar nerve.

(d) Lateral plantar nerve.

(e) Deltoid ligament.

Question 14

A 24-year-old man was shot in the popliteal fossa in a hunting accident. The man was carried to the Emergency Department where the attending surgeon recognised that the bullet had severed the tibial nerve. Which of the following would have most likely been seen during a physical examination of this patient?

(a) Inability to extend the knee.

(b) Inability to flex the knee.

(c) Inability to stand from a seated position.

(d) A dorsiflexed and everted foot.

(e) Foot drop.

Appendix A
Answers to questions

Chapter 2

Q1 Answer: (c).
See Carpal bones (p. 22, 26).

Q2 Answer: (b).
See Tarsal bones (p. 30).

Q3 Answer: (d).
See Vertebrae (p. 16).

Q4 Answer: (b).
See Introduction (p. 11).

Q5 Answer: (a).
See Introduction (p. 11).

Q6 Answer: (a).
The scaphoid is the most commonly fractured carpal bone. In forceful extension of the wrist, such as when falling on an outstretched hand, the 'waist' of the scaphoid is levered over the styloid process of the radius, resulting in a fracture. The 'anatomical snuffbox' (p. 119) is an area at the lateral base of the thumb formed by the tendons of the extensor pollicis longus and the superimposed tendons of the extensor pollicis brevis and abductor pollicis longus. The radial artery traverses the snuff box, but more importantly for this case the scaphoid forms the floor of the snuff box. Tenderness in the snuff box is indicative of a fractured scaphoid. This is confirmed by radiography.

Q7 Answer: (c).
The fibula is a non-weight bearing bone that is not essential for ambulation. All the other bones are weight bearing or essential for forearm function. It has been observed that the main blood supply of the fibula, the fibular artery and vein, are relatively large. This fact would make it easier to re-anastomosis the blood supply in a new location, such as the forearm. Studies have shown that when the fibula has been harvested to be used as a free vascularized graft, there is no resultant abnormality in the patient's gait.

Q8 Answer: (c).
A major structure securing the clavicle to the scapula is the coracoclavicular ligament (pp. 101–102) that runs from the coracoid process of the scapula to the inferior surface of the clavicle near its lateral end. It consists of two parts, the conoid and the trapezoid ligaments, either of which could be torn in a shoulder dislocation. Generally, it is not important to determine if one or both of these ligaments are torn as treatment is usually the same in either case. Dislocation of the glenohumeral joint (p. 107) would create a step between the acromion and the upper humerus.

Chapter 3

Q1 Answer: (c).
See Pituitary gland (p. 37).

Q2 Answer: (d).
See **Fig. 3.4** and Head and neck in sagittal section (p. 39).

Q3 Answer: (e).
See Precentral gyrus, Postcentral gyrus and Lateral sulcus (p. 45).

Q4 Answer: (a).
See pp. 45–50.

Q5 Answer: (c).
See Cranial nerves (pp. 52–55).

Q6 Answer: (a).
See sections on Tracts in the spinal cord (pp. 56–58).

Q7 Answer: (e).
See Teeth (p. 68).

Q8 Answer: (b).
See pp. 42, 86 and 87 and **Fig. 3.5**.

Q9 Answer: (a).
The pituitary stalk has most likely been ruptured during the head trauma. The pituitary stalk conducts antidiuretic hormone (ADH; and oxytocin, which is not relevant in this case) to the posterior pituitary where it is released into the bloodstream to regulate kidney function. Specifically, ADH increases reabsorption of water in the distal convoluted tubules of the nephron, thereby concentrating the urine. Loss of ADH results in diabetes insipidus, which is what is described in this patient.

Q10 Answer: (a).
Thrombosis (blood clot) in the cavernous sinus is usually caused by the spread of bacteria (such as *Staphylococcus aureus*) from the front of the face to the cavernous sinus through veins. Symptoms include those experienced by this patient. The adduction of the right eye suggests that the thrombus is in the right cavernous sinus. The abducent nerve (cranial nerve VI) passes through the cavernous sinus. Since this nerve innervates the lateral rectus muscle, paralysis of this muscle results in an adducted eye.

Q11 Answer: (d).
The finding is referred to as 'pupils fixed and dilated' and this is a bad prognostic sign. Head trauma often results in increased intracranial pressure and this impairs brain function. In this case, specifically the oculomotor nucleus is no longer functioning. Most likely cardiac and respiratory activity have also ceased.

Q12 Answer: (c).
Middle ear infection (otitis media) is often associated with upper respiratory tract infections. It is relatively common in children because the auditory (Eustachian) tube is relatively wide and short and infections easily spread from the nasopharynx to the tympanic cavity. The inflammatory process often results in fluid accumulating in the cavity. This exerts an outward pressure on the tympanic membrane and the membrane can no longer vibrate freely.

Q13 Answer: (e).
A pyramidal lobe of the thyroid gland is an occasional finding. In itself it is not indicative of pathology but rather reflects the migratory path of thyroid tissue during development. When present, it may cause bleeding problems during a cricothyrotomy.

Q14 Answer: (a).
The piriform recesses are lateral to the aryepiglottic folds and form part of the pathway for swallowed solids and liquids to be shunted around the larynx. They are a common site for foreign objects to lodge. In this case, most likely a fish bone lodged in a piriform recess.

Chapter 4

Q1 Answer: (d).
See Brachial plexus (Chapter 3, p. 60 and **Fig. 3.18**) and Cords of the brachial plexus (p. 109).

Q2 Answer: (a).
See Shoulder joint (p. 107–108).

Q3 Answer: (b).
See Muscles in the arm (pp. 111–113). Four of the descriptions do not accurately match any known muscle:
a) no muscle attaching to the medial epicondyle is a main elbow flexor;
b) is brachioradialis;
c) brachialis passes from the anterior humerus to the coronoid process, not the posterior humerus;
d) biceps does not attach to the humerus but passes to radial tuberosity;
e) supinator passes from the ulna to the radius.

Q4 Answer: (e).
See Median nerve (p. 117 and **Fig. 4.13**).

Q5 Answer: (b).
See Small muscles of the hand and First carpometacarpal joint (pp. 121–124).

Q6 Answer: (e).
The axillary nerve, along with the posterior circumflex humeral artery, wraps around the surgical neck of the humerus to pass posteriorly. This nerve innervates the deltoid and teres minor muscles. The deltoid is easily palpated. The nerve also supplies a small patch of skin inferior to the acromion. Loss of sensation in this cutaneous distribution is an additional sign that the axillary nerve is compromised.

Q7 Answer: (d).
The shoulder capsule is very lax (pp. 107, 108) (compared with the hip joint (p. 217) to allow for a wide range of motion.

Generally, the rotator cuff muscles compensate for the laxness of the capsule but shoulder dislocations are relatively common. There are some thin bands on the interior surface of the capsule that can be 'tightened' by shortening them during shoulder arthroplasty.

Q8 Answer: (d).
The radial nerve wraps around the midshaft of the humerus and is vulnerable to injury from a fracture in this location. The radial nerve innervates all of the extensors of the wrist and fingers so the physical examination also indicates a lesion of the radial nerve. The other choices are not indicated by the physical examination results or the radiological finding.

Q9 Answer: (b).
Infection of the synovial sheath of a digit is called tenosynovitis. The synovial sheath of the flexor pollicis longus is called the radial bursa. The tendons of the flexor digitorum superficialis and flexor digitorum profundus are surrounded by a common sheath called the ulnar bursa. A communication may occur between the radial and ulnar bursae, which would allow a 'horseshoe abscess' to form in this case. The flexor carpi radialis and the flexor pollicis brevis do not have synovial sheaths.

Q10 Answer: (b).
The scaphoid (old name, navicular) is one of the most frequently fractured bones in the body. The narrow 'waist' of the scaphoid is levered over the distal radius of the radius where it usually fractures. The styloid process of the ulna is infrequently fractured and not particularly stressed in such a fall. Fracture of the distal radius was described by Abraham Colles and is a common fracture. It could have been fractured in such a fall but the scaphoid is more likely. The capitate bone was not at risk and is infrequently fractured. The first

metacarpal is only fractured when the force is directly on the thumb.

Q11 Answer: (a).
A lesion of the deep branch of the ulnar nerve results in paralysis of the lumbrical muscles of the fourth and fifth digits and all of the interosseous muscles. Extension of the metacarpophalangeal joints is intact because extensors in the forearm innervated by the deep branch of the radial nerve remains unharmed. Extension of the IP joints of the fourth and fifth digits is lost because the lumbrical and interosseous muscles to those fingers have been paralysed. Lumbrical muscles to the second and third digits are innervated by the medial nerve and remain functional. The interosseous muscles to those fingers are paralysed, so some weak extension is still possible. The recurrent branch of the median nerves innervates thenar muscles, which are not injured in this case. The deep branch of the radial nerve is in the forearm and not injured. The superficial branch of the radial nerve provides some sensation on the dorsum of the hand but does not innervate any hand muscles. The median nerve in the carpal tunnel is vulnerable to lesion when the wrist is lacerated, but the thenar and first two lumbrical muscles would be paralysed, which did not happen in this case.

Q12 Answer: (a).
The median nerve, which lies within the carpal tunnel, innervates the thenar muscles and the first and second interossei. Due to compression of the median nerve in carpal tunnel syndrome, these muscles are compromised. The other listed muscles are innervated by the ulnar nerve and that nerve does not traverse the carpal tunnel.

Q13 Answer: (e).
The ulnar nerve passes behind the medial epicondyle and is vulnerable to injury in a fracture of this structure. The ulnar nerve innervates most of the intrinsic muscles of the hand, including the interosseous muscles that abduct and adduct the fingers. None of the other nerves pass close to the medial epicondyle.

Q14 Answer: (d).
The sensory innervation of joints follows Hilton's Law (see Chapter 2, Introduction). Since the median nerve innervates several flexors that act on the wrist joint (e.g. flexor carpi radialis), then we know the median nerve carries sensation from the wrist joint. The other nerves listed do not innervate muscles acting on the wrist joint.

Chapter 5

Q1 Answer: (b).
See Lungs and pleura (pp. 148–151).

Q2 Answer: (d).
See Chambers and great vessels (p. 140) and Borders (p. 145).

Q3 Answer: (b).
See heart blood supply (pp. 147–148).

Q4 Answer: (e).
See Lobes and Surface markings (p. 148–149).

Q5 Answer: (a).
See Lobes and Surface markings (p. 148–149).

Q6 Answer: (c).
See Oesophagus (p. 134).

Q7 Answer: (c).
The serratus anterior is innervated by the long thoracic nerve and this nerve is susceptible to iatrogenic (physican-induced) injury during mastectomy because the nerve runs on the superficial aspect of the muscle, not the deep side as is the case in most nerve/muscle relationships. The serratus anterior rotates the scapula laterally

and this is needed to raise the arm past 90 degrees. The trapezius is also important in scapular rotation and injury to the spinal accessory nerve (cranial nerve XI) can cause similar symptoms.

Q8 Answer: (c).
Most of the lymph from the breast flows to the axillary lymph nodes, which are palpable and are accessible for surgical removal. A lesser amount of lymph from the breast also flows to the parasternal nodes, which are not palpable and are not as accessible. The other lymph nodes are not in the region of the breast.

Q9 Answer: (d).
A tumour at the apex of the lung is likely to impinge on structures passing between the neck and the thorax. The sympathetic nerves originating in the thorax ascend through the thoracic inlet to ultimately supply smooth muscle and sweat glands in the head. These include the superior tarsal muscle (of Müller; responsible for keeping the eyelid from drooping), the dilator papillae and sweat glands in the face. This combination of symptoms is known as Horner's syndrome and is often caused by an interruption of sympathetic nerves to the head, as seen in this case. A tumour in this location is called a Pancoast tumour because it was first described in 1924 by the American radiologist Henry Pancoast.

Q10 Answer: (c).
Heart sounds are best heard (auscultated) not directly over the valve but along the line of blood flow 'downstream' from the valve. The mitral valve is best auscultated at the apex of the heart, as in this patient.

Q11 Answer: (b).
The phrenic nerves pass anteriorly to the hilum of the lung to innervate the diaphragm. Compression of either phrenic nerve compromises the role of the diaphragm in respiration. The vagus nerves pass posterior to the hilum. The other nerves do not have a direct relationship to the hilum of the lung.

Q12 Answer: (a).
The left recurrent laryngeal nerve innervates all of the muscles in the left side of the larynx except the cricothyroid muscle. This nerve passes back superiorly (hooking) around the aortic arch just distal to the ligamentum arteriosum. A tumour in the left lung may compromise this nerve. The right recurrent laryngeal nerve recurs around the right subclavian artery and does not enter the thorax. The other nerves do not innervate the larynx.

Q13 Answer: (b).
The anterior interventricular artery (often referred to clinically as the left anterior descending or simply LAD) supplies the anterior portions of the right and left ventricles and the anterior two-thirds of the interventricular septum, as well as the right and left bundle branches.

Q14 Answer: (e).
During pericardiocentesis the needle may be inserted in the left fifth intercostal space in the mid-clavicular line with little risk of piercing the pleura and causing a pneumothorax. This also provides access to the lowest portion of the pericardial cavity where fluid accumulates. Another favoured approach for pericardiocentesis is below the xiphoid process, approaching the pericardial cavity from below.

Chapter 6

Q1 Answer: (c).
See Inguinal canal (p. 158).

Q2 Answer: (b).
See Inguinal canal (p. 158).

Q3 Answer: (c).
See Surface features (p. 159). The aorta divides at L4 and the femoral artery forms at the inguinal ligament.

Q4 Answer: (d).
See Adrenal gland (p. 182), Stomach (p. 169).

Q5 Answer: (c).
See Stomach (p. 169), Large intestine (p. 172).

Q6 Answer: (d).
See Abdominal aorta (pp. 164–165 and **Fig. 6.6**).

Q7 Answer: (b).
See Abdominal aorta (pp. 164–165 and **Fig. 6.6**).

Q8 Answer: (c).
See Kidneys and ureters, Blood supply (p. 181) and **Figs. 6.5** and **6.7**.

Q9 Answer: (a).
The liver and gallbladder are located in the upper right quadrant of the abdomen. On the anterior abdominal wall this region is known as the right hypochondrium. The term 'hypochondrium' refers to the location of this region deep to the costal cartilages of ribs 7 to 10. Interestingly, the term 'hypochondriac' (a person complaining of a pain for which no organic cause can be identified) is thought to be related to hypochondrium. A few hundred years ago, gallbladder disease was not recognised by the 'medical' community. A patient complaining of pain in the hypochondrium was dismissed as a complainer who had no illness. A lesson for current times is that patients who are labelled hypochondriacs may simply have a pathology that is not yet detectable or recognised.

Q10 Answer: (b).
During descent of the testis, the gonad in accompanied by a peritoneal pouch called the processus vaginalis, which extends the length of the inguinal canal, from the deep inguinal ring to the superficial ring. Normally, the processus vaginalis obliterates later. When it remains patent, contents of the peritoneal cavity, often a loop of the small intestine, can be pushed into the processus vaginalis (which is now called a hernia sac), and thereby into the scrotum, when abdominal pressure is increased. Since the processus vaginalis begins at the deep inguinal ring, this is where the hernia sac begins.

Q11 Answer: (e).
An enlarged, palpably hard liver suggests cirrhosis of the liver, a fibrotic 'scarring' of the liver parenchyma. Cirrhosis can be caused by several factors, including hepatitis or chronic alcoholism, relatively common conditions in the homeless population. Portal hypertension is a result of cirrhosis. When blood is prevented from flowing freely through a fibrotic liver, pressure is increased in the portal venous system and blood is forced into alternate channels. One of these channels is blood from the left gastric vein that is diverted into veins in the submucosa of the oesophagus, ultimately draining into the azygous vein. These oesophageal veins become dilated (varicose) and fragile. When these veins rupture the patient vomits venous blood, which is dark red as in this case.

Q12 Answer: (c).
Jaundice is a symptom, not a disease. Whereas jaundice can be caused by many diseases, a tumour in the head of the pancreas is the most likely of those choices. The common bile duct passes through the head of the pancreas and a tumour in this location is able to block the duct, causing bile to 'back up' into the bloodstream and resulting in jaundice.

Q13 Answer: (c).
The appendix receives its sensory input from the tenth thoracic nerve. Distension

of an inflamed appendix causes referred pain to the dermatome to T10, which is the epigastric region. As the inflammation progresses, it involves parietal peritoneum adjacent to the appendix. Since sensation from the parietal (but not visceral) peritoneum is localised, the patient perceives the pain as coming from the area of the appendix, usually the right lower quadrant of the abdominal wall.

Q14 Answer: (d).
The third part of the duodenum crosses in front of the aorta behind the SMA. Following dramatic weight loss, the angle between the aorta and the SMA can become more acute, compressing the third part of the duodenum and causing SMA syndrome, as described in this patient. As for surface anatomy, the third part of the duodenum usually crosses the aorta at the level of the third lumbar vertebra. Mnemonic: third part of duodenum, third lumbar vertebra.

Chapter 7

Q1 Answer: (e).
See Levator ani (p. 193).

Q2 Answer: (d).
See Testis and epididymis (p. 200).

Q3 Answer: (b).
See Ovary (p. 202).

Q4 Answer: (e).
See Urethra to Penis (pp. 200–201).

Q5 Answer: (c).
See Prostate (p. 199).

Q6 Answer: (e).
See Vagina (p. 204), Levator ani (p. 193).

Q7 Answer: (a).
See Rectum and anal canal (blood supply, p. 197).

Q8 Answer: (b).
See Testis and epididymis (p. 200).
Varicoeles can be due to a disruption of flow arising from the abrupt angulation occurring where the left testicular vein meets the left renal vein. Alternatively, it could arise due to defective venous valves in the testicular veins or, finally, due to a renal abnormality causing obstruction of the normal venous drainage.

Q9 Answer: (b).
See Vagina (p. 204).

Q10 Answer: (c).
Soon before a woman is to give birth, a hormone called relaxin is released by the placenta and ovaries. One of the effects of relaxin is that the cartilaginous joint at the pubic symphysis is loosened so that it may separate a small amount during delivery, allowing the birth canal to enlarge. There is no pathology (dislocated hips or torn ligaments) and it is clearly not psychosomatic. The woman's hip bones actually 'wobble'. Her centre of gravity has shifted forward but this causes lordosis (swayback) in the spine, not wobbly hips.

Q11 Answer: (c).
The obturator nerve is formed from branches from L2 to L4 (p. 61) and passes from the pelvis through the obturator canal to enter the medial compartment of the thigh. This compartment contains the adductors of the thigh that are paralysed in this patient (p. 214). The femoral nerve (p. 210) innervates the anterior compartment, which contains the quadriceps femoris that extends the leg at the knee. The sciatic nerve (p. 215) innervates the posterior compartment of the thigh that contains the hamstrings. The sciatic nerve divides into the tibial and common fibular (peroneal) nerves that innervate all the muscles below the knee.

Chapter 8

Q1 Answer: (b).
See Femoral triangle, Femoral nerves, Femoral artery and vein, Great saphenous vein and Femoral canal (pp. 210–213).

Q2 Answer: (b).
See Muscles that produce movements of the hip joint (p. 217–218).

Q3 Answer: (c).
See Sciatic nerve (p. 215), Tibial nerve (p. 223) and Common fibular (peroneal) nerve (p. 225).

Q4 Answer: (d).
See Knee joint (p. 218) and Lateral, medial and cruciate ligaments (p. 222).

Q5 Answer: (d).
See Popliteal fossa (p. 223).

Q6 Answer: (c).
See Muscle sections (pp. 227–231 and 235).

Q7 Answer: (a).
See Ligaments (p. 236), Plantar aponeurosis (p. 234) and Foot ligaments (p. 236).

Q8 Answer: (b).
A lesion of the superior gluteal nerve results in paralysis of the gluteus medius and minimus (and the tensor fascia lata, but that does not play a role in this case). These gluteal muscles are known as abductors of the thigh, but more importantly they are stabilisers of the pelvis when the weight is on one limb. When the woman is asked to stand on her right foot the gluteus medius and minimus are unable to maintain the distance between the ilium and the greater trochanter of the femur and the left side of her pelvis droops. The gluteus maximus, innervated by the inferior gluteal nerve, is largely responsible for extending the hip, such as during standing from a seated position. The iliopsoas and rectus femoris, innervated by lumbar nerves, are responsible for flexion of the thigh at the hip.

Q9 Answer: (c).
The deep fibular (peroneal) nerve innervates the muscles in the anterior compartment of the leg. These muscles dorsiflex the foot. Paralysis of these muscles result in foot drop. The saphenous nerve is a cutaneous branch of the femoral nerve. The superficial fibular (peroneal) nerve innervates the lateral compartment of the leg and these muscles evert the foot. The tibial nerve innervates the posterior compartment of the leg and these muscle plantarflex the foot. The sciatic nerve divides in the thigh into the tibial and common fibular (peroneal) nerves.

Q10 Answer: (b).
The piriformis muscle is considered the key to the gluteal anatomy. It originates from the anterior surface of the sacrum and inserts on the greater trochanter after passing through the greater sciatic foramen. The superior gluteal nerve and blood vessels pass above the piriformis. The inferior gluteal nerve and blood vessels, the sciatic nerve and several other structures pass below the piriformis. The other listed structures are not landmarks.

Q11 Answer: (c).
When the tibia can be pulled anteriorly from under the femur, this is a 'positive drawer sign' (as in pulling out a drawer from a cabinet). An intact anterior cruciate ligament would not allow this movement. If the posterior cruciate ligament is torn, the tibia can be moved posteriorly relative to the femur, a 'positive posterior drawer sign'. An injured meniscus does not result in a positive drawer sign.

Q12 Answer: (d).
The lateral plantar nerve innervates the interosseous muscles in the foot, which are responsible for abduction of the toes.

The superficial and deep fibular (peroneal) nerves innervate muscles that move the foot, not the toes. The saphenous nerve is a cutaneous branch of the femoral nerve. It does supply cutaneous innervation to the medial side of the foot.

213 Answer: (a).
The anterior talofibular ligament (often called the 'anterior talofib'). This ligament is commonly injured in an inversion injury of the ankle. The posterior talofibular ligament is rarely injured. The medial and lateral plantar nerves would not be injured in an ankle sprain. The deltoid ligament is more commonly injured in an eversion injury.

Q14 Answer: (d).
The tibial nerve innervates muscles that plantarflex and invert the foot. The muscles that dorsiflex the foot would be unopposed. These muscles are in the anterior compartment of the leg and are innervated by the deep fibular (peroneal) nerve. Injury to the deep fibular (peroneal) nerve would result in foot drop. The knee is extended by the quadriceps femoris nerve, which is innervated by the femoral nerve. The knee is flexed by the hamstrings, which are innervated by the sciatic nerve. Extending the hip during standing from a seated position is mostly done by the gluteus maximus, which is innervated by the inferior gluteal nerve.

Appendix B
Glossary: derivation of anatomical and other terms

Most anatomical (and medical) terms have Latin (L) or Greek (G) origins. The following list indicates derivations/meanings.

abdomen L — probably meaning to hide

abducent L — leading from

acetabulum L — little vinegar cup

acoustic G — related to hearing

acromion G — extremity of shoulder

adenoid L — gland-like

aditus L — opening or entrance

adrenal L — towards the kidney

afferent L — carrying to

ampulla L — globular flask

anastomosis G — towards a mouth; joining together

annulus L — ring

antrum L — cave

anus L or Anglo-Saxon — to sit

aorta G — to lift or heave

aponeurosis G — derived from a sinew

arachnoid G — spider-like

arrector (also erector) L — to stand up

artery G — keeping air (arteries were thought to contain air)

arytenoid G — like a ladle

atlas G — Greek god, bearing the earth on his shoulders

axilla L — armpit

azygos G — unpaired, not yoked

basilic G — important or prominent

biceps L — two heads

brachium L — arm

brevis L — short

bronchus G — windpipe

buccal L — cheek

buccinator L — trumpeter

bulla L — large vesicle

bursa L — purse

caecum L — (cecum) blind

calcaneus L — heel

calcarine L — spur-shaped

callosum L — thick

canaliculus L — little canal

canine L — dog-like

canthus G — niche or corner

capitate L — head-like

capitulum L — little head

cardiac G/L — heart

carina L — keel (of boat), projecting ridge

carotid G — heavy sleep (from the Greek belief that the carotid arteries caused drowsiness)

carpus G/L	wrist	
caudate L	tail	
cephalic G	head	
cerebellum L	little brain	
cerebrum L	brain	
cervix L	neck	
chiasma G	crossed lines, like the Greek letter chi, X	
choana G/L	funnel	
choroid G	like a vascular membrane	
cilia L	eyelashes	
circumflex L	bending round	
clavicle L	little key	
clitoris G	shut up	
clivus L	slope	
cloaca L	sewer	
coccyx G	cuckoo, whose beak the bone resembles	
cochlea L	snail or snail shell	
coeliac G/L	(celiac) belly	
colliculus L	little hill	
colon G/L	large intestine	
concha L	shell	
condyle L	joint or knuckle	
conjunctiva L	join togther	
conoid G	cone-like	
coracoid G	crow-like, beak like a crow's	
cornea L	horn	
coronal L	crown or garland used to describe frontal suture (on which garland sat) and then for a vertical transverse section parallel to this suture	
coronary L	encircling like a crown	
corpus L	body	
cortex L	bark or shell	
cranium G/L	upper part of head	
cremaster G/L	hang or suspend	
cribriform L	sieve-like	

cricoid G	ring-like	
cruciate L	crossed	
cruciform L	cross-shaped	
cubital L	elbow	
cuneate, cuneiform L	wedge-shaped	
cusp L	pointed tip	
cutaneous L	skin	
cyst G/L	sac or bladder	
decussation G	crossing like the letter X	
defaecation L	(defecation) purification or cleansing	
deferens L	carrying away	
deltoid G	triangular like the capital fourth letter of the Greek alphabet, delta	
dens L	tooth	
dermatome G	cutting skin	
diaphragm G	through a fence; a partition	
dorsum L	back	
duct L	to lead	
duodenum L	twelve (length of 12 fingerbreadths)	
dura mater L	tough mother	
efferent L	carrying out	
ejaculation L	throwing out	
embryo G	to swell	
endocrine G	to secrete inside	
endolymph G	water inside	
epidermis G	upon skin	
epididymis G	upon the testicle	
epiglottis G	upon the tongue	
epiploic G	floating	
epithelium G	upon the nipple	
erythrocyte G	red cell	
ethmoid G	sieve-like	
faeces L	(feces) sediment or dregs	
falciform L	sickle-shaped	

fascia L	bandage or sash		**hallux** L	great toe
femur L	thigh		**hamate** L	hooked
fibula L	buckle or brooch, especially the pin of		**hepatic** G	liver
			hernia L	protrusion through an opening
fimbria L	fringe, border			
fissure L	cleft or groove		**hiatus** L	gape
flexion L	bending		**hilum** L	a small bit or trifle
foetus L	(fetus) offspring – now used for unborn		**hormone** G	to excite
			humerus L	shoulder
follicle L	leather ball or money bag		**humour** G	liquid
foramen L	small opening		**hyaline** G	glassy
fornix L	arch		**hyoid** G	U-shaped, from the Greek letter upsilon
fossa L	ditch			
fovea L	small pit		**hypophysis** G	undergrowth
fundus L	bottom of a cavity		**hypothenar** G	under the palm
			ileum G/L	small intestine, twisting
galli L	cock		**ilium** L	loin
ganglion G	knot or swelling		**incisor** L	cut into
gastric G	stomach		**index** L	forefinger, point out
gastrocnemius G	stomach of the leg		**infundibulum** L	funnel
gemellus L	a twin		**inguinal** L	groin
genitalia L	reproductive organs, belonging to birth		**innominate** L	unnamed
			iris G/L	rainbow
genu L	knee		**ischium** G/L	hip
gingiva L	gum			
glans L	acorn		**jejunum** L	empty, hungry
glenoid G	socket-like		**jugular** L	neck, throat or collar bone
glomerulus L	little ball			
glottis G	vocal apparatus		**keratin** G	horn
gluteus L	rump			
goitre F/L	(goiter) throat or gullet		**labium,**	
gonad G	seed		**labrum** L	lip
gracile L	slender		**labyrinth** G	maze
gyrus G/L	ring or circle		**lacerum** L	jagged
			lacrimal L	tear
haemorrhage L/G	(hemorrhage) bleeding violently		**lactation** L	milk
			lamina L	plate or layer
haemorrhoid L/G	(hemorrhoid) a flow of blood		**larynx** G	upper windpipe
			lateral L	side or flank
			latissimus L	widest

lemniscus G/L	ribbon		**nephron** G	kidney
leucocyte G	white cell		**neuron** G	nerve or sinew
levator L	lifter		**node** L	knot
lienal L	spleen, splenic		**nucleus** L	kernel, small nut
lingual L	tongue			
lumbar L	loin		**obturator** L	plug an opening
lumbrical L	earthworm		**occiput** L	back of the head
lunate L	crescent-shaped		**oculomotor** L	eye mover
lutea L	yellow		**oesophagus** G	(esophagus) carrying food
lymph L	clear water		**oestrogen** G	(estrogen) from oestrus (G, gadfly) + gen
			olecranon G	head of the elbow
magnus L	great		**olfactory** G	make smell
malleolus L	little hammer		**omentum** L	fatty membrane, to clothe
malleus L	hammer		**ophthalmic** G	eye
mamillary L	nipple		**opponens** L	placing against
mamma L	breast		**optic** G/L	sight
mandible L	lower jaw; chew		**oral** L	mouth
manubrium L	handle		**orthopaedic** G	(orthopedic) ortho = straight; pedis = children
manus L	hand		**os** L	mouth (plural ora)
masseter G	chewer		**os** L	bone (plural ossa)
mastoid G	breast-like		**ostium** L	door or opening
maxilla L	jawbone		**otic** G	ear
maximus L	biggest		**ovum** L	egg
meatus L	passage			
medial L	towards the midline		**palate** L	palate
median L	in the midline		**palpebra** L	eyelid
mediastinum L	median partition		**pampiniform** L	tendril-shaped
medius L	middle		**pancreas** G	all flesh
medulla L	marrow		**papilla** L	nipple
meninges G	membranes		**paralysis** G	loosen alongside
meniscus G/L	crescent		**parietal** L	wall
mental L	chin		**parotid** G	near the ear
mesentery G	middle intestine		**patella** L	flat dish
micturition L	desire to pass urine		**pectinate** L	like a comb
minimus L	smallest		**pectoral** L	breast
molar L	mill for grinding		**pedicle** L	little foot
motor L	mover		**peduncle** L	stalk
myenteric G	intestinal muscle		**pelvis** L	basin
			penis L	tail
nares L	nostril			
navicular L	small boat			

perilymph G	water around	**punctum** L	sharp point
perineum G	evacuate around	**pupil** L	doll (from image reflected in cornea)
periodontal G	around tooth		
peripheral G	carry around	**pylorus** G	gatekeeper
peristalsis G	constriction around		
peritoneum G	stretch around	**quadrate** L	four-sided
peroneal G	brooch, pointed for piercing	**quadriceps** L	four-headed
pes L	foot	**radius** L	a spoke
petrous G	stony	**ramus** L	a branch
phalanx G	line of soldiers	**raphe** G	a seam
pharynx G	throat	**rectus** L	straight
philtrum L	love charm	**recurrent** L	run back
phrenic G	mind or heart as centre of emotions	**renal** L	kidney
		retina L	net
pia mater L	soft mother	**rima** L	cleft
pineal L	pine cone	**rotundum** L	round
pituitary L	mucus (the gland was thought to secrete nasal mucus)	**sagittal** L	arrow
		salpinx G	tube, trumpet
		saphenous G	apparent, not hidden
placenta L	cake	**sartorius** L	tailor (sitting cross-legged)
plantar L	sole of foot		
platysma G	broad	**scala** L	staircase
pleura G	rib, side	**scalene** G	triangle with unequal sides
plexus L	network		
pollex L	thumb	**scaphoid** G	boat-shaped
pons L	bridge	**scapula** L	shoulderblade
popliteus L	ham	**sciatic** G	hip
porta L	entrance	**sclera** G	hard
prepuce L	foreskin	**scrotum** L	bag
profundus L	deep	**sebaceous** L	grease
pronation L	bend forward	**sella turcica** L	Turkish saddle
proprioceptive L	take one's own	**seminiferous** L	carrying seed
prostate G	stand before	**serratus** L	toothed
psoas G	loin muscle	**sesamoid** G	like a sesame seed
pterion G	wing	**sigmoid** G	like the letter S
pterygoid G	wing-like	**sinus** L	curve or hollow
ptosis G	falling	**spermatozoa** G	seed animals
pubis L	secondary sex hair	**sphenoid** G	wedge-like
pudendal L	ashamed	**sphincter** G	tight binder
pulmonary L	lung	**splanchnic** G	organ

squamous L	scale-like	
stapes L	stirrup	
sternum G/L	breast, breast bone	
stroma G	bed, framework	
styloid G	pillar-like	
sulcus L	groove	
supination L	bend backwards	
sural L	calf	
suture L	seam	
symphysis G	growing together	
synovial G	with egg (like white of egg)	
taeniae L/G	(teniae) band or ribbon	
talus L	ankle	
tarsus G	flat surface	
temporal L	time (temples, where hair first goes grey)	
tegmen L	covering	
tendon G	stretch out	
teres L	round/long	
testicle L	diminutive of testis	
testis L	witness	
thalamus G	chamber, bedroom	
thenar G	palm of hand	
thorax G/L	breastplate	
thrombus G	curd, clot	
thymus G	sweetbread (like a bunch of thyme flowers)	
thyroid G	shield-like	
tibia L	flute	
trachea G	rough air channel	
tragus G	goat (goat-like hairs in front of the ear)	

trapezium G	four-sided figure with no two sides parallel
trapezoid G	like trapezium
triceps G	three-headed
triquetral L	three-cornered
trochanter G/L	runner
trochlea G/L	pulley
tuber L	protuberance
tumour L	(tumor) swelling
turbinate L	child's top
tympanum G/L	drum
ulna L	elbow
umbilicus L	navel
uncinate L	hooked
ureter G/L	urinary canal
uvula L	little grape
vagina L	sheath
vagus L	wandering
vallecula L	little hollow
vas deferens L	vessel carrying away
ventricle L	little belly
vermiform L	worm-like
vertebra L	turning joint
vesicle L	little bladder
viscus L	internal organ
vomer L	ploughshare
vulva L	wrapper
xiphoid G	sword-like
zygmomatic G	yoke

Index

Note: Page references in *italic* refer to figures

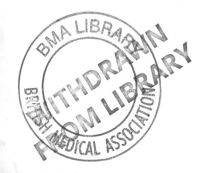